Peter V. Giannoudis

Editor

# Practical Procedures in Elective Orthopaedic Surgery

## Pelvis and Lower Extremity

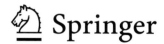

Springer

*Editor*
Peter V. Giannoudis, B.Sc., M.B., M.D., FRCS
Academic Department of Trauma
and Orthopaedic Surgery
School of Medicine
University of Leeds
Leeds
UK

ISBN 978-0-85729-813-3          e-ISBN 978-0-85729-814-0
DOI 10.1007/978-0-85729-814-0
Springer London Dordrecht Heidelberg New York

British Library Cataloguing in Publication Data
A catalogue record for this book is available from the British Library

Library of Congress Control Number: 2011933720

Printed on acid-free paper

Springer is part of Springer Science+Business Media (www.springer.com)

*To my wife Rania, my children Marilena and Vasilis*
*Whom*
*I have missed so much during my medical career.*
*I thank them for providing me with ongoing inspiration and support.*
*Their love has been a source of endless energy and creativity.*

# Preface

A plethora of Orthopaedic Textbooks have been produced over the years presenting the advances made in this ever evolving discipline. Some of them being colossal cover the entire practice of orthopaedic surgery, whereas others include only regional orthopaedics by focusing into a specific anatomical site of the musculoskeletal system.

The idea of the book was conceived during the beginning of my residency program in Orthopaedic Surgery. Moving every 6 months to a different subspecialty, it became clear that I had to obtain different textbooks in order to use them as a quick, yet comprehensive reference, prior to performing a surgical procedure.

Following the development and the popularity of the trauma textbook, I felt obliged to also develop a similar book in elective orthopaedic surgery that would contain a stepwise approach related to these types of surgical procedures. In this textbook, the most common procedures that a surgeon in training is expected to perform during his residency program for the pelvic ring and the lower extremity have been included. Each procedure has been written by an expert or under a supervision of an expert. Each chapter provides such useful information to the trainee as indications, clinical and radiological assessment, surgical approach, implant positioning, tips and tricks, postoperative complications to be aware of, mode of mobilisation and the time intervals of outpatient follow up. Intra-operative pictures have been incorporated to allow the surgeon to be aware of all the important issues and steps involved for each procedure.

This book by no means covers all the procedures to be performed during a residency program. The objective was not to become cumbersome, but rather the textbook to be easy to carry and simple to read. It is expected to be the companion for the resident in training and to improve the standard of care of our patients that we care so much about.

Leeds, UK                                  Peter V. Giannoudis B.Sc., M.B., M.D., FRCS

# Acknowledgments

Without the dedication and the hard work of my Hospital Staff and my colleagues it would not have been possible to complete this project.

I would also personally like to thank all the contributors who have shared with me their expertise.

# Contents

# Contributors

**John Antoniou, M.D., Ph.D., FACS, FRCSC (Orth)** Division of Orthopaedic Surgery, School of Medicine, McGill University, Montreal, QC, Canada

**George C. Babis, M.D., Ph.D.** First Department of Orthopaedics, School of Medicine, University of Athens, ATTIKON University General Hospital, Athens, Greece

**Peter Bobak, M.D., FEBOT** Department of Trauma and Orthopaedic Surgery, Leeds Teaching Hospitals NHS Trust, Leeds, UK

**Stuart J. Calder, MBChB, M.D., FRCS (Orth)** Department of Trauma and Orthopaedic Surgery, Leeds Teaching Hospitals NHS Trust, Leeds, UK

**Giorgio Maria Calori, M.D.** Academic Department of Trauma & Orthopaedic Surgery, Instituto Ortopedico Gaetano Pini, Milan University, Milan, Italy

**Peter V. Giannoudis, B.Sc., M.D., FRCS-Eng** Academic Department of Trauma and Orthopaedic Surgery, School of Medicine, University of Leeds, Leeds, UK

**Alexandra Dimitrakopoulou, M.D.** The London Hip Arthroscopy Centre, The Wellington Hospital, London, UK

**Rozalia I. Dimitriou, M.D.** Department of Trauma and Orthopaedic Surgery, Leeds Teaching Hospitals NHS Trust, Leeds, UK

**Kurt Haendlmayer, FRCS (Orth)** Department of Trauma and Orthopaedic Surgery, Leeds Teaching Hospitals NHS Trust, Leeds, UK

**Nick Harris, FRCS (Orth)** Department of Trauma and Orthopaedic Surgery, Leeds Teaching Hospitals NHS Trust, Leeds, UK

**Fernando de la Huerta, M.D.** Orthopaedic Division, Hospital de Especialidades, Instituto Mexicano del Seguro Social, Guadalajara, Mexico

**Nikolaos K. Kanakaris, M.D., Ph.D.** Department of Trauma and Orthopaedic Surgery, Leeds Teaching Hospitals NHS Trust, Leeds, UK

**Efthimios J. Karadimas, M.D., Ph.D.** Department of Trauma and Orthopaedic Surgery, Leeds Teaching Hospitals NHS Trust, Leeds, UK

**Athanasios E. Karamitros, M.D.** Third Academic Department of Trauma and Orthopaedic Surgery, School of Medicine, University of Athens, Athens, Greece

**George M. Kontakis, M.D., Ph.D.** Academic Department of Trauma and Orthopaedic Surgery, School of Medicine, University of Crete, Crete, Greece

**Robert G. Middleton, FRCS (Orth)** Department of Trauma and Orthopaedic Surgery, Royal Bournemouth Hospital, Bournemouth, UK

**Vassilios S. Nikolaou, M.D., Ph.D.** Division of Orthopaedic Surgery, School of Medicine, McGill University, Montreal, QC, Canada

**Christos Plakogiannis, M.D.** Department of Trauma and Orthopaedic Surgery, Royal Bournemouth Hospital, Bournemouth, UK

**Vasileios I. Sakellariou, M.D.** First Department of Orthopaedics, School of Medicine, University of Athens, ATTIKON University General Hospital, Athens, Greece

**Panayotis N. Soucacos, M.D., FACS** Professor of Orthopaedic Surgery, University of Athens, School of Medicine, Director, Orthopaedic Research & Education Center (OREC), Athens, Greece

**Ernest Schilders, FRCS (Orth)** The London Hip Arthroscopy Centre, The Wellington Hospital, London, UK
Faculty of Health, Leeds Metropolitan University, Leeds, UK

**Lorenzo Tagliabue, M.D.** Department of Trauma & Orthopaedic Surgery, Instituto Ortopedico Gaetano Pini, Milan, Italy

**Peter Templeton, M.D., FRCS (Orth)** Department of Trauma and Orthopaedic Surgery, Leeds Teaching Hospitals NHS Trust, Leeds, UK

**Theodoros I. Tosounidis, M.D., EEC (Orth)** Department of Trauma and Orthopaedic Surgery, Leeds Teaching Hospitals NHS Trust, Leeds, UK

**George Tselentakis, M.D., FRCS (Orth)** Department of Trauma and Orthopaedics, East Surrey Hospital, Surrey, UK

**Ram Venkatesh, M.Sc., FRCS (Orth)** Department of Trauma and Orthopaedic Surgery, Leeds Teaching Hospitals NHS Trust, Leeds, UK

**Fragkiskos N. Xypnitos, M.D., M.Sc., Ph.D., EEC (Orth)** Department of Trauma and Orthopaedics Surgery, Leeds Teaching Hospitals NHS Trust, Leeds, UK

# Part I

# Pelvis: Osteotomies

# The Periacetabular Osteotomy

1

Fernando de la Huerta and Peter V. Giannoudis

## Indications

- The periacetabular osteotomy (PAO) is a hip pre-serving procedure performed to correct a congenital deficiency of the acetabulum.
- The goal is to mobilize the acetabulum in order to cover adequately the femoral head.

## Preoperative Planning

### Clinical Assessment

- Walking capacity is compromised due to pain.
- Antalgic gait pattern is frequently present.
- Range of motion of the affected hip is usually full but is associated with pain.
- Neurological examination is mandatory as well as assessment of the presence of muscular wasting.
- The ideal case for this surgery is the patient with spherical joint surfaces with no osteoarthritis.
- Obtain baseline blood investigations including clotting screen and group and safe.

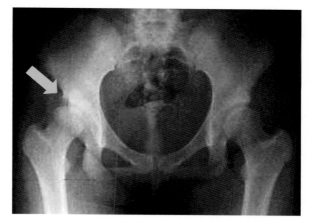

**Fig. 1.1** Radiograph AP pelvis. Bilateral hip dysplasia is noted with the right hip (*arrow*) being the most affected. PAO is performed

### Radiological Assessment

- Radiographs (AP (anteroposterior) of the pelvis and a lateral hip X-ray) allow evaluation of the degree of the dysplasia of the acetabulum.
- Comparison to the opposite healthy hip joint can also be performed as part of the preoperative plan-ning (Fig. 1.1).
- MRI scan can provide a more detailed picture of the state of the cartilage of the hip joint.

## Operative Treatment

### Anaesthesia

- General anaesthesia plus epidural or regional triple block.

F. de la Huerta(✉)
Orthopaedic Division, Hospital de Especialidades,
Instituto Mexicano del Seguro Social,
Guadalajara, Mexico
e-mail: delahuertafernando@hotmail.com

P.V. Giannoudis
Academic Department of Trauma and Orthopaedic Surgery,
School of Medicine, University of Leeds,
Leeds, UK
e-mail: pgiannoudi@aol.com

P.V. Giannoudis (ed.), *Practical Procedures in Elective Orthopaedic Surgery*,
DOI 10.1007/978-0-85729-814-0_1, © Springer-Verlag London Limited 2012

- Insert urinary bladder catheter.
- Administer one dose of prophylactic antibiotics as per local unit protocol.

## Table and Patient Positioning

- Patient is positioned supine on a radiolucent table.
- Place a sandbag to elevate the affected hip.
- Place a pillow under the ipsilateral knee to keep it flexed thus relaxing the anterior neuromuscular structures of the hip.
- Image intensifier is positioned at the contralateral side.
- The patient should be draped in such a way that the leg can be moved during the course of the procedure.

## Surgical Tools

- Standard orthopedic tray.
- Use angled chisel to perform ischium osteotomy.
- Use Gigli saw to perform pubis osteotomy.
- Use reciprocating saw for the transverse osteotomy of the ilium.
- Use Schanz screws to move the acetabulum after performing the osteotomy.
- Use K-wires to fix the acetabulum in the desired position under fluoroscopic control.
- Large fragment set (4.5-mm cortical screws).

## Landmarks and Surgical Approach

- Identify and mark the anterior superior iliac spine (ASIS) (Fig. 1.2a).
- Mark the skin incision starting from ASIS (2-cm slighted curve incision) extending distally approximately 12 cm (Fig. 1.2b).
- An anterior Smith-Petersen approach allows good access to perform the osteotomy.
- Using a skin knife, cut through the skin, fat, and the fascia lata of the thigh.
- Split the fascia in the line of the vertical component of the skin incision and identify sartorius, tensor fascia lata, and rectus femoris.
- Expose the intermuscular plane between the tensor fasciae latae and the sartorius (Fig. 1.3a).

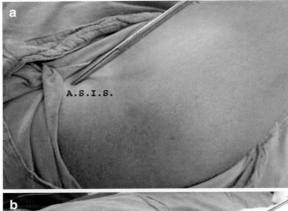

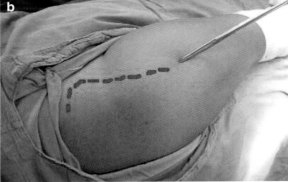

**Fig. 1.2** (a) Identify and mark with a sterile marking pen the anterior superior iliac spine (ASIS). (b) An anterior Smith-Petersen approach is performed from a 2-cm slighted curve incision over the anterior superior iliac spine and extending distally 12 cm

- Identify the lateral femoral cutaneous nerve and avoid damaging it during the dissection and retraction of the soft tissue (Fig. 1.3b).
- Open the interval between sartorius and tensor fascia lata all the way up to the anterior superior iliac spine.
- Detach the origins of the tensor fasciae latae from the outer lip of the anterior half of the iliac crest (outer pelvic portal) (Fig. 1.4).
- Detach the origins of the iliac muscle from the inner lip of the anterior half of the iliac crest (inner pelvic portal).
- Using a 3.5-mm drill, perform a perforation in the ASIS then tap and introduce a 6–0 mm cancellous screw with a washer. Then remove screw until the first thread (Fig. 1.5a).
- After setting up the screw for later use, make use of an oscillating saw to osteotomise the ASIS in a block of 1.5 cm (Fig. 1.5b).

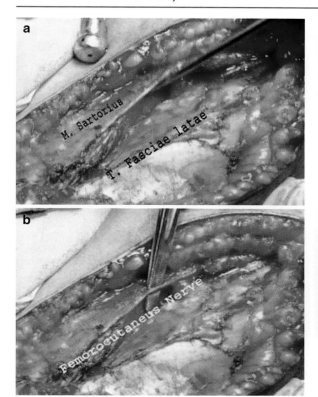

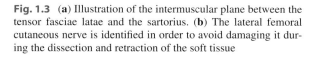

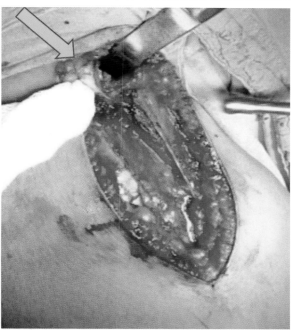

Fig. 1.4 Detachment of the origins of the tensor fasciae latae from the outer lip of the anterior half of the iliac crest (outer pelvic portal) (*arrow* points to iliac crest)

Fig. 1.3 (**a**) Illustration of the intermuscular plane between the tensor fasciae latae and the sartorius. (**b**) The lateral femoral cutaneous nerve is identified in order to avoid damaging it during the dissection and retraction of the soft tissue

- Detach and mobilize medially the fragment of bone with the lateral inguinal ligament attachment (Fig. 1.5c).
- Using Cobb retractor detach periosteum from the inner and outer surfaces of the iliac crest, this subperiosteal dissection prevents damage to the nearby vital structures.
- Identify the plane between joint capsule and the surrounding structures (Fig. 1.6).
- Place a retractor in the ischial tuberosity (Fig. 1.7a, b).
- Having exposed the lower end of the acetabulum, perform the osteotomy of the ischium in the frontal plane (Fig. 1.8a, b).
- Perform proximal dissection of the obturator foramen to prepare the introduction of the Gigli saw in order to cut the pubic ramus (Fig. 1.9a, b).
- Perform a transverse osteotomy of the superior pubic ramus (Fig. 1.10).

- The biplanar osteotomy of the ilium (just below the anterosuperior iliac spine to the region of the pelvic brim) to be performed is illustrated on the plastic pelvic bone model (Fig. 1.11).
- Opposite side (inner pelvis) of transverse osteotomy of the Ilium is demonstrated (Fig. 1.12).
- The continuity of the posterior column of the acetabulum is preserved and remains intact (Fig. 1.13).
- The final osteotomy is done across the posterior portion of the ischium underneath the acetabulum in order to complete the separation of the acetabulum from the remaining pelvis (Fig. 1.14a).
- Use two Schanz screws as handles in order to mobilize the free acetabulum to the intended position (Fig. 1.14b).
- The joint should be routinely opened and evaluated for labral lesions (torn labral fragments are usually excised) (Fig. 1.15). Care should be taken to avoid impingement between the anterior femoral neck and the anterior acetabulum. This can be checked by flexing and internally rotating the hip.

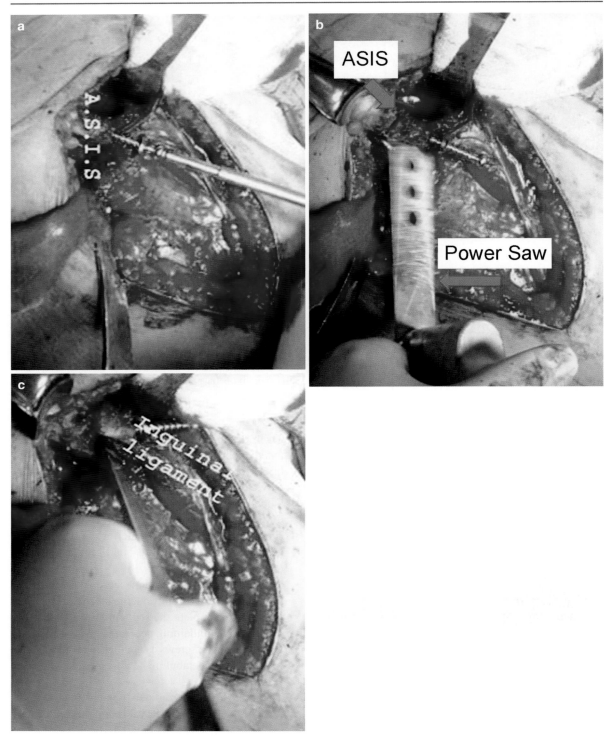

**Fig. 1.5** (**a**) Perform a perforation with a 3.5-mm drill in the ASIS then tap and introduce a 6.0-mm cancellous screw with a washer continuing to remove screw until the first thread. (**b**) After setting up the screw for later use, use an oscillating saw to remove the ASIS in a block of 1.5 cm. (**c**) Detach and mobilize medially the fragment of bone with the lateral inguinal ligament attachment

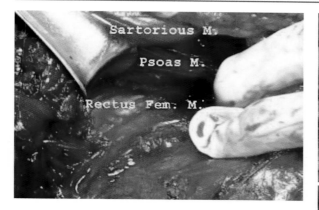

**Fig. 1.6** Identify the plane between joint capsule and the surrounding structures

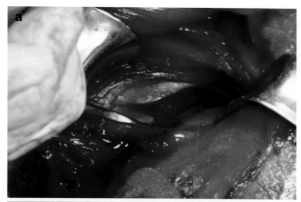

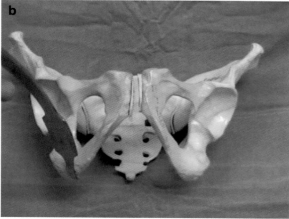

**Fig. 1.7** (**a**) A retractor is placed in the ischium tuberocity. (**b**) Plastic pelvic model illustrates the point of placement of the retractor

- The most challenging aspect of the operation is making sure that the proper correction and coverage of the femoral head can be achieved.

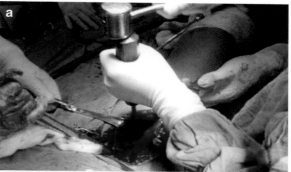

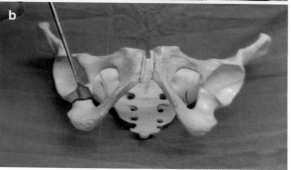

**Fig. 1.8** (**a**) Having exposed the lower end of the acetabulum, perform an osteotomy of the ischium in the frontal plane. (**b**) A plastic pelvic model is used to illustrate the osteotomy of the ischium

- For adequate coverage, displace the periacetabular segment medially and rotate it anteriorly and laterally (maintaining proper anteversion). Flex the limb to 90° to check the free ROM of the femoral neck and the anterior border of the acetabulum prior of temporarily stabilizing the desirable position with k-wiring.
- The segment is then provisionally fixed with two smooth K-wires (Fig. 1.16a).
- The acetabular fragment is then fixed with two or three long 4.5-mm cortical screws from distal to proximal. The first cortical screw is applied to the medial part of the acetabulum; otherwise, the lateral screw can modify the corrected position of the acetabulum (Fig. 1.16b). Position of screws should be checked with the image intensifier.

## Closure

- The anterosuperior iliac spine is reattached to its original place with the previous placed screw, and the integrity of the inguinal ligament is restored (Fig. 1.17).

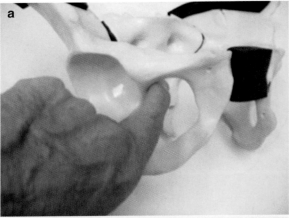

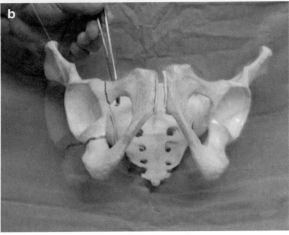

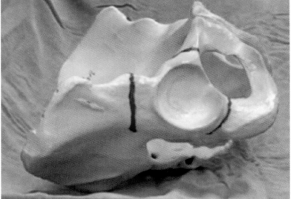

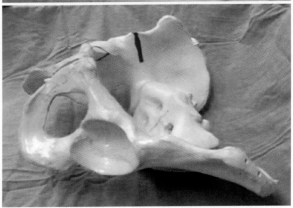

**Fig. 1.11** The biplanar osteotomy of the ilium (just below the anterosuperior iliac spine to the region of the pelvic brim) to be performed is illustrated on the plastic pelvic bone model

**Fig. 1.9** (**a**) This image indicates how the Gigli saw pass through the obturator foramen. (**b**) This image indicates the use of a curved forceps and how it can be passed through the obturator foramen to grip the Gigli saw

- A drain is applied to the depth of the incision.
- Closure the layers with 1/0 and 2/0 Vicryl. Skin is closed with 3/0 s/c suture.
- The fasciae compartment is close with 1/0 Vicryl. The iliac muscle fascia is attached with the tensor fascia lata over the applied screw in the ASIS. This suture covers the head of this screw (Fig. 1.18).
- Skin closure is made with surgical staples.

## Postoperative Rehabilitation

- *First day*
  - Request routine postoperative bloods. Evaluate need for blood transfusion.
  - Start mechanical VTE prophylaxis at admission and continue until the patient no longer has significantly reduced mobility, based on an assessment of risks. Start pharmacological VTE

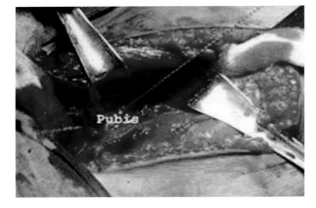

**Fig. 1.10** Performed a transverse osteotomy of the superior pubic ramus

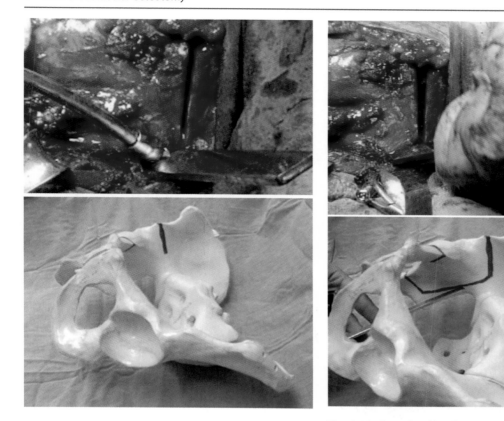

**Fig. 1.12** Opposite side (inner pelvis) transverse osteotomy of the Ilium is demonstrated

**Fig. 1.13** Opposite side of (inner pelvis) oblique iliac osteotomy is shown. A retroacetabular osteotomy was performed from the pelvic brim, along the inside of the pelvis behind the acetabulum, continuing along the posterior column

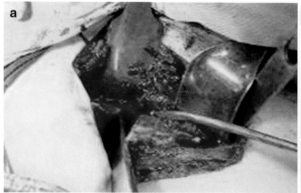

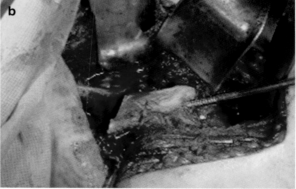

**Fig. 1.14** (**a**) The final osteotomy was done across the posterior portion of the ischium underneath the acetabulum in order to complete the separation of the acetabulum from the remaining pelvis. (**b**) Use two Schanz screws as handles in order to mobilize the free acetabulum to the intended position

prophylaxis after surgery and continue until the patient no longer has significantly reduced mobility.

- The patient is encouraged to sit on the bed while moving the operated limb, bending the hip to 90°.

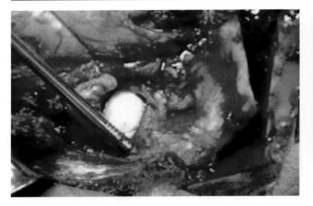

**Fig. 1.15** The joint should be routinely opened and evaluated for labral lesions (torn labral fragments are usually excised)

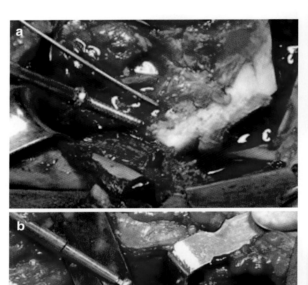

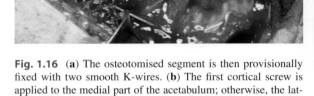

**Fig. 1.16** (**a**) The osteotomised segment is then provisionally fixed with two smooth K-wires. (**b**) The first cortical screw is applied to the medial part of the acetabulum; otherwise, the lateral screw can modify the corrected position of the acetabulum

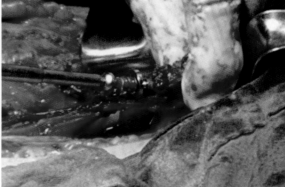

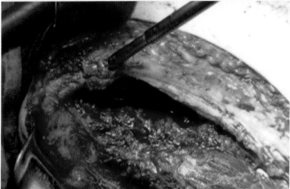

**Fig. 1.17** The anterosuperior iliac spine is reattached in its original place with the previous placed screw, and the integrity of the inguinal ligament is restored

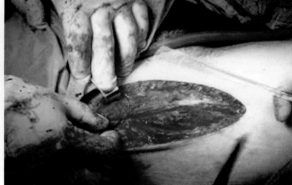

**Fig. 1.18** The fasciae compartment is close with 1/0 Vicryl

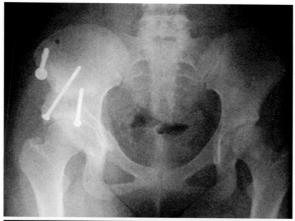

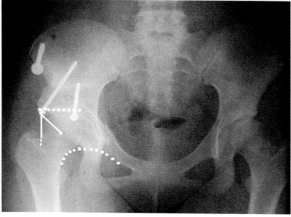

**Fig. 1.19** Postoperative radiograph revealing the correction and the coverage of the right femoral head following the PAO osteotomy

- The drainage tube is removed.
- *Second day*
  - The patient can sit out in a chair.
- *Third day*
  - Using elbow crutches toe-touch weight-bearing is encouraged.
  - Discharge home.

- For 3 weeks, the patient walks T/T weight-bearing with two crutches.
- At the beginning of the 4th week, the patient progresses to partial weight-bearing.
- At the end of the 6th week, the patient stops using the ipsilateral crutch.
- Three weeks later, the patient stops using the second crutch.
- The patient is encouraged to do exercise in a stationary bike during the rehabilitation process.

## Follow-Up

- Outpatient appointments in the clinic should be performed at 6 and 12 weeks and at 6 and 12 months for clinical and radiological assessment. Radiograph at 6 months revealing the correction and the coverage of the right femoral head following the PAO osteotomy, femoral head is medialized to within 5–15 mm of the ilioischial line and Shenton's line is near normal (Fig. 1.19).

## Further Reading

Troelsen A, Elmengaard B, Søballe K. Medium-term outcome of periacetabular osteotomy and predictors of conversion to total hip replacement. J Bone Joint Surg Am. 2009;91(9):2169–79.

Ganz R, Klaue K, Vinh TS, et al. A new periacetabular osteotomy for the treatment of hip dysplasias. Technique and preliminary results. Clin Orthop Relat Res. 1988;232:26–36.

Clohisy JC, St John LC, Nunley RM, et al. Combined periacetabular and femoral osteotomies for severe hip deformities. Clin Orthop Relat Res. 2009;467(9):2221–7.

Teratani T, Naito M, Shiramizu K, et al. Modified pubic osteotomy for medialization of the femoral head in periacetabular osteotomy: a retrospective study of 144 hips. Acta Orthop. 2008;79(4):474–82.

Kim YJ, Ganz R, Murphy SB, et al. Hip joint-preserving surgery: beyond the classic osteotomy. Instr Course Lect. 2006; 55:145–58.

# Triple Pelvic Osteotomy

## Peter Templeton and Peter V. Giannoudis

## Indications

- Acetabular dysplasia with point loading, lateral migration, and painful limp.
- Hip joint should be reasonably congruent in abduction and internal rotation.

## Preoperative Planning

### Clinical Assessment

- May have a short leg on the ipsilateral side.
- Trendelenburg positive.
- Painful hip, thigh, or knee.
- Confirm females are not on contraceptive pill for 4 weeks before surgery.

### Radiological Assessment

- AP pelvis standing.
- AP pelvis with hips abducted and internal rotation.
- CT 3D reconstruction to determine where acetabulum is deficient (Fig. 2.1).
- CT through femoral neck and femoral condyles to determine femoral neck anteversion compared to the opposite side.

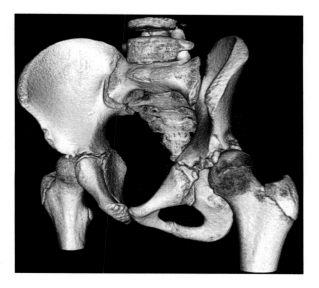

**Fig. 2.1** CT 3D reconstruction presenting the hip dysplasia

- Use information to judge
  - Amount of femoral head coverage required.
  - Amount of femoral neck anteversion and size of AO 90° blade plate if femoral neck osteotomy is required.

## Operative Treatment

### Anesthesia

- General anesthesia plus epidural or regional triple block.
- Prophylactic intravenous antibiotics administered at the time of induction.

P. Templeton
Department of Trauma and Orthopaedic Surgery,
Leeds Teaching Hospitals NHS Trust,
Leeds, UK

P.V. Giannoudis (✉)
Academic Department of Trauma and Orthopaedic Surgery,
School of Medicine, University of Leeds,Leeds, UK
e-mail: pgiannoudi@aol.com

**Fig. 2.2** Surgical tray with the respective tools

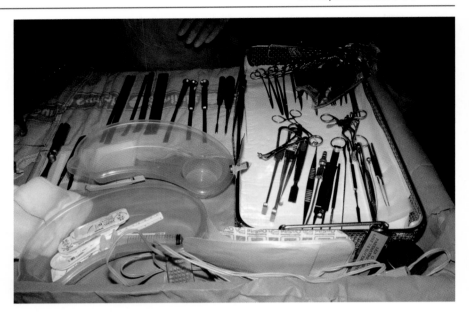

## Equipment (Fig. 2.2)

- Periosteal elevators.
- Lahey clamps.
- Osteotomes and mallet.
- Nibblers.
- Rang retractors.
- Gigli saw.
- Bone-holding forceps.
- Laminar spreaders.
- Travers self-retaining retractors.
- Cannulated screws that are 6.5 mm in diameter. Using a cannulated screw that requires a 3.2-mm-diameter guide wire makes accurate placement much easier.
- Image intensifier.

## Table Set Up

- Radiolucent table allowing unobstructed AP view of the pelvis. Consider extension for standard table or OSI table (Fig. 2.3a).

## Patient Positioning

- Patient supine, sandbag, or "jelly" under lumbar region of affected side.

- Check that it is possible to perform AP view of pelvis with image intensifier (Fig. 2.3b).

## Draping

- Place a "U-shaped" isolation drape before preparing the skin with aqueous betadine or chlorhexidine. Make sure ischium is exposed.
- Then drape as per hip operation leaving thigh, buttock, and iliac crest freely accessible.
- Use a waterproof "sock" for the leg up to the knee.

## Incision

- *Transverse incision* in gluteal fold of buttock. With hip flexed and knee both flexed to 90° in neutral rotation and abduction, expose ischial tuberosity. Reflect gluteus maximus laterally. Hamstrings are attached to the ischial tuberosity. Sciatic nerve is situated lateral to semimembranosus. Clear tendon attachments from site of osteotomy and place Lahey clamps on each side of ischium to protect the pudendal nerve and vessels in obturator foramen (Fig. 2.4).
- *Anterior oblique incision* centered on a point 2 cm distal to the anterior superior iliac spine. Explore the interval between sartorius and tensor fascia

**Fig. 2.3** (**a**) Radiolucent table allowing unobstructed AP view of the pelvis. (**b**) Patient positioning and marked leg

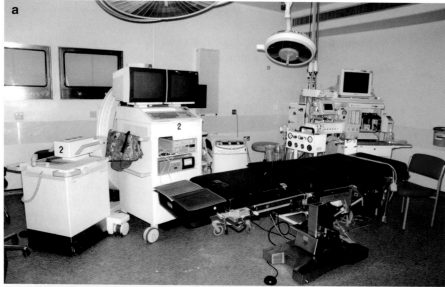

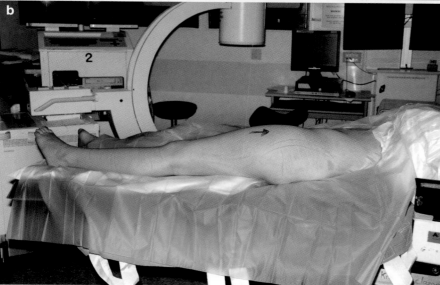

lata muscles, protecting the lateral cutaneous nerve of the thigh which should be retracted medially. Conjoint tendon of rectus does not need to be reflected if joint capsule is not going to be opened. In immature patients, split iliac crest with knife from anterior superior iliac spine backwards to the middle third of the crest at least. Reflect crest medially and laterally using a broad periosteal elevator down to greater sciatic notch. Keeping close to medial and lateral cortices of ilium, aim 45° distally and not vertically downwards for fear

of injuring superior gluteal vessel and sciatic nerve. Pack with a swap on each side (Fig. 2.5).

## Procedure

- *Ischial osteotomy.* Isolate ischium and protect contents of obturator foramen. Use osteotome to divide ischium from lateral to medial. Consider using nibblers to broaden the osteotomy to ensure ease of displacement (Fig. 2.6).

- *Superior pubic osteotomy.* Via the anterior oblique approach, the pubis is exposed subperiosteally. Flexing and adducting the hip will make this exposure easier. I release psoas at the brim by performing an intramuscular tenotomy to reduce tension in the psoas. Again the pubis is isolated using Lahey clamps, one superior and one inferior to ensure that the osteotomy is performed in the correct place and not intra-articularly. Curved osteotomes are used to complete the osteotomy under image intensifier control (Fig. 2.7a, b).

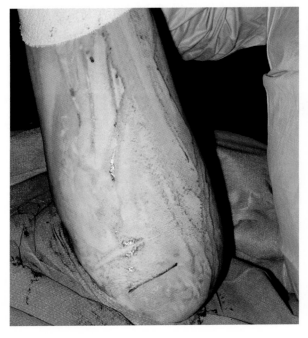

**Fig. 2.4** Transverse incision marked

- *Salter pelvic osteotomy.* A routine Salter osteotomy is performed from the greater sciatic notch to the anterior inferior iliac spine or 0.5 cm above it to allow crossed cannulated screws if necessary. The contents of the greater sciatic notch are protected with Rang retractors, and a Gigli saw is passed from medial to lateral using the curved Lahey clamps. The Rang retractors should be positioned perpendicular to the plane of the ilium. While the Gigli saw is being used, it is important to keep one's hands as far apart as possible to prevent the saw "binding" in the middle of the manoeuvre. Once complete, the anterior third of the iliac crest is harvested with an oscillating saw to be used as a graft. It may as well need to be fashioned into a 25° wedge with the saw. The iliac osteotomy is opened to provide improved anterior and lateral coverage by placing the lower limb in a "figure of 4" position and pulling the distal iliac fragment forward and inferiorly with a bone-holding forceps and a laminar spreader. It is essential not to allow the distal fragment to drop backwards, and the posterior edges of the iliac osteotomy must be touching at the greater sciatic notch to prevent injury to the sciatic nerve and to prevent overlengthening of the lower limb. The graft is inserted and then held with two guide wires under image intensifier control (Fig. 2.8a–c).

## Implant Positioning

- Either 2 proximal to distal 6.5-mm cannulated screws or a crossed configuration can be used to give the

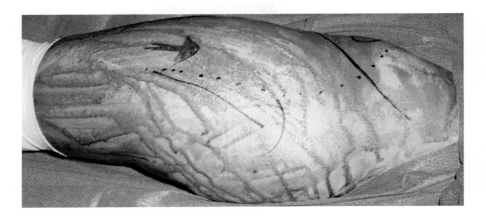

**Fig. 2.5** Anterior oblique incision marked

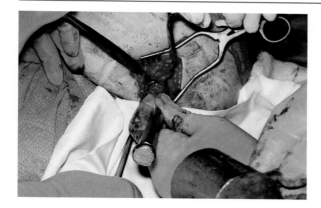

**Fig. 2.6** Ischial osteotomy with the osteotome

most stable fixation. One can expect a 15° improvement in the center-edge angle (Figs. 2.9a, b and 2.10).

- If the coverage obtained is not sufficient then consider a femoral osteotomy as well (Fig. 2.11).

## Closure

- Wash with saline.
- Close ischial wound at time of procedure.
- Anterior wound requires iliac crest to be brought together with towel clips and then sutured with 1.0 Vicryl interrupted sutures.
- External oblique and fascia closed with 2.0 Vicryl taking care not to trap lateral cutaneous nerve of the thigh. Fat closed with 2.0 Vicryl and 3.0 Vicryl subcuticular for skin (Fig. 2.12).

## Postoperative Rehabilitation

- I do not use a spica in adolescents or adults.
- An epidural for 48 h postop provides excellent pain relief.
- Mobilize once comfortable after removal of epidural.
- Start mechanical VTE prophylaxis at admission and continue until the patient no longer has significantly reduced mobility based on an assessment of risks. Start pharmacological VTE prophylaxis after surgery and continue until the patient no longer has significantly reduced mobility.
- Toe-touch weight-bearing for 6 weeks then partial weight-bearing for another 6 weeks.
- Encourage a range of movement exercises after osteotomies have united, 6–8 weeks after surgery.
- If satisfactory at 12 weeks, consider full weight-bearing.

## Outpatient Follow-Up

- Review wounds by district nurse or practice nurse at 2 weeks.
- Review in the clinic at 6 weeks for an AP pelvic X-ray and then at 12 weeks (Fig. 2.13).

## Implant Removal

- I leave the cannulated screws in situ unless they will cause a problem with future total hip replacement.

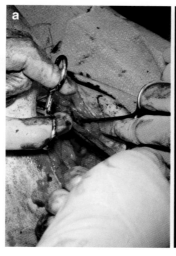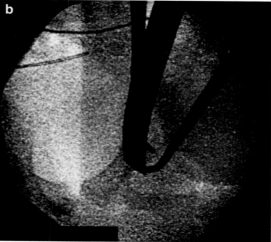

**Fig. 2.7** (**a**) Superior pubic osteotomy. (**b**) Superior pubic osteotomy performed under image intensifier

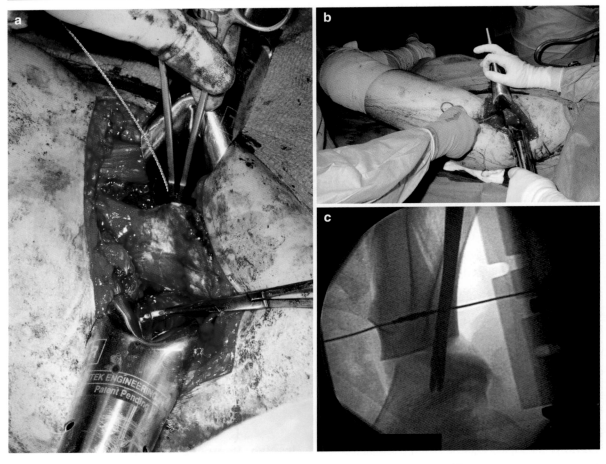

**Fig. 2.8** (**a**, **b**) Salter pelvic osteotomy. (**c**) Salter pelvic osteotomy performed under image intensifier

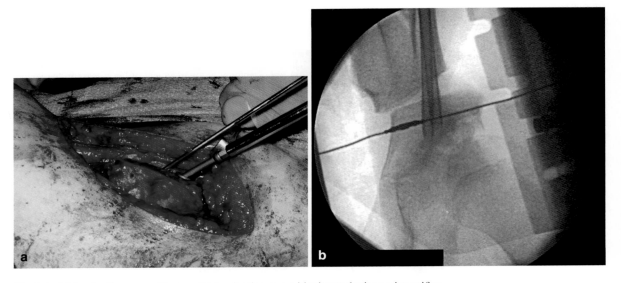

**Fig. 2.9** (**a**) Implant/screw positioning. (**b**) Implant/screw positioning under image intensifier

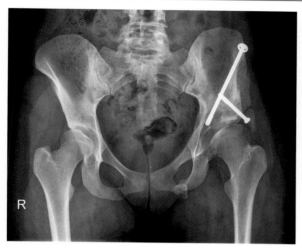

Fig. 2.10 Postoperative X-ray

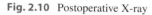

Fig. 2.12 Skin closure

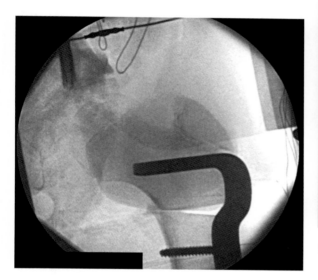

Fig. 2.11 Femoral osteotomy if it necessary

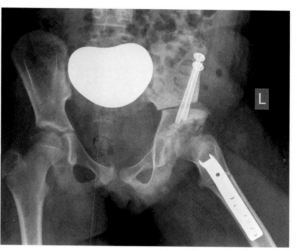

Fig. 2.13 X-rays are necessary during the follow-up period

## Further Reading

Vukasinovic Z, Pelillo F, Spasovski D, et al. Triple pelvic osteotomy for the treatment of residual hip dysplasia. Analysis of complications. Hip Int. 2009;19(4):315–22.

Santore RF, Turgeon TR, Phillips 3rd WF, et al. Pelvic and femoral osteotomy in the treatment of hip disease in the young adult. Instr Course Lect. 2006;55:131–44.

Gillingham BL, Sanchez AA, Wenger DR, et al. Pelvic osteotomies for the treatment of hip dysplasia in children and young adults. J Am Acad Orthop Surg. 1999;7(5):325–37.

De Kleuver M, Kooijman MA, Pavlov PW, et al. Triple osteotomy of the pelvis for acetabular dysplasia: results at 8 to 15 years. J Bone Joint Surg Br. 1997;79(2):225–9.

# Pubic Symphysis Fusion

Peter V. Giannoudis and Nikolaos K. Kanakaris

**3**

## Introduction

- Chronic pain secondary to osteitis pubis.
- Postpartum pelvic instability.
- Chronic pain due to degeneration of the cartilage.
- Previous traumatic diastasis that failed to unite and mobility is associated with abnormal movement of the joint and pain.
- Exclude painful visceral pathologies of the pelvis (urogenital, gastrointestinal), lower back pain syndromes (lumbar disc lesion/prolapse, radiculopathies, spondylolisthesis, rheumatism, sciatica, spinal stenosis, or lumbar spine arthritis), urinary tract infections, femoral vein thrombosis and obstetric complications (preterm labor, abruption, round ligament pain).

## Preoperative Planning

### Clinical Assessment

- Obtain detailed history of presenting complaint (number of pregnancies, trauma sustained and presence of underlying systemic inflammatory diseases).

P.V. Giannoudis (✉)
Academic Department of Trauma and Orthopaedic Surgery,
School of Medicine, University of Leeds, Leeds, UK
e-mail: pgiannoudi@aol.com

N.K. Kanakaris
Department of Trauma and Orthopaedic Surgery,
Leeds Teaching Hospitals NHS Trust, Leeds, UK

- Assess intake and frequency of painkillers and other treatment modalities (i.e., physiotherapy, injections), which were prescribed without success.
- Note essential symptoms – pain of the pubic symphysis on walking or at standing on one leg, or while climbing stairs or turning over in bed. Pain may radiate to the groin, perineum or posterior thigh.
- Alteration of the gait patterns or a temporary "catching" sensation or clicking on hip flexion, located mostly anteriorly.
- Tenderness to deep palpation of the suprapubic area and palpable step of the pubic symphysis joint may be evident.
- Signs of local inflammation (erythema, edema, warmth) may exist in a small percentage of the cases.
- Request baseline blood investigations to exclude an infectious process.

### Radiological Assessment

- Standard anteroposterior (AP), inlet, and outlet pelvic films are used to measure the degree of symphyseal separation and to identify cortical sclerosis, spurring, or rarefaction.
- The use of single-limb stance AP or flamingo views delineates more subtle cases of pubic symphysis separation and appears useful in quantifying the degree of pelvic girdle instability.
- The detection of a step-off of more than 2 mm at the standard AP or flamingo views, respectively, is considered by some authors as the threshold of pelvic instability (Fig. 3.1).

P.V. Giannoudis (ed.), *Practical Procedures in Elective Orthopaedic Surgery*,
DOI 10.1007/978-0-85729-814-0_3, © Springer-Verlag London Limited 2012

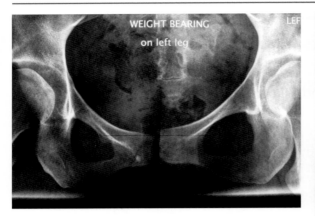

**Fig. 3.1** Flamingo view illustrating abnormal movement of the pubis symphysis

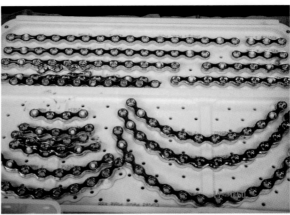

**Fig. 3.2** Matta plating system

- CT scans and scintigraphy can be used to evaluate joint pathology and to exclude other causes.
- MRI is recommended for the differential diagnosis of pelvic instability and for the detection of bone oedema and early joint degeneration.
- Guided local anesthetic injections to the pubis symphysis joint...offer significant diagnostic specificity reaching 100%; however, this diagnostic specificity reflects only to intra-articular pathologies.

## Operative Treatment

### Anesthesia

- Prophylactic antibiotics are given as per local hospital protocol.
- General anesthesia is administered with the patient in the supine position.

### Table and Equipment

- The Matta plating system and osteotomes (Fig. 3.2).
- Image intensifier is required from the beginning, and a radiolucent table (OSI).
- The equipment tray is set up on the site of the operation.
- The image intensifier is on the opposite side of the surgeon.

## Draping and Surgical Approach

- The skin is prepared with the usual antiseptics.
- The draping of the patient is in the usual fashion from two fingers below the pubis symphysis to two fingers superior to the umbilicus.
- A transverse Pfannenstiel incision is used for the approach (Fig. 3.3a).
- Following incision of the skin and subcutaneous fat layer, the linea alba is identified (Fig. 3.3b) and divided longitudinally (Fig. 3.3c) with careful elevation of the insertion of the abdominis muscle laterally from each superior pubic ramus.
- Hohmann retractors are placed in the obturator foramen, allowing enhancement of the exposure.
- Using a small osteotome and bone nibblers, the symphyseal cartilage is removed, and the joint is exposed (Fig. 3.4a, b).
- Part of the superior pubic ramus cortex is removed from each side to expose the cancellous part of the bone forming a T-shaped bed (Fig. 3.5).
- A well-vascularised bed has now been developed for the implantation of the T-shaped tricortical graft, which can be harvested from the iliac crest (Fig. 3.6a, b).

## Implant Positioning

- A 3.5-mm 8-hole plate is applied superiorly over the pubis symphysis (over the graft), precontoured as per the shape of the anterior pelvic ring.

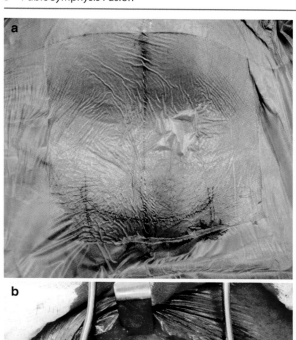

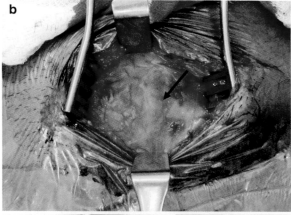

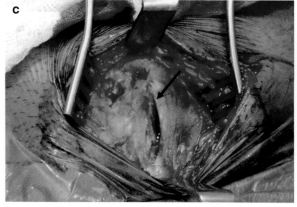

**Fig. 3.3** (**a**) Pfannenstiel incision is used for the approach. (**b**) After dissection of skin and the underlying subcutaneous fat layer, the linea alba (*black arrow*) is identified and (**c**) divided longitudinally (*black arrow*)

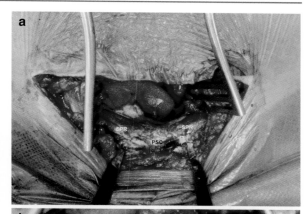

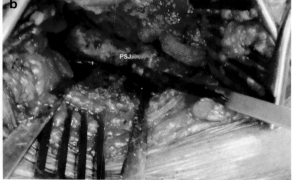

**Fig. 3.4** (**a**) Exposure of pubis symphysis and visualization of cartilage (*PSC* pubis symphysis cartilage, *SPR* superior pubic rami). (**b**) By using a small osteotome and bone nibblers, the symphyseal cartilage is removed for exposure of the joint (*PSJ* pubis symphysis joint)

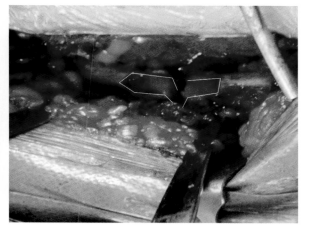

**Fig. 3.5** Part of the superior pubic ramus cortex is removed from each side to expose the cancellous part of the bone forming a T-shaped bed (outlined with the *white lines*)

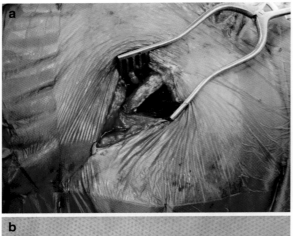

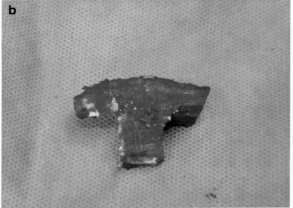

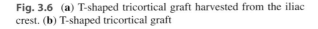

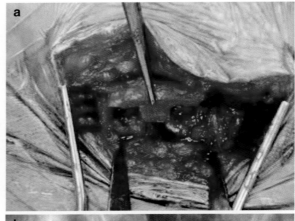

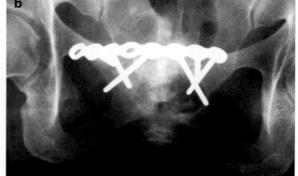

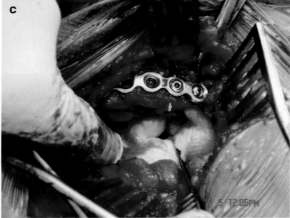

**Fig. 3.6** (**a**) T-shaped tricortical graft harvested from the iliac crest. (**b**) T-shaped tricortical graft

- Four 3.5-mm cortical screws are inserted through the plate in each superior pubic ramus. One of them secures the graft to each superior pubic ramus, inserted in an oblique direction to optimize the purchase and compression of the T-shaped tricortical graft (Fig. 3.7a–c).
- Primary bone healing is the expected method of fusion. This is the best way to minimize the risk of impaired bone healing, which can be as high as 50% for the pubis symphysis.
- Intraoperatively screening with an image intensifier and obtaining AP, inlet and outlet views will confirm the appropriate screw length and implant positioning.

**Fig. 3.7** (**a**) Compression of the T-shaped tricortical graft within the bed previously prepared. (**b**) Screws are inserted in an oblique direction to optimize the purchase and stability of the graft. (**c**) Plate is placed superiorly over the graft and pubic rami

## Closure

- Irrigate the wound thoroughly.
- A drain should be placed in the space of Retzius.

- Any detachment of the abdominis from the pubis symphysis should be reattached with 1.0 Vicryl sutures.

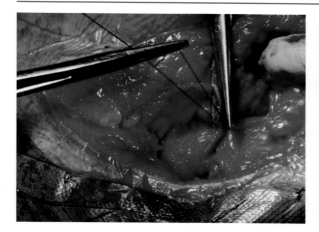

**Fig. 3.8** Closure of linea alba with 1/0 Vicryl suture

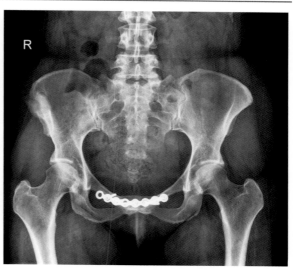

**Fig. 3.9** AP pelvic radiograph revealing fusion of pubis symphysis a year after surgery

- The linea alba should be repaired with interrupted sutures with 1.0 Vicryl sutures (Fig. 3.8).
- The fat layer should be approximated with 2.0 Vicryl sutures.
- The skin should be closed with either surgical staplers or 3.0 S/C PDS suture in continuous manner.

## Postoperative Management

- Start mechanical VTE prophylaxis at admission and continue until the patient no longer has significantly reduced mobility based on an assessment of risks. Start pharmacological VTE prophylaxis after surgery and continue until the patient no longer has significantly reduced mobility.
- At home, the authors prefers the prescription of 75 mg of aspirin for 6–8 weeks.
- Perform routine blood tests and radiography of the pelvis in 24 hours, including AP, inlet, and outlet views.
- Postoperatively watch for DVT and infection.
- Mobilization (weight-bearing) should be restricted for 6 weeks (until fusion has been confirmed on the radiographs). A wheelchair can be used for this period of time.
- When full weight-bearing is allowed, physiotherapy is indicated.
- Physiotherapy should be indicated at increasing hip abductor strength.

- Restoration of a normal gait; lower back strengthening exercises should be the focus of the rehabilitation program.

## Postoperative Complications

- Pneumonia, deep vein thrombosis, pulmonary embolism, and dehiscence of the wound.
- Loss of fixation is usually associated with failed fusion. If this occurs, the entire procedure requires revision.

## Outpatient Follow-up

- Follow-up should be taken in 2 weeks, 6 weeks, and 12 weeks after surgery and then in 6 months and a year later (Fig. 3.9).
- Patient can be discharged and seen again following the request of general practitioner.

## Implant Removal

- Implant removal is not indicated unless there is good evidence to suggest that any ongoing symptoms are secondary to the presence of the implant.

## Further Reading

Giannoudis PV, Chalidis BE, Roberts CS. Internal fixation of traumatic diastasis of pubic symphysis: is plate removal essential? Arch Orthop Trauma Surg. 2008;128(3):325–31.

Bagchi K, Uhl RL. Fixation of pubic symphyseal disruptions: One or two plates? Orthopedics. 2009;32(6):427.

Haider NR, Syed RA, Dermady D. Osteitis pubis: an important pain generator in women with lower pelvic or abdominal pain: a case report and literature review. Pain Physician. 2005;8(1):145–7.

# Sacroiliac Joint Fusion

**4**

Peter V. Giannoudis, Fragkiskos N. Xypnitos, and Nikolaos K. Kanakaris

## Introduction

- The sacroiliac (SI) joint is a complex, synovial, diarthrodial joint that transmits forces from the pelvis to the spine and allows 2–4° of movement in the sagittal plane.
- Receives innervation from the lumbosacral nerve roots.
- The SI joint is unable to function in isolation; anatomically and biomechanically, it shares all of its muscles with the hip joint.
- Causes of SI joint pain:
    - SI joint dysfunction.
    - Inflammatory arthritis.
    - SI joint osteoarthritis.
    - Posttraumatic arthritis.
    - Infection.
    - Postpartum SI instability.
    - Crystal arthropathy (gout or pseudogout).
    - Osteitis condensans ilii.
    - Tumor or tumor-like conditions.

P.V. Giannoudis (✉)
Academic Department of Trauma and Orthopaedic Surgery,
School of Medicine, University of Leeds,
Leeds, UK
e-mail: pgiannoudi@aol.com

F.N. Xypnitos • N.K. Kanakaris
Department of Trauma and Orthopaedic Surgery,
Leeds Teaching Hospitals NHS Trust,
Leeds, UK

## Indications

- The mainstay of therapy for disorders of the SI has been nonoperative treatment, including rest, physiotherapy, nonsteroidal anti-inflammatory agents, radiofrequency neurotomy, and intra-articular injections. When these modalities fail, SI fusion is recommended.
- Various techniques have been proposed to achieve SI joint arthrodesis, including the anterior approach and the percutaneous fixation.
- These techniques include:
    - Noninstrumented arthrodesis with bone graft.
    - Instrumented arthrodesis with or without bone graft.
    - Percutaneous instrumented arthrodesis guided by fluoroscopy or computed tomography with or without bone graft.
- SI joint fusion through an anterior approach is authors' method of choice.

## Preoperative Planning

### Clinical Assessment

- Clinical evaluation consists of:
    - Patrick's test.
    - Gaenslen's test.
    - Yeoman's test.
    - Gillet's test.
    - Iliac compression test.

- Unfortunately, the main characteristic that these tests share is that none has been proven to be sensitive or specific enough on its own.
- A fluoroscopically guided intra-articular injection represents the gold standard test to confirm the diagnosis.

## Radiological Assessment

- Plain radiographs of the pelvis (Fig. 4.1a–c) and lumbosacral spine and specific views of the SI joint are used to identify signs of arthritis or sclerosis.
- CT scan of the SI joint will confirm the extent of arthritis of the joint. It will also demonstrate the precise anatomy of the patient. This enhances the safety of iliosacral screw placement.
- MR scan of both the lumbosacral spine and the SI joint can be used in order to identify coexisting neurological pathology or compression in the lumbosacral spine.

## Operative Treatment

### Anesthesia

- General anesthesia.
- Administration of prophylactic antibiotics as per local hospital protocol at induction.

### Table and Equipment

- Radiolucent table.
- Image intensifier.

### Table Setup

- The instrumentation is set up at the site of the operation.
- Image intensifier is from the contralateral site.
- Position the table diagonally across the operating room so that the operating area lies in the clean air field.

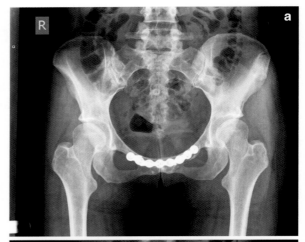
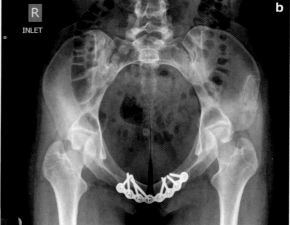
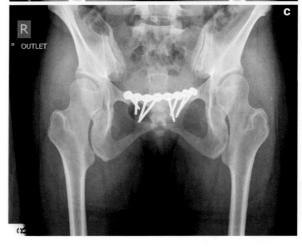

**Fig. 4.1** Preoperative radiographs of the pelvis. (**a**) AP, (**b**) inlet, (**c**) outlet

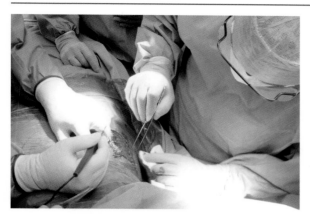

**Fig. 4.2** Skin incision

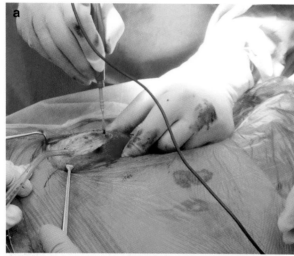

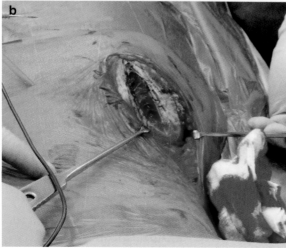

**Fig. 4.3** (**a, b**) Detachment of the abdominal muscles and the fascia of the iliacus from the ilium

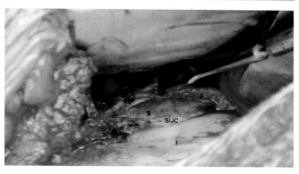

**Fig. 4.4** Subperiosteal elevation and revelation of SI joint (*S* sacrum, *I* ilium, *SIJC* sacroiliac joint cartilage, *P* periosteum)

## Patient Positioning

- Supine.
- The patient is positioned so that four radiologic views of the pelvis can be obtained: lateral, antero-posterior, inlet, and outlet views.

## Draping and Surgical Approach

- Prepare the perineum, abdomen, part of the flanks, and lower extremities with the usual antiseptic solutions (aqueous/alcoholic povidone-iodine).
- Skin incision (Fig. 4.2).
- The first window of the ilioinguinal approach is utilized.
- The abdominal muscles and the fascia of the iliacus are detached from the ilium (Fig. 4.3a, b) following subperiosteal elevation (Fig. 4.4). Access is made to the SI joint.
- Care has to be taken to avoid any injury to the lumbar sacral nerve root L5, which runs very close by, approximately 1.5 cm across the ala of the sacrum.
- Thorough debridement of the SI joint cartilage using a chisel (Fig. 4.5a) and a burr (Fig. 4.5b).
- Removal of articular cartilage (Fig. 4.6a).
- Introduction at the SI joint space (Fig. 4.6b) of the bone graft (Fig. 4.7a–c).
- A narrow DCP 4.5 or 3.5 are the preferred implants (Fig. 4.8).
- Two plates enable fixation in areas of dense bone and prevent shearing.

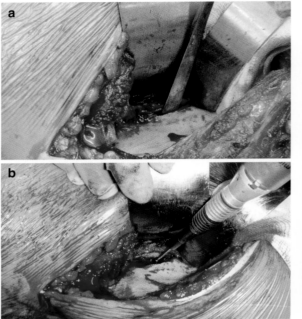

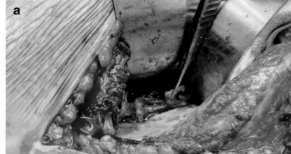

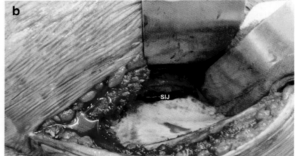

**Fig. 4.5** (**a**) SI joint debridement with a chisel. (**b**) SI joint debridement with a burr

**Fig. 4.6** (**a**) Removal of articular cartilage. (**b**) SI joint (*SIJ*) after debridement

- Alternatively, the combination of a 7.3-mm cannulated cancellous screw and a plate can be used (Fig. 4.9a).
- The holes of the sacral screws are drilled under direct vision and parallel to the joint.

## Closure

- Irrigate the wound thoroughly and achieve hemostasis.
- The fascia is closed with No.1 PDS or Vicryl over one drain.
- Subcutaneous fat is closed with absorbable sutures 2.0 PDS or Vicryl.
- Skin is closed with stainless steel surgical staples or monofilament nylon sutures in an interrupted manner.

## Pitfalls to Avoid and Tips

- Noninstrumented arthrodesis relies on the intact SI joint ligaments to secure stability.
- Arthrodesis via anterior or posterior approaches can cause major complications, such as injury to the erector spinae muscle insertions, the dorsal sensory nerve roots, the sacral plexus, and the internal iliac vessels.
- Percutaneous instrumented arthrodesis without bone graft relies on the strength of the screws to secure long-term stability.
- The initial iliosacral screw is positioned in such a way as to allow the insertion of a second screw, if required.
- The planned screw location should avoid the anterior sacral slope.
- The sacroiliac joint is L-shaped, and care is required when introducing the guidewire. The safe zone lies between the alar cortex superoanteriorly and the sacral neural foramen posteriorly.
- The inlet view shows the orientation of screws relative to the coronal plane and will show any screw tip perforating the ala anteriorly, and the outlet view will show those extending into the sacral foramina or superior to the ala.

## Postoperative Rehabilitation

- Two further doses of prophylactic antibiotics, routine bloods, and radiographs of the pelvis in 24 h, including AP pelvis and inlet/outlet views.

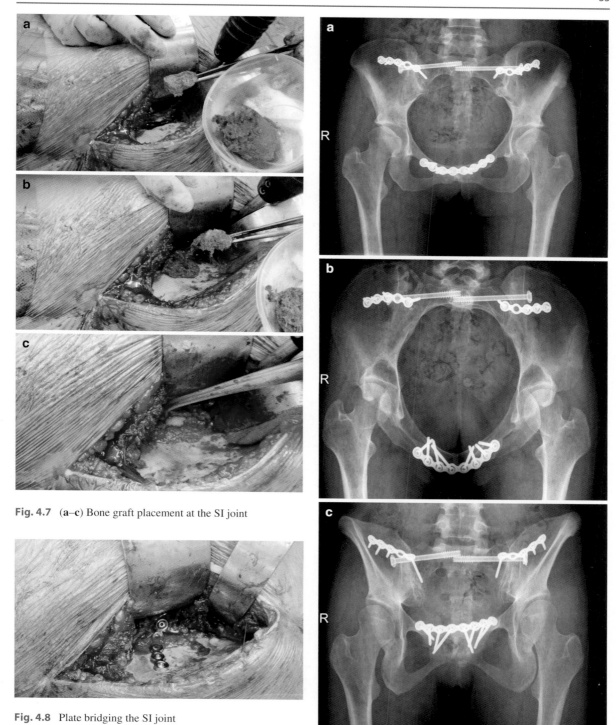

**Fig. 4.7** (**a–c**) Bone graft placement at the SI joint

**Fig. 4.8** Plate bridging the SI joint

**Fig. 4.9** Postoperative radiographs at 12-month follow-up. (**a**) AP, (**b**) inlet, (**c**) outlet

- Start mechanical VTE prophylaxis at admission and continue until the patient no longer has significantly reduced mobility based on an assessment of risks. Start pharmacological VTE prophylaxis after surgery and continue until the patient no longer has significantly reduced mobility.
- Postoperatively watch for DTV, PE, and infection.
- The drains are removed in 24 h.
- The patient is mobilized with toe-touch weight-bearing on the affected side.

## Outpatient Follow-up

- Review at 3 weeks, 6 weeks, 3 months, 6 months, and 12 months with both clinical and radiographic assessments of the pelvis (Fig. 4.9a–c).
- Further radiological evaluation is performed only if patients report continuing symptoms. In these cases, a CT scan to determine whether or not fusion had occurred and an MR scan to identify any alternative source of pain are obtained.
- Discharge from follow-up after clinical and radiological evidence of fusion. The absence of clinical symptoms and signs and the absence of any radiological signs of metal failure or lucency indicate fusion of the sacroiliac joint – usually after 12–18 months from the time of the surgery.
- Review again at the request of the GP.

## Implant Removal

- No removal is indicated unless there is a good evidence of soft tissue irritation.

## Further Reading

Buchowski JM, Kebaish KM, Sinkov V, Cohen DB, Sieber AN, Kostuik JP. Functional and radiographic outcome of sacroiliac arthrodesis for the disorders of the sacroiliac joint. Spine J. 2005;5:520–8.

Giannoudis PV, Tsiridis E. A minimally-invasive technique for the treatment of pyogenic sacroiliitis. A case report. J Bone Joint Surg Br. 2007;89-B:112–4.

Khurana A, Guha AR, Mohanty K, Ahuja S. Percutaneous fusion of the sacroiliac joint with hollow modular anchorage screws. Clinical and radiological outcome. J Bone Joint Surg Br. 2009;91-B:627–31.

# Part III

# Lower Extremity: Hip – Femur

# Hip Arthroscopy for Femoroacetabular Impingement (FAI)

## 5

Ernest Schilders and Alexandra Dimitrakopoulou

## Introduction

- Femoroacetabular impingement (FAI) is a condition reintroduced by Ganz in 2003. The overall incidence has been estimated to be around 10–15%, and there is growing scientific evidence that FAI leads to arthritis of the hip.
- There are three types of FAI: cam deformity, pincer deformity, and a mixed type.
- A cam deformity refers to an increased offset of bone at the anterolateral aspect of the head–neck junction of the femur. The femoral head has lost its spherical shape. When the hip is flexed and internally rotated, the abnormal head impinges against the labrum and acetabulum. Because of the shear forces, delamination of the articular cartilage occurs gradually leading to full thickness cartilage lesions. The delamination typically starts at the junction between labrum and articular cartilage. Cam abnormalities can occur after a silent slipped femoral capital epiphysis or after a malunion of a neck of femur fracture or through genetic predisposition.
- A pincer abnormality means that there is an acetabular overcoverage of the femoral head. There are two types of pincer abnormalities: a more focal type and coxa profunda when there is global overcoverage. With 90° flexion and internal rotation, the labrum and acetabulum abuts against the femoral neck. This may lead to tearing, degeneration and ossification of the labrum and often there is associated articular cartilage damage.
- A cam deformity is more common in young males, whilst a pincer abnormality is more common in middle-aged females, although most hips show a mixed femoroacetabular impingement pattern with cam predominance.

## Clinical Findings

### Clinical Examination

- Deep-seated pain in the groin area with sports activities and activities such as sitting, walking, putting on socks and shoes.
- Reduced ROM of the hip predominantly affecting internal rotation, flexion, and abduction.
- A positive impingement test (Fig. 5.1a). A reduced Faber distance (Fig. 5.1b).

### Radiographic Assessment

- X-ray true pelvis (Fig. 5.2a) to demonstrate a pincer (crossover sign) or cam abnormality. To ensure accurate pelvic rotation, the coccyx should be centered over the symphysis. The cross-table lateral (Fig. 5.2b) enables better assessment of the anterior profile of the femoral neck.

E. Schilders (✉)
The London Hip Arthroscopy Centre,
The Wellington Hospital, London, UK

Faculty of Health, Leeds Metropolitan University,
Leeds, UK
e-mail: ernest.schilders@onehealth.co.uk

A. Dimitrakopoulou
The London Hip Arthroscopy Centre,
The Wellington Hospital, London, UK
e-mail: alexdimitr@yahoo.gr

P.V. Giannoudis (ed.), *Practical Procedures in Elective Orthopaedic Surgery*,
DOI 10.1007/978-0-85729-814-0_5, © Springer-Verlag London Limited 2012

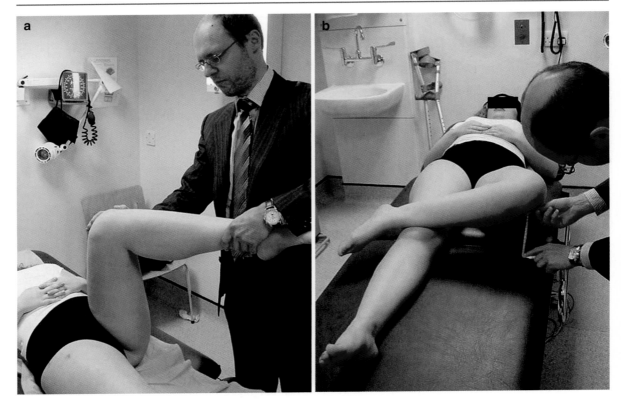

Fig. 5.1 (a) Anterior Impingement test. (b) Measurement of the Faber distance

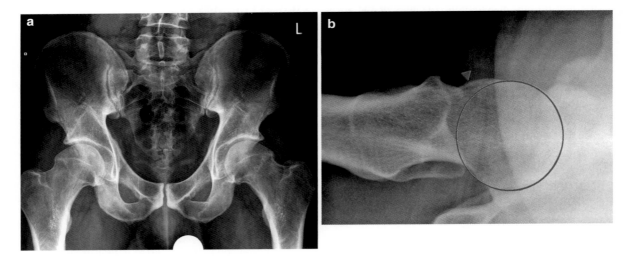

Fig. 5.2 (a) An anteroposterior X-ray, (b) Lateral X-ray (cross-table view), and

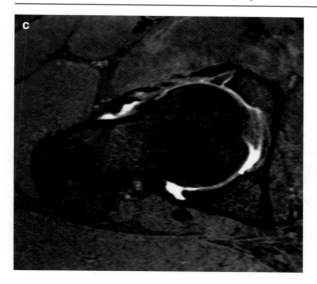

**Fig. 5.2** (**c**) MRI arthrogram, demonstrating a labral tear

- Image intensifier guided diagnostic injection of the hip with a local anaesthetic.
- MRI arthrogram (Fig. 5.2c) with a local anesthetic to detect labral tears and articular cartilage lesions or other associated pathology.

## Operative Treatment

### Instruments/Equipment

- An image intensifier.
- A hip positioning system or traction table.
- Fluid management system. It is important to have a system which has an inflow and outflow system. A pump which only has an inflow should not be used because of the risk of excessive swelling.
- A 70° arthroscope
- Hip arthroscopy cannula system
- Radiofrequency probes
- Long shaver blades
- Half pipes
- Arthroscopic knife
- Microfracture set
- Labral repair set

## Anaesthesia

- Muscle relaxant at induction (Atracurium 0.6 mg/kg)
- Remifentanyl infusion during surgery for blood pressure control, muscle relaxation, and analgesia
- Multimodal analgesia at the end of the surgery. NSAID/paracetamol and morphine
- Postoperative pain relief consists of codeine, paracetamol, and NSAID
- Antibiotics administration at induction

## Patient Positioning (Fig. 5.3)

- Supine position
- The C arm is positioned on the contralateral side of the patient, so we can screen when required
- The television screen is positioned on the opposite operated site of the patient
- The fluoroscopy monitor at the foot end
- Intermittent calf compression, DVT prophylaxis

## Hip Distraction

- Traction table or hip positioning system to distract the hip. The hip is positioned in a slightly flexed position and maximal internal rotation. The sciatic nerve is at risk when traction is applied with the hip in too much flexion.
- The post is positioned against the medial aspect of the operated leg to achieve lateral and axial directing forces of distraction. Use a large perineal post to avoid pudendal nerve injuries. The scrotum can be taped away, so it is not interpositioned between the post and perineum. Slight countertraction is applied on the contralateral leg.
- Distraction is applied under image intensification until the vacuum phenomenon (Fig. 5.4a) is observed.
- To access the hip joint safely, approximately 1 cm of distraction is required to ensure safe introduction of instruments into the central compartment.
- Draw the anatomical landmarks (Fig. 5.4b) of the greater trochanter and the anterior superior iliac

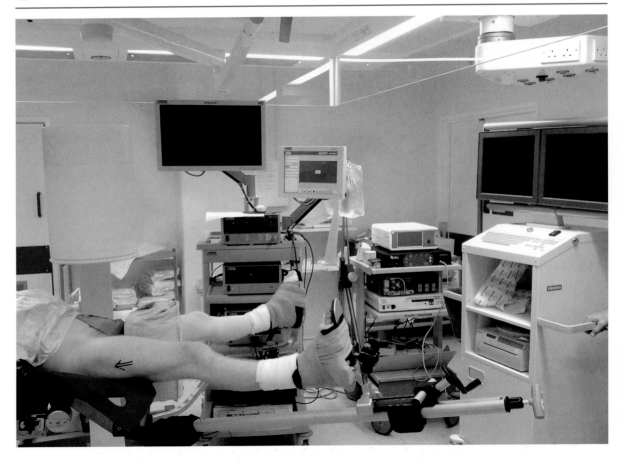

**Fig. 5.3** Patient's positioning

spine (ASIS) and mark the anterior and anterolateral portal. Draw a vertical line from the ASIS, the main femoral neurovascular bundle lies medial to this line.

- It is important that traction should not be excessive and be kept to a minimum period of time; guidelines suggest not more than 90 min.
- Once proceed to the peripheral compartment, the traction is released, and the perineal post is removed. This stage of the procedure is dynamic and requires flexion, rotation, and abduction to assess impingement. When using a traction table, the amount of flexion that can be achieved is limited, and the foot will have to be taken out of the boot to allow 90° of hip flexion. With commercial hip positioning systems, dynamic assessment can be accomplished without taking the foot out of the boot.

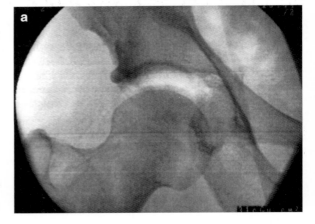

**Fig. 5.4** (a) The traction is applied, and the vacuum phenomenon is evident in the X-ray

**Fig. 5.4** (b) Marking the anatomical landmarks

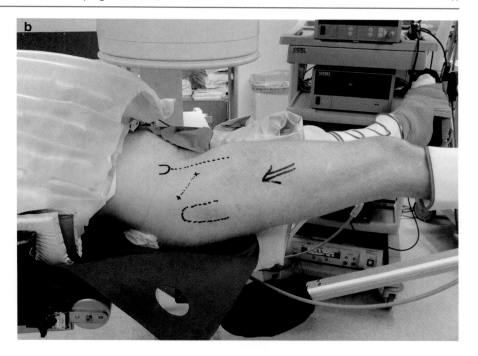

## Portal Placement

- Anterolateral portal is positioned 1 cm anterior and superior to the tip of the greater trochanter.
- An arthroscopic needle is inserted parallel to femoral neck just above the femoral head to avoid labral damage (Fig. 5.5a).
- Remove the guide wire from the needle and inject 40 mL saline, which will further distend the hip joint (Fig. 5.5b).
- The needle can then be repositioned just above the femoral head. A Nitinol guidewire is inserted, the needle removed, and a small skin incision made. A deeper incision puts the lateral cutaneous nerve at risk.
- A 5-mm cannula with obturator is inserted over the guidewire (Fig. 5.5c). It is preferable to use a 5-mm cannula initially as it provides optimum fluid inflow which improves visibility.
- The anterior portal is positioned 7 cm medial and slightly more distal than previous portal. This portal is made under direct vision. Look for the capsule in the triangle formed by the femoral head and the anterior labrum and position the needle in the center (Fig. 5.5d).

## Steps of the Procedure

- The hip joint can be divided in two compartments: the central compartment and the peripheral compartment.
  - The central compartment is the area between acetabulum and femoral head and is accessed under traction.
  - The peripheral compartment refers to the extra-articular yet intracapsular part of the hip around the femoral neck. The peripheral compartment is accessed without traction.

## Central Compartment Arthroscopy

- Both portals are used as working and viewing portals, and therefore to appropriately inspect the entire anatomy of the central compartment, generous capsulotomies will enable easier and safer use of instruments.
- At the stage of the procedure, it is important to monitor the traction time.
- Develop a standardized approach in viewing the normal hip anatomy.

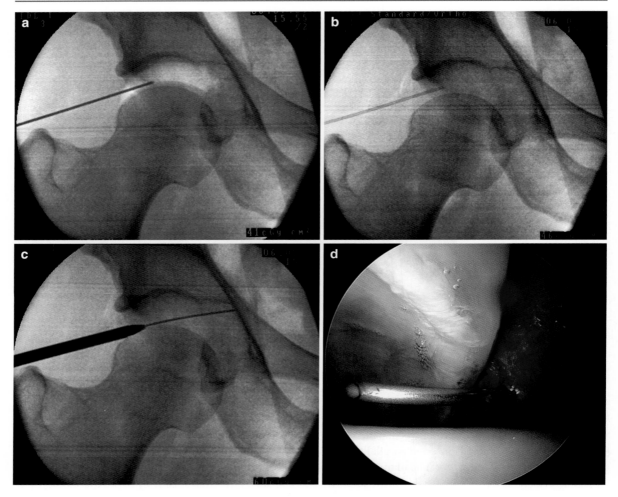

**Fig. 5.5** (**a**) The needle is inserted into the joint through the anterolateral portal. (**b**) Saline is injected for further joint's distraction. (**c**) The cannula is inserted into the joint following the guidewire and (**d**) an arthroscopic view of the joint through the anterior portal

- Inspect structures for the common pathology, often associated with impingement such as labral tears, articular cartilage lesions.

### Chondral Lesions
- A number of patterns of chondral damage exist.
- The initial stage of chondral cartilage delamination is the wave sign (Fig. 5.6a), progressing to partial and full thickness chondral tears (Fig. 5.6b).

- Unstable chondral flap tears should be resected, and full-thickness chondral lesions treated with microfracture.

### Labral Tears
- The majority of labral tears associated with impingement occur at the chondrolabral junction (Fig. 5.7) and can be treated with a labral debridement or labral repair.

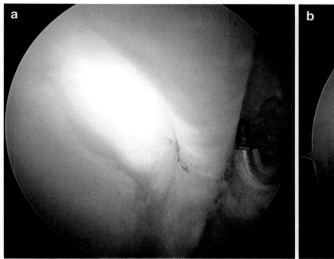

**Fig. 5.6**  (**a**) The wave sign. (**b**) Full-thickness cartilage tear

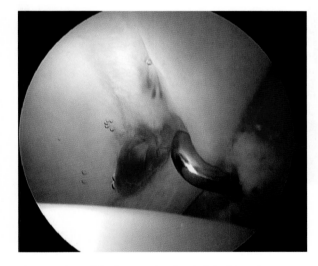

**Fig. 5.7**   Acute labral tear at the chondrolabral junction

## Acetabular Recession

- To correct a pincer abnormality, an acetabular rim recession is performed (Fig. 5.8a, b).
- To perform an acetabular recession, the labrum is detached.
- Debridement of the lateral gutter.
- Identification of the bony labral junction.
- Detach the labrum with an arthroscopic knife or shaver (Fig. 5.8c).

- Resection of the pincer abnormality is performed until reaching stable articular cartilage but avoid excessive resection (Fig. 5.8d).
- Reattachment of the labrum with suture anchors (Fig. 5.8e).

## Peripheral Compartment

- The peripheral compartment can be accessed directly from the central compartment without repositioning the portals.
- It is important at this stage to assess the remaining impingement attributable to the cam lesion. The extent of the impingement is dynamically assessed with flexing, rotation, and abduction of the hip.

### Femoral Osteoplasty
- The capsulotomy can be extended anterolaterally to improve visualization of the head–neck junction of the femur. Orientation in the peripheral compartment is challenging for inexperienced hip arthroscopists.
- First step is to increase the fluid pump pressure to about 90 mmHg.
- Orientation points include the medial synovial fold, the labrum, and the head–neck junction (Fig. 5.9a).
- The camera can be positioned through the antero-lateral or anterior portal.

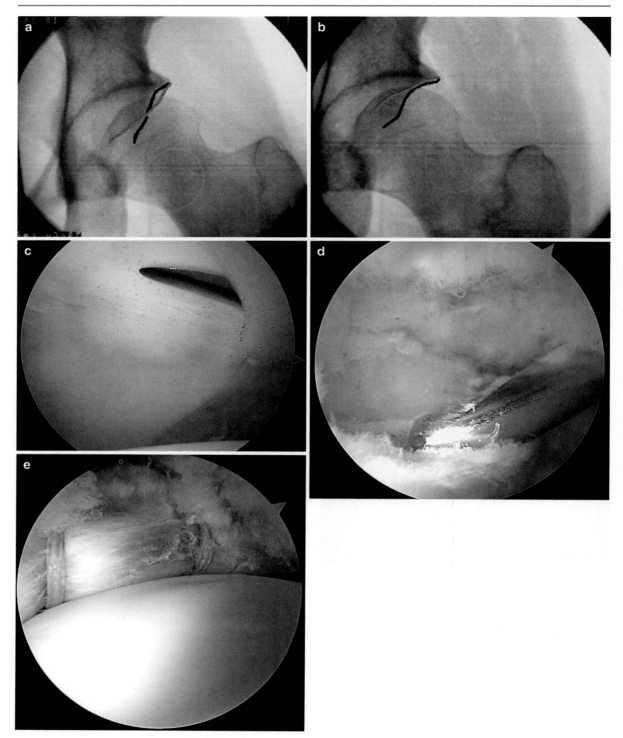

**Fig. 5.8** (**a**) Pincer abnormality before resection (crossover sign). (**b**) Pincer abnormality resected. (**c**) Labral detachment with banana blade. (**d**) Acetabular rim resection and (**e**) labral repair

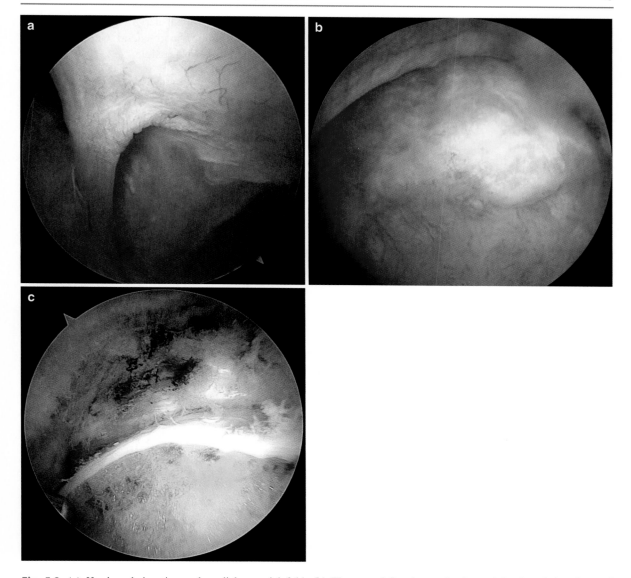

**Fig. 5.9** (**a**) Head–neck junction and medial synovial fold. (**b**) The cam deformity at the femoral head-neck junction and (**c**) complete osteoplasty with hip in full flexion

- Inspect the cam lesion. The articular cartilage within the impingement zone is well demarcated and appears degenerative compared to the rest of the femoral head (Fig. 5.9b).
- The image intensifier can be utilized to confirm the position of the shaver and burr.
- A 4- or 5.5-mm burr is preferable to perform the femoral osteoplasty.
- Dynamic assessment of impingement is repeated and further osteoplasty performed as required (Fig. 5.9c).

## Postoperative Rehabilitation

- Start mechanical VTE prophylaxis at admission and continue until the patient no longer has significantly reduced mobility, based on an assessment of risks. Start pharmacological VTE prophylaxis after surgery and continue until the patient no longer has significantly reduced mobility.
- Cycling on a static bicycle.
- Stretching and passive range of motion exercises.

- Passive rotation exercises to avoid capsular adhesions.
- Crutches partial weight bearing for a 2–4 week period and extended to 6 weeks if microfracture has been performed.
- Generally, a return to sports can be expected around 3–5 months.

## Complications

- Although hip arthroscopy is a relatively safe procedure, some potential complications can occur.
- Informed consent should include the following uncommon but important complications such as infection, DVT, neck of femur fracture, avascular necrosis, and ankle pain.

- Nerve injury to sciatic nerve (traction), pudendal nerve (positioning), and lateral cutaneous nerve (portal placement) is possible.

## Further Reading

Dienst M, Kohn D. Arthroscopic treatment of femoroacetabular impingement. Technique and results. Orthopade. 2009;38(5): 429–43.

Ilizaliturri Jr VM. Complications of arthroscopic femoroacetabular impingement treatment: a review. Clin Orthop Relat Res. 2009;467(3):760–8.

Shindle MK, Voos JE, Nho SJ, et al. Arthroscopic management of labral tears in the hip. J Bone Joint Surg Am. 2008;90 Suppl 4:2–19.

Lee HH, Klika AK, Bershadsky B, et al. Factors affecting recovery after arthroscopic labral debridement of the hip. Arthroscopy. 2010;26(3):328–34.

# Cemented Total Hip Arthroplasty (THA): Posterior Approach

Peter Bobak , Fragkiskos N. Xypnitos, and Peter V. Giannoudis

## Indication

- Painful arthritis of the hip resulting in loss of function and/or progressive deformity

## Preoperative Planning

### Clinical Assessment

- When the patient walks into the examination room, a careful observation of the gait should be performed; note any limp/antalgic, drop foot gait, abductor lurch, broaden gait, etc.
- Look at the patient from the front and behind to observe any deformity of the leg, back, and pelvis; note any pelvic tilt/increased lumbar lordosis suggesting fixed flexion deformity (FFD) of the hip.
- Check for swelling, discoloration, temperature, and scars around the hip.
- Feel for bony landmarks: ASIS, iliac crest, greater trochanter, and ischial tuberosity.
- Determine the presence/absence of leg length discrepancy.
- Assess ROM: flexion/extension, internal/external rotation, and abduction/adduction.

- Specific tests – Thomas: FFD and Trendelenburg: abductor function.
- Examine the distal vascular supply and neurological function of the limb.
- Check for spine/knee pathology.
- General preoperative medical assessment and routine blood tests: FBC, urea and electrolytes, group and save/cross-matched blood, ECG, and MRSA screening.
- Thromboembolic risk should always be considered and prophylaxis used according to agreed protocol.

### Radiological Assessment

- Good quality and adequate X-rays (AP pelvis and lateral of the hip view) are required for accurate preoperative planning.

## Operative Treatment

### Anesthesia

- Regional or general anesthesia ± nerve blocks

### Theatre Preparations

- Confirm the correct patient and hip to be operated on.
- Operating theater should use ultra clean air systems for surgery.
- Implants and instruments specific to the operation must be available.
- Antibiotic prophylaxis according to agreed protocol.

P. Bobak • F.N. Xypnitos
Department of Trauma and Orthopaedic Surgery,
Leeds Teaching Hospitals NHS Trust, Leeds, UK

P.V. Giannoudis (✉)
Academic Department of Trauma and Orthopaedic Surgery,
School of Medicine, University of Leeds, Leeds, UK
e-mail: pgiannoudi@aol.com

P.V. Giannoudis (ed.), *Practical Procedures in Elective Orthopaedic Surgery*,
DOI 10.1007/978-0-85729-814-0_6, © Springer-Verlag London Limited 2012

**Fig. 6.1** Patient positioning to allow adequate access. Stability is achieved with ASIS and sacral supports. T mark represents Greater Trochanter

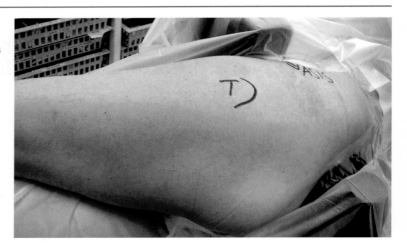

## Patient Positioning

- Should be performed by the operating surgeon.
- Lateral position: patient's pelvis is stabilized by specific supporting posts to the sacrum-LS spine and ASIS with protective gel pads; ensure flexion of the hip above 90° (Fig. 6.1).
- Check correct placement of diathermy plate, calf pumps (mechanical thromboprophylaxis) and pressure sore prevention gel pad to the contralateral leg.
- Sandbag or foot support to stabilise contralateral side.
- Pillow can be used between the legs to prevent adduction of the affected hip and aid leg length assessment.

## Draping and Surgical Approach

- Highest standard in antiseptic preparation is essential.
- The surgical site is isolated with sterile drapes to keep out the perineum.
- Posterolateral skin incision over the posterior half of the greater trochanter is curved toward PSIS; hemostasis of perforating vessels (Fig. 6.2).
- Protect the skin edges.
- Deep fascia incised in line of the skin incision.
- Deep retractors put in place to identify the short external rotators; feeding vessels cauterized.
- Using cutting diathermy, the short external rotators are detached as a single layer including piriformis

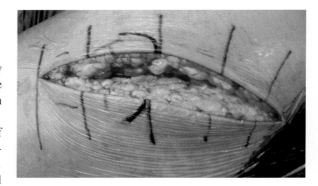

**Fig. 6.2** Posterolateral skin incision over the posterior half of the greater trochanter curved towards PSIS

proximally and part of quadratus femoris distally; this soft tissue cuff is used to protect the sciatic nerve during the procedure (Fig. 6.3).
- Hip is dislocated by flexion, adduction, and careful internal rotation.
- Femur is positioned horizontal, knee is flexed, and tibia should be vertical.
- Level of neck resection dictated by the femoral system used, usually just in the middle of lesser trochanter and the head-neck junction (Fig. 6.4).
- Femoral neck sealed with bone wax to minimize bleeding (Fig. 6.5).
- Anterior retractor placed carefully in front of the acetabulum; positioning may be facilitated by incising the anterior capsule.
- Obturator retractor and additional self retractors used to achieve circumferential view of the acetabulum (Fig. 6.6a).

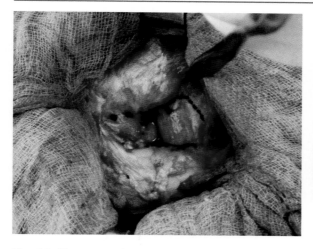

Fig. 6.3 Short external rotators incised in line of the dotted line

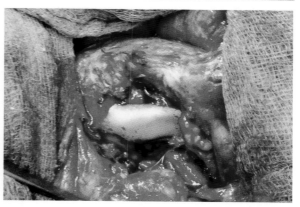

Fig. 6.5 Femoral neck sealed with bone wax to minimize bleeding

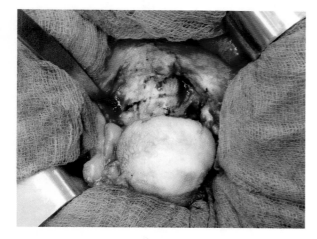

Fig. 6.4 Neck resection halfway between lesser trochanter and head-neck junction

- Acetabulum is prepared with gouges and reamers to explore sufficient cancellous bone for cement injection and maintain subchondral plate at the periphery of the acetabulum for better mechanical support to the socket.
- Determine the correct size of the acetabular component to achieve full bony containment and allow sufficient volume of cement to be used for fixation.
- Use pulse-lavage system to remove fat and debris from the acetabulum.
- Dry surface must be achieved to optimize cement penetration.

- Half of the volume of cement delivered to the acetabulum and pressurized.
- Second volume is placed over the cement, and the component is placed into its anatomical position using bony – posterior and anterior rim, teardrop – and soft tissue – transverse ligament – landmarks (Fig. 6.6c).
- Cup must be held until cement is set and the socket is firm.
- Unsupported cement must be removed.
- Knee is flexed; femur internally rotated to facilitate exposure to the proximal femur.
- Piriformis fossa identified; medullary canal approached.
- Bone block is taken for closure of the canal.
- Correct access to the medullary canal identified by advancing the long Charnley curette or T-handle reamers bypassing the isthmus of the femur (Fig. 6.7a).
- Femur is prepared with broaches in increasing sizes (Fig. 6.7b).
- Correct size identified and dictated by preoperative planning; intraoperative observations: size of the medullary canal, femoral offset, stability, and leg length.
- Trial reduction to confirm stability and correct leg length.
- Previously harvested bone block is implanted in order to close the medullary canal (bone restrictor).
- Use pulse-lavage system to remove fat and loose debris from the femur.
- Dry surface must be achieved to facilitate cement penetration.

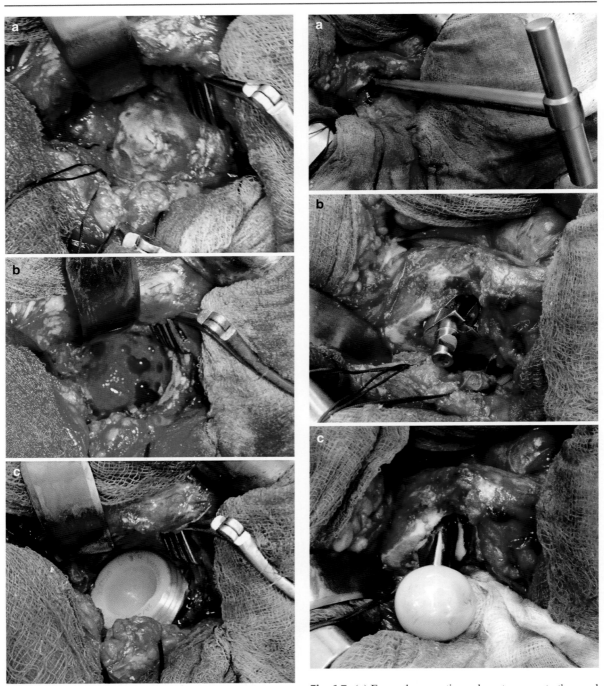

**Fig. 6.6** (**a**) Circumferential view of the acetabulum must be achieved, short external rotators held by stay sutures. (**b**) Acetabulum prepared, several different sizes of anchor holes and grooves made to enhance cement injection, and (**c**) flanged socket is sitting on the rim, its position dictated by bony and soft tissue landmarks

**Fig. 6.7** (**a**) Femoral preparation: adequate access to the canal is reproduced by advancing a long T-handle reamer bypassing the isthmus of the femur. (**b**) Femur is prepared with broaches and (**c**) stem cemented in situ, ceramic head component in place

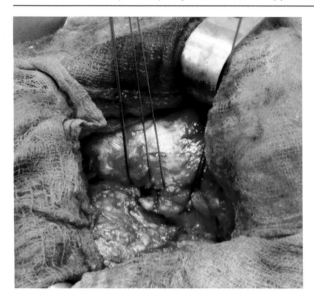

**Fig. 6.8** Short rotators reattached with sutures through the trochanter

- Retrograde and rapid cement delivery with proximal seal to pressurize cement.
- Stem introduced slowly, focusing on position to the required depth; cement pressurized at the medial neck using a thumb.
- Stem should be between neutral position and 10° anteversion and avoid retroversion.
- Leg position must be maintained by the assistant.
- Stem must be held firmly until cement is set (Fig. 6.7c).

- Excess of cement around the neck of the implant removed.
- Assess stability and leg length to confirm head size.
- Hip relocated.
- Short rotator cuff reattached with transtrochanteric sutures to increase stability of the hip joint, (Fig. 6.8).
- Irrigation, further hemostasis if required, and infiltration with local anesthetic and epinephrine.

## Closure

- In layers: deep fascia with Vicryl 0 or 1, subcutaneous tissues with Vicryl 2/0 and skin with absorbable sutures and/or 3/0 nylon.
- Drain is optional and its use is usually dictated by the surgeon's view and preference.

## Postoperative Care

- Observe blood loss and requirements for analgesia.
- Monitor vascular and neurological status of the leg.
- Start mechanical VTE prophylaxis at admission and continue until the patient no longer has significantly reduced mobility. Start pharmacological VTE prophylaxis after surgery and continue for 28–35 days.

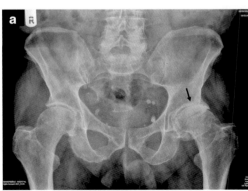

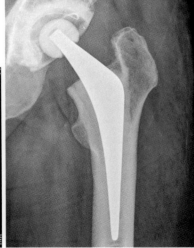

**Fig. 6.9** (**a**) Pre-operative AP pelvic radiograph demonstrating degenerative changes of the left hip (*black arrow*). (**b**) post-operative radiograph following left total hip replacement

- Mobilize weight-bearing and start ROM exercises with physiotherapist as early as possible – usually day 1 after surgery; Various walking aids /stick, crutches/frame can be used to support rehabilitation for 6-12 weeks.
- Check X-ray (Fig. 6.9) and FBC.

## Complications

- Wound healing
- Dislocation
- Neurovascular
- Infection
- Fractures
- Thromboembolic
- Ectopic ossification
- Loosening
- Residual pain, Leg length discrepancy (LLD)

## Follow-up

- Patients are assessed clinically and radiographically at 3/12 and 12/12 post surgery. Ideally indefinitive clinical and radiological follow-up is required. However, it's frequency is influenced by local and national guidelines.

## Further Reading

Panesar SS, Cleary K, Bhandari M, et al. To cement or not in hip fracture surgery? Lancet. 2009;374(9695):1047–9.

Hulleberg G, Aamodt A, Espehaug B, et al. A clinical and radiographic 13-year follow-up study of 138 Charnley hip arthroplasties in patients 50–70 years old: comparison of university hospital data and registry data. Acta Orthop. 2008;79(5):609–17.

Parker MJ, Gurusamy K. Arthroplasties (with and without bone cement) for proximal femoral fractures in adults. Cochrane Database Syst Rev. 2006;3:CD001706.

Morshed S, Bozic KJ, Ries MD, et al. Comparison of cemented and uncemented fixation in total hip replacement: a meta-analysis. Acta Orthop. 2007;78(3):315–26.

British Orthopaedic Association publication: Primary total hip replacement: A guide to good practice, August 2006.

# Cementless Total Hip Arthroplasty (THA): Posterior Approach

**7**

George C. Babis, Vasileios I. Sakellariou, and Panayotis N. Soucacos

## Indications

- Primary osteoarthritis (OA) of the hip joint
- Secondary OA following acetabular dysplasia [hip dysplasia, developmental dysplasia of the hip (DDH), or congenital disease of the hip (CDH)]
- Rheumatoid arthritis (RA)
- Osteonecrosis (ON)
- Legg-Calve-Perthes' disease (LCP disease)
- Slipped capital femoral epiphysis (SCFE)
- Deteriorated or failed pelvic osteotomy (deteriorated cases)
- Traumatized hip with deformity and malalignment (posttraumatic arthritis)

## Preoperative Planning

### Clinical Assessment

- Pain
- Limited and painful range of motion
- Abductors sufficiency/deficiency
- Demands for walking supports

G.C. Babis (✉) • V. I. Sakellariou
First Department of Orthopaedics, School of Medicine,
University of Athens, ATTIKON University General Hospital,
Athens, Greece
e-mail: george.babis@gmail.com

P.N. Soucacos
Professor of Orthopaedic Surgery,
University of Athens, School of Medicine, Director,
Orthopaedic Research & Education Center (OREC),
Athens, Greece
e-mail: psoukakos@ath.forthnet.gr

- Leg length discrepancy (LLD), true or apparent
- Pelvic obliquity
- Lumbar spine curvatures (stiff or flexible)
- Patient's expectancies

### Radiological Assessment

- Anteroposterior (AP) radiograph of pelvis
- AP and lateral views of the affected hip
- AP and lateral views of the lumbar spine
- Hip to ankle standing radiograph in case of severe LLD, congenital disease of the hip, mechanical axis abnormalities
- Further imaging investigations include:
  - CT +/− 3D reconstruction (severe hip deformities, definition of altered anatomy, defects, need for specific implants, design of custom made prostheses)
  - MRI (avascular necrosis, evaluation of contralateral hip)
  - Bone scans (history of infection, septic loosening, tumors, and metabolic diseases)

### Preoperative Templating

- Useful in all cases of hip arthroplasties.
- Assessment of implant design/type, size, positioning.
- Evaluation of femoral offset, improve biomechanics of reconstructed hip, decrease of wear.
- Templating always performed after clinical evaluation (LLD, gait, abductors sufficiency). Always estimate apparent LLD using the "block" method. Blocks of different heights are placed under the shorter leg until the pelvis is horizontal and the patient feels the legs as comfortably equal.

- Draw a horizontal line through two points at the inferior aspect of the ischial tuberosities or a horizontal line between the inferior aspects of the acetabular teardrops (more reliable points of reference than the ischia).
- A vertical line from the horizontal reference to the estimated center of each femoral head or to the center of the lesser trochanters represents a radiographic estimate of the limb-length discrepancy.
- All measurements should be reduced by a factor of approximately 20% to account for the enlargement of the osseous anatomy on the radiographs. Special magnification markers are used for accurate measurement of magnification.
- Orientation of the acetabular shell: 45° relative to the horizontal plane (AP radiograph) and 20° of anteversion (cross table lateral radiograph). The apex should be positioned just lateral to the teardrop and covered at its superolateral margin.
- Positioning of the acetabular component defines the new centre of rotation of the reconstructed hip.
- At the AP radiograph with the femur internally rotated approximately 20° (so that the true neck-shaft angle is in the same plane as the radiograph), the femoral template is superimposed on the radiograph.
- The optimal femoral component size is then established parallel to the anatomic axis of the proximal part of the femur.
- Align to the anticipated center of rotation by a distance that is equal to the measured LLD.
- Neck length and varus/valgus positioning are marked.

## Operative Treatment

### Anesthesia

- Regional (spinal/epidural) and/or general anesthesia.
- One hour prior to anticipated skin incision, administer intravenously prophylactic antibiotics as per local hospital protocol (e.g., combination of a second generation cephalosporin and aminoglycoside, or vancomycin in >50% MRSA hospitals).

### Table and Equipment

- THA instrumentation set – ensure availability of the complete set of proper implants, according to preoperative templating.

- The instrumentation is set up on the side of the operation.
- Position the table diagonally across the operating room so that the operating area lies in the clean air field.

## Patient Positioning

- Place the patient in the true lateral position with the affected limb uppermost. The unaffected limb is secured at 90° of knee flexion for intraoperative assessment of leg length (Fig. 7.1).
- Protect the bony prominences with pads. Place a pillow between the knees.

## Draping and Surgical Approach

- Prepare the skin over the buttock, hip, femur, and tibia up to the malleoli with the usual antiseptic solutions (aqueous/alcoholic povidone-iodine, alcoholic chlorhexidine).
- Drape the limb using adhesive single-use U-drapes.
- Cover the foot, ankle, and tibia with a socket.
- Isolate the proximal femur using Iobane sterile drapes.
- Drape the affected limb free to leave room for movement during the procedure. Hip flexion of at least 90° is essential for intraoperative assessment of stability.
- Palpate greater trochanter on the outer aspect of the thigh. It is easier to palpate the posterior edge of the trochanter, which is more superficial than the anterior and lateral portions.
- Make a 9–12 cm curved incision centered on the posterior aspect of the greater trochanter. In obese patients, a longer incision may be required.
- Begin the incision 4–6 cm above and posterior to the posterior aspect of the greater trochanter (Fig. 7.2).
- Curve the incision across the buttock, cutting over the posterior aspect of the trochanter, and continue distally along the shaft of the femur.
- If the hip is flexed to 90° and a straight longitudinal incision is made over the posterior aspect of the trochanter, it will curve into a "Moore style" incision when the limb is straight.
- Incise fascia lata on the lateral aspect of the femur to uncover vastus lateralis.

**Fig. 7.1** True lateral position of the patient on the operative table. A nurse is holding the leg for aseptic preparation

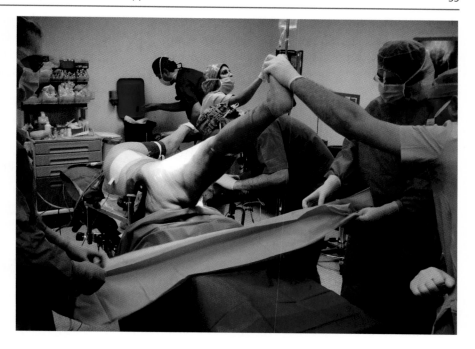

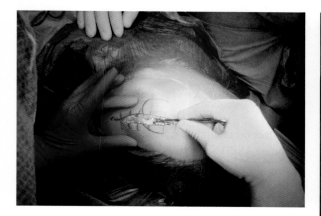

**Fig. 7.2** Skin incision in relation to the greater trochanter

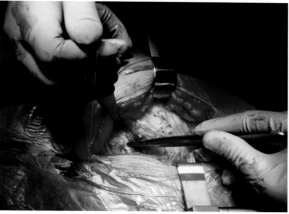

**Fig. 7.3** A Hoffman's retractor under the gluteus medius. The pickup is showing the piriformis muscle before its detachment

- Lengthen the fascial incision superiorly in line with the skin incision and split the fibers of gluteus maximus by blunt dissection.
- Split the muscle gently, so you may be able to pick up, cauterize, and cut the crossing vessels before they are stretched and avulsed by the blunt dissection of the split.
- Retract the fibers of the split gluteus maximus and the deep fascia of the thigh using Charnley's self-retaining retractor.

- Place a Hoffman's retractor and elevate the tendon of gluteus medius to uncover the short external rotator muscles.
- Internally rotate the hip to put the short external rotator muscles on a stretch and to pull the operative plane farther from the sciatic nerve (Fig. 7.3).
- Insert stay sutures into piriformis and obturator internus tendons just before their insertion into the greater trochanter.

- Detach the muscles close to their femoral insertion using electrocautery device and reflect them backward, laying them over the sciatic nerve to protect it during the rest of the procedure.
- Incise the posterior joint capsule in an L-shaped fashion to expose the femoral head and neck. The one leg of this capsular incision should run parallel to the proximal border of piriformis.
- Dislocation of the femoral head is achieved by internally rotating, flexing, and adducting the hip.

## Implant Positioning

- Place two Hoffman's retractors at each side of the femoral neck. The medial retractor should be placed at the level of the lesser trochanter, whereas the other one should protect the gluteus medius tendon.
- The resection level of the femoral head-neck is determined by the preoperative templating and marked accordingly using electrocautery or by a methylene blue marker.
- The calcar planer may be used to adjust the neck cut.
- Four Hoffman's retractors are placed at each side of the acetabulum, at the anterior wall, the posterior wall, the upper rim, and distal to the transverse ligament (Fig. 7.4a).
- The joint capsule, the acetabular labrum, and any osteophytes of the upper rim are removed so to reveal the true size of the acetabulum.
- Progressively ream the acetabulum until bleeding subchondral bone is revealed (Fig. 7.4b).
- The angle of orientation should match that recorded during preoperative templating, which is normally 45° of lateral opening (abduction) and 15–30° of anteversion which can be confirmed by external alignment instrumentation.
- Using the cup impactor, place a trial cup sizer into the reamed acetabulum and assess its position and bone contact.
- The inferior rim of the trial cup should be level with the bottom of the teardrop.
- The acetabular shell is placed in situ with adequate primary stability. Additional screws may be used according to surgeons' preference. These screws are preferably placed at the posterior superior and posterior inferior quadrants of the acetabulum which are formed by two lines: line A connecting the center

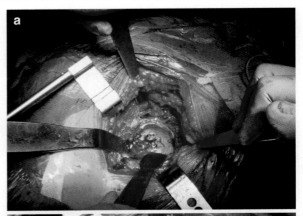
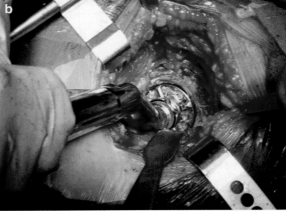

**Fig. 7.4** (**a**) Exposure of the acetabulum. (**b**) Reaming of the acetabulum with the special offset reamer

of the acetabulum and the anterior superior iliac spine (ASIS) and line B perpendicular to line A.
- A trial insert is placed into the acetabular shell during preparation of the femur.
- Initiate the pilot femoral hole opening with the stepped IM initiator which should be aligned with the femoral canal.
- Use a box osteotome to enter the femoral canal at the junction of the femoral neck and the greater trochanter (Fig. 7.5a).
- Attach the trochanteric reamer to the T-handle or a power reamer and insert it into the canal. Proper alignment of the reamer along the long axis of the femur is important to ensure correct component positioning. Sequential reaming beginning two or three sizes below the preoperatively templated size is recommended. Resistance and chatter from cortical engagement may be used as a signal to stop tapered reaming.

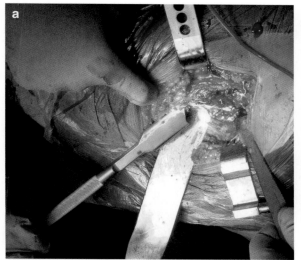

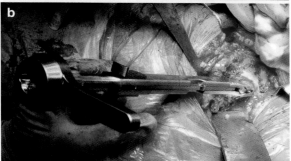

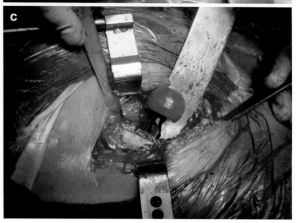

Fig. 7.5 (a) Preparation of the femoral canal. A starter box osteotome is used to open the metaphyseal entry of the femoral canal. (b) A broach inside the femoral canal. Note the cut neck of the femur, and (c) trial stem, trial modular neck (*black*), and head (*blue*) in place before trial reduction

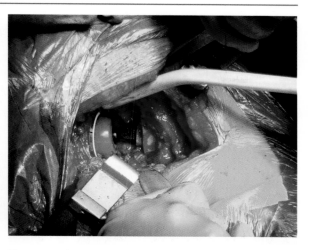

Fig. 7.6 After trial reduction, the combined anteversion is determined. The hip is placed in 15° of flexion and 30° of internal rotation. The equator of the femoral head is the same as of the cup insert. In this case, the combined anteversion is 45° which is optimal

down the medullary canal, ensuring proper alignment and anteversion are achieved. To ensure proper alignment, orient the broach laterally toward the greater trochanter. The final broach should fit and fill the proximal femur, with the top of the cutting teeth resting at the point of the desired neck resection. The final broach should look and feel rotationally stable (Fig. 7.5b).

- Trial neck segments and modular heads are tested to assess proper component position, joint stability, range of motion, and leg length (Fig. 7.5c).
- Perform a final trial reduction using the trial acetabular liner and trial femoral head, selecting the optimal liner and modular head for implant stability and leg length.
- Range of motion, presence of femoroacetabular impingement, LLD, and hip stability are assessed.
  - With the hip in 90° of flexion and 0° of abduction, internal rotation should be at least 45° with no tendency to dislocate.
  - In extension, there should be full external rotation with no tendency to dislocate or impinge.
  - Combined anteversion of the socket and femoral head should be approximately 45° (Fig. 7.6). The combined anteversion is defined by co-equatorial placement of the femoral head in respect to the acetabular liner when the leg is in 15° of flexion and 30° of internal rotation.

- Broaching of the proximal femur should begin two to three sizes smaller than the preoperatively templated size. Sequentially, advance the broaches

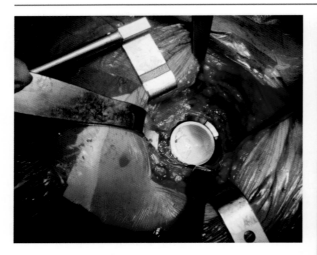

**Fig. 7.7** A delta ceramic insert of 36 diameter in place

- – Longitudinal pull of the limb with a single triceps force should not lead to telescoping of the hip.
- – Abductors are assessed with the drop-kick test (if abductors are too tight, adduction of the hip leads to extension of the knee).
- Following the final trial reduction, remove the trial acetabular liner and insert the appropriate acetabular liner. When inserting a ceramic liner, extreme caution should be taken to avoid fracture or chipping (Fig. 7.7).
- Choose the stem size that matches the final broach, thread it to the inserter, and introduce it to the medullary canal.
- Rotate the stem into its proper orientation and advance the stem into the canal using hand pressure. When resistance is met, usually 10–15 mm above the desired final seating position, advance the stem into position with multiple moderate blows using a mallet.
- Clean and dry the taper and introduce the appropriate femoral head by firmly pushing and twisting the femoral head into place. Using the head impactor, engage the head with several mallet taps.
- Reduce the hip and make a final assessment of leg length, tension of hip abductors, and hip stability (Fig. 7.8).

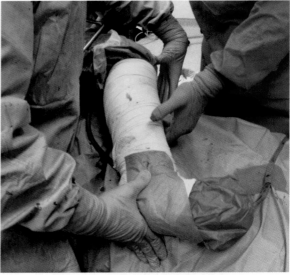

**Fig. 7.8** Intraoperative estimation of the leg length

## Closure

- Irrigate the wound thoroughly and achieve hemostasis.
- Reattachment of small external rotator tendons: Using a 3.2-mm drill, make two tunnels at the posterior ridge of the greater trochanter (Fig. 7.9a). With loop wires, pass the stay sutures which have been already inserted to the piriformis and obturator internus tendons through the osseous tunnels and ligate them together over the posterolateral aspect of the trochanter (Fig. 7.9b). Reconstruct the quadratus femoris muscle if possible.
- Close fascia lata (No 2 PDS, Vicryl) over a drain (14/16F) and the subcutaneous fat with absorbable sutures (No 0 PDS, Vicryl).
- Skin closure – stainless steel surgical staples, monofilament non-absorbable sutures, or absorbable sutures placed in the subcuticular layer.
- Secure the position of the leg by using special abduction triangle shaped pillows.

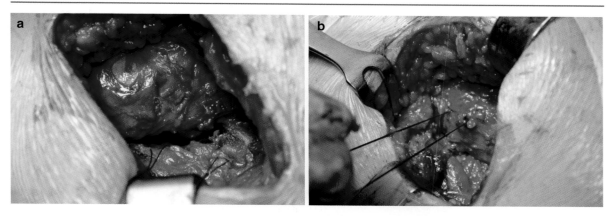

**Fig. 7.9** (**a**) Drilling of the greater trochanter for passage of sutures. (**b**) Sutures attached to the piriformis muscle and the posterior capsule passed through the greater trochanter

## Postoperative Rehabilitation

- One further dose of prophylactic antibiotics is sufficient. Use of antibiotics can be extended until removal of the drains or 48 h postoperatively.
- Start mechanical VTE prophylaxis at admission and continue until the patient no longer has significantly reduced mobility. Start pharmacological VTE prophylaxis after surgery and continue for 28–35 days.
- Routine AP radiograph of the pelvis within 24 h. Cross table lateral hip X-ray for assessment of cup anteversion.
- Routine blood counts at 6 and 12 h postoperatively.
- Use special abduction pillow.
- Remove drains in 48 h otherwise when drainage is less than 30 mL/24 h.
- Hip range of motion and general muscle strength in the operative extremity.
- Sitting exercises.
- Mobilize with partial weight bearing.
- Refine gait pattern and instruct in stair climbing.
- Review home instructions/exercise program with emphasis on hip dislocation/precautions.
- A Zimmer frame, an elevated toilet seat, and follow-up physical therapy are required.

## Follow up

- Patients are assessed clinically and radiographically at 1, 3, 6, and 12 months and every 5 years thereafter, unless GPs request (Fig. 7.10).
- Range of motion, impingement, abductor sufficiency, need for assistive devices, level of residual pain, independence, and quality of life parameters are evaluated.
- Orientation of acetabular and femoral components, progressive insert wear, signs of osteolysis, and radiolucent lines around implants are assessed with sequential plain radiographs of the pelvis and the hip.

**Fig. 7.10** Postoperative
X-ray after cementless THA
with posterior approach

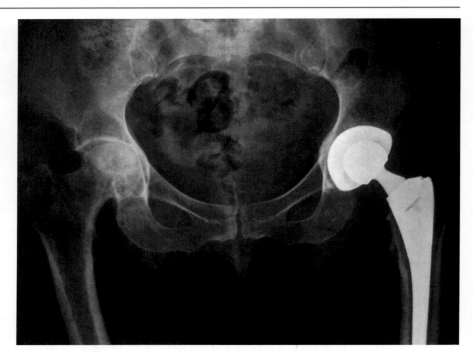

## Further Reading

Anseth SD, Pulido PA, Adelson WS, et al. Fifteen-year to twenty-year results of cementless Harris-Galante porous femoral and Harris-Galante porous I and II acetabular components. J Arthroplasty. 2010;25(5):687–91.

Springer BD, Connelly SE, Odum SM, et al. Cementless femoral components in young patients: review and meta-analysis of total hip arthroplasty and hip resurfacing. J Arthroplasty. 2009;24(6 Suppl):2–8.

Aldinger PR, Jung AW, Breusch S, et al. Survival of the cementless Spotorno stem in the second decade. Clin Orthop Relat Res. 2009;467(9):2297–304.

Yamada H, Yoshihara Y, Henmi O, et al. Cementless total hip replacement: past, present, and future. J Orthop Sci. 2009; 14(2):228–41.

Dutton A, Rubash HE. Hot topics and controversies in arthroplasty: cementless femoral fixation in elderly patients. Instr Course Lect. 2008;57:255–9.

# Hip Resurfacing Arthroplasty

**8**

Christos Plakogiannis and Robert G. Middleton

## Introduction

The results of resurfacing depend on three factors:
- Patient selection
- Surgical technique
- Implant selection

This is a more technically demanding procedure than total hip replacement. A surgeon should complete 200 hip replacements before attempting resurfacing. The learning curve is between 20 and 50 cases.

Component placement is critical. Notching of the femoral neck can lead to fracture. Ideal acetabular component position is 40° of abduction and 20° of anteversion. A cup left open and too anteverted will lead to edge loading, increased wear, increased risk of ALVAL (aseptic lymphocytic vasculitis-associated lesions), and failure.

Not all implants are the same. Component design, particularly the cup varies, so do the jigs for component positioning. Training in a particular implant is required in addition to resurfacing technique. The outcomes of different implants vary considerably in joint registries. Some are being withdrawn from the market or being redesigned. Therefore, choose an implant with care and up-to-date outcome data and review it regularly.

C. Plakogiannis (✉) • R.G. Middleton
Department of Trauma and Orthopaedic Surgery,
Royal Bournemouth Hospital,
Bournemouth, UK

## Indications

- Osteoarthritis in young active patients (under 65 years)

## Contraindications

- Infection
- Gross deformity of the hip (developmental or traumatic)
- Cysts in the femoral head and neck >1 cm
- Poor bone quality – osteoporosis

## Relative Contraindications

- Women (increased risk of failure)
- Women of childbearing age (metal ions circulating in the bloodstream cross the placenta during pregnancy, with unknown effects)
- Renal disease (metal ions excreted by kidneys)
- Avascular necrosis
- Metal sensitivity
- Age >65
- Femoral head size <46 mm
- Leg length or offset inequality >1 cm

## Preoperative Planning

### Clinical Assessment

- Leg length
- Neurovascular status

P.V. Giannoudis (ed.), *Practical Procedures in Elective Orthopaedic Surgery*,
DOI 10.1007/978-0-85729-814-0_8, © Springer-Verlag London Limited 2012

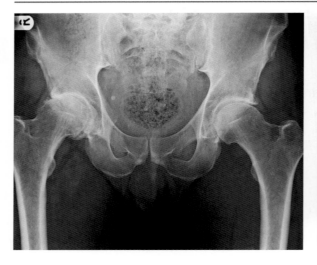

**Fig. 8.1** Preoperative AP pelvis X-ray. It is evident the arthritis of the right hip

- ROM
- Physical activity and demands

## Radiological Assessment

- AP pelvis (Fig. 8.1) and lateral of the involved hip. Assess the head-neck ratio, presence of cysts, and deformity of the hip joint.
- Templating will give the surgeon an estimate of the implant sizes and leg length and offset.

Informed consent of the patient is of paramount importance as this is a newer technique and has increased risks over standard total hip replacement.

- General risks
  - Death, medical and anesthetic complications
  - Infection 1%
  - DVT and PE
  - Neurovascular injury <1%
  - Dislocation
  - Leg length inequality requiring a shoe raise
  - Wear and failure requiring revision <10% at 10 years
- Specific risks
  - Unknown results >10 years.
  - Femoral neck fracture.
  - Squeaking.
  - Unknown long-term (decades) effect of metal ions in the body.

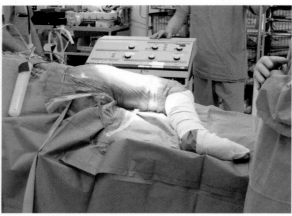

**Fig. 8.2** Patient positioning

- Local allergic/hypersensitivity reaction to components and metal ions (ALVAL) leading to fluid and soft tissue swellings (pseudotumors) causing muscle and bone necrosis requiring revision surgery.
- Intraoperative conversion to total hip replacement.

## Operative Treatment

### Anesthesia
- Spinal and/or general anesthetic
- Perioperative antibiotic prophylaxis as per local protocol

### Theater Setup and Equipment
- Laminar flow theater
- Standard orthopedic table
- Hip instruments set
- Hip resurfacing instruments set
- Total hip replacement set and implants should be available
- Low viscosity antibiotic-loaded cement

### Table Setup
- The instrumentation is set up at the far end of the table.

### Patient Positioning
- Lateral position (Fig. 8.2).
- Patient should be positioned and secured on the table by the operating surgeon himself.
- Flexion of the hip >90° should be allowed.

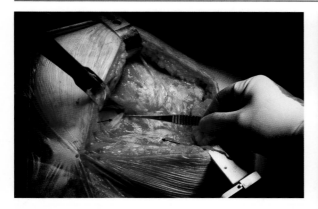

**Fig. 8.3** Posterolateral approach: *arrows* pointing the tendon of the piriformis and the fat covering the sciatic nerve

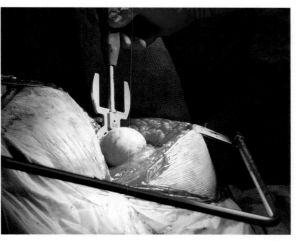

**Fig. 8.4** Head sizing

## Draping and Surgical Approach

- The skin is prepped with the usual antiseptic solution.
- The limb is drape-free.
- The operative field is isolated by an adhesive membrane.

## Surgical Procedure and Implantation

- Skin incision for a posterolateral approach (resurfacing can be performed through a lateral approach but this is less commonly used since is not as good).
- Split the fascia lata in line with the skin incision.
- Identify the sciatic nerve and place a stay suture through the short rotators and the capsule (Fig. 8.3).
- Divide the tendon of the gluteus maximus.
- Expose the hip joint taking down the short rotators and the capsule as a full thickness flap.
- Dislocate the hip and perform a circumferential capsulotomy leaving a cuff (1 in.) of capsule attached anteriorly to protect the iliopsoas tendon from impinging on the front of the cup.
- Femoral head implants come in 2 mm increments, and the outer diameter of the corresponding cups is 6 and 8 mm larger (i.e., for 52 mm head, one can use either 58 or 60 mm OD cup).
- Head-neck templates are applied on the widest part of the neck after this has been cleared off the osteophytes. This determines the smallest femoral head size that can be used (Fig. 8.4).

- Using either a lateral or medial reference, jig pass a guide wire through the center of the femoral neck (Fig. 8.5a–c).
- The position of the wire is checked with a stylus.
- Overdrill and central guide bar insertion (Fig. 8.6a, b).
- Central positioning is checked again.
- Femoral head is prepared with peripheral cutters from larger to smaller sizes.
- It is advisable to stop reaming one size larger than the minimum templated.
- If the bone quality is poor or if the femoral neck is notched during the preparation, one should proceed with total hip replacement.
- Acetabulum is then prepared to the predetermined size (for most designs, underream 2 mm from the implant size).
- If the surgeon feels that excessive bone needs to be removed, attention should be taken back to the femur and decide whether this can be downsized.
- If this is not possible and reaming to the desired size would compromise the acetabular walls, the procedure should be abandoned and a total hip arthroplasty should be performed instead.
- When the acetabular reaming is completed, a trial shell should be implanted. This should have good stability, and the surgeon should reproduce its position with the definitive implant (Fig. 8.7).
- The acetabular cup should be adequately anteverted to avoid impingement in flexion (the transverse acetabular ligament is a fairly reliable landmark),

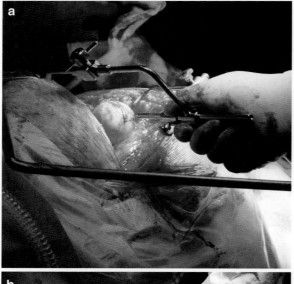

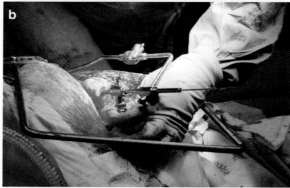

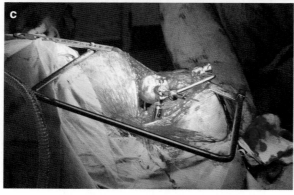

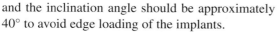

**Fig. 8.5** (**a–c**) Femoral head jigging and drilling

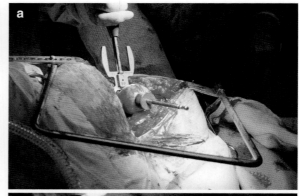

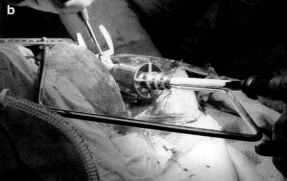

**Fig. 8.6** (**a, b**) Femoral head preparation

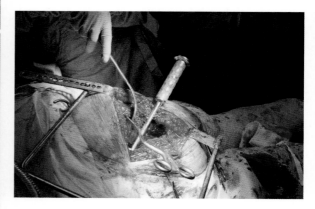

**Fig. 8.7** Acetabular cup trial

and the inclination angle should be approximately 40° to avoid edge loading of the implants.
- The definitive acetabular cup is press fitted (Fig. 8.8a, b).
- Remove any anterior impinging osteophytes.

- Preparation of the femoral head is completed with the chamfer reamer (Fig. 8.9a).
- Keyholes drilled on the superior aspect of the head (Fig. 8.9b, c).
- The femoral component is implanted with one mix of low viscosity antibiotic-loaded cement while the

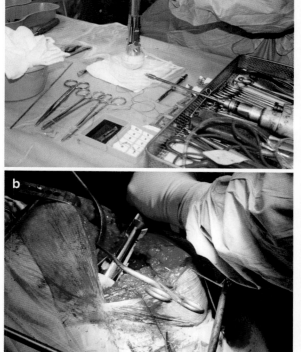

**Fig. 8.8** (**a, b**) Acetabular implantation

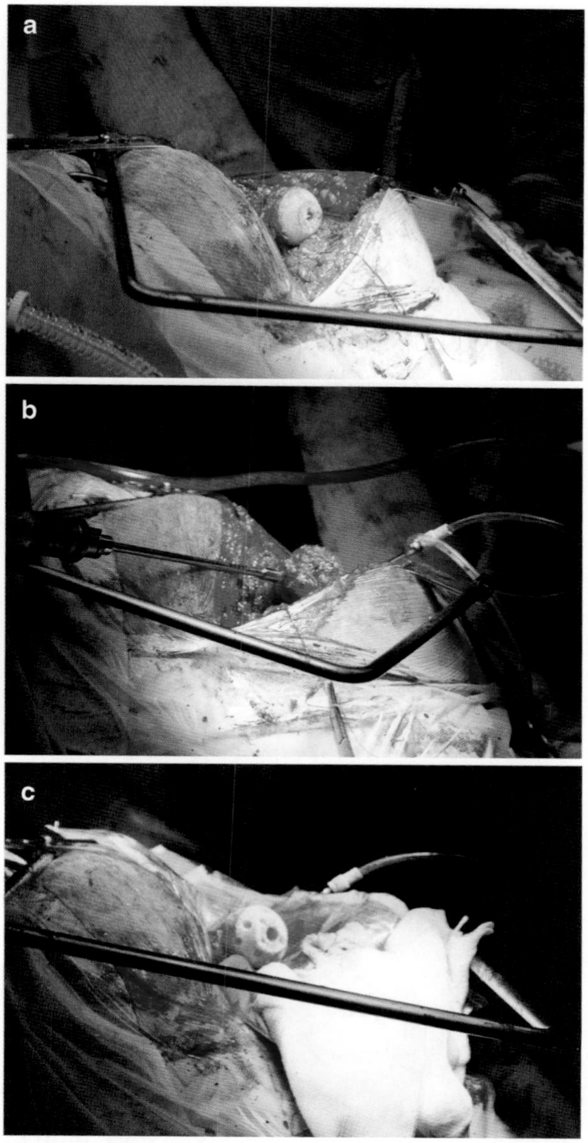

proximal femur is vented through a cannula connected to the suction (Fig. 8.10a, b).

- Reduce the hip carefully to prevent capsule becoming trapped between the articulating surfaces. Fill the cup with saline so on reduction the saline either pushes the capsule out or hold the capsule back manually and reduce under direct vision (Fig. 8.11).
- The hip is reduced; leg length and stability are checked.

**Fig. 8.9** (**a–c**) Femoral head chamfer cut and keyholes drilled

## Closure

- The wound is irrigated and haemostasis is achieved.
- Short rotators and capsule are attached to bone through drill holes.
- The tendon of the gluteus maximus is repaired.
- The fascia lata and the subcutaneous fat are closed with absorbable sutures.
- The skin is closed with clips.

## Postoperative Management

- Start mechanical VTE prophylaxis at admission and continue until the patient no longer has significantly reduced mobility. Start pharmacological VTE prophylaxis after surgery and continue for 28–35 days.
- Routine blood tests.
- Check radiograph, pelvis AP (Fig. 8.12), and lateral of the hip.
- Mobilize full weight-bearing.

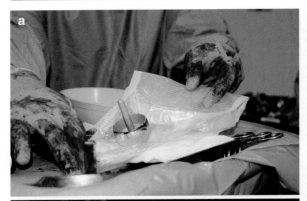

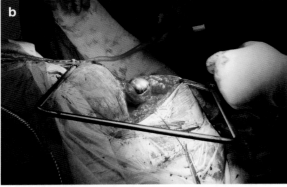

**Fig. 8.10** (**a, b**) Low viscosity cement poured in the femoral component (*arrow*) and implanted while the proximal femur is vented

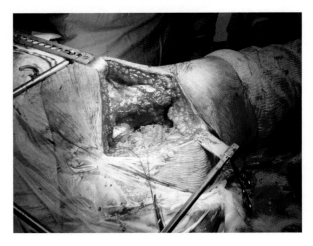

**Fig. 8.11** Joint reduced and trialed for leg length and stability

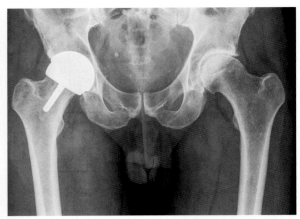

**Fig. 8.12** The post operative AP X-ray from the same case as in Fig. 8.1

- If all satisfactory return to driving, office, and light manual work.
- Return to sport and manual work at 3–6 months.

## Further Reading

Beaule PE, Dorey FJ, LeDuff M, Gruen T, Amstutz HC. Risk factors affecting outcome of metal-on-metal surface arthroplasty of the hip. Clin Orthop Relat Res. 2004;418:87–93.

Hart AJ, Sabah S, Henckel J, Lewis A, Cobb J, Sampson B, et al. The painful metal-on-metal hip resurfacing. J Bone Joint Surg Br. 2009;91(6):738–44.

Archbold HAP, Mockford B, Molloy D, McConway J, Ogonda L, Beverland D. The transverse acetabular ligament: an aid to orientation of the acetabular component during primary total hip replacement: a preliminary study of 1000 cases investigating postoperative stability. J Bone Joint Surg Br. 2006; 88(7):883–6.

Glyn-Jones S, Pandit H, Kwon Y-M, Doll H, Gill HS, Murray DW. Risk factors for inflammatory pseudotumour formation following hip resurfacing. J Bone Joint Surg Br. 2009;91(12): 1566–74.

Shimmin A, Beaulé PE, Campbel P. Metal-on-metal hip resurfacing arthroplasty. J Bone Joint Surg Am. 2008;90:637–54.

Langton DJ, Jameson SS, Joyce TJ, Hallab NJ, Natu S, Nargol AVF. Early failure of metal-on-metal bearings in hip resurfacing and large-diameter total hip replacement. J Bone Joint Surg Br. 2010;92(1):38–46.

## Outpatients Follow-up

Patients are assessed clinically and radiographically at 1, 3, 6, and 12 months and every 5 years thereafter, unless GP's request.

# Revision Total Hip Arthroplasty

Vassilios S. Nikolaou and John Antoniou

**9**

## Indications

- Consider revision of total hip arthroplasty (THA) when patient has pain or functional disability due to:
  - Implant loosening
  - Implant fracture
  - Advanced bearing surface wear
  - Periprosthetic fracture
  - Infection
  - Recurrent dislocation – Implant mal-positioned
- Do not proceed to revision unless you have a clear idea about patient's cause of symptoms!

## Preoperative Planning

- Especially for revision, THA adequate preoperative planning is of paramount importance.

## Clinical Assessment

- A detailed history should be obtained. Ensure that patient is fit for surgery. Consult medicine, cardiology, urology, vascular surgery as appropriate.
- Observe patient's gait. Marked trendelenburg gait indicates abductors damage or insufficiency.
- Assess limb length discrepancy (LLD).

V.S. Nikolaou (✉) • J. Antoniou
Division of Orthopaedic Surgery,
School of Medicine, McGill University,
Montreal, Canada
e-mail: vassilios.nikolaou@gmail.com

- Ensure that you know the mechanism of THA failure.
- Learn as much as you can regarding the previous installed implants (company, size, and extraction tools).
- Exclude infection! Check ESR, CRP, and WBC. Perform hip aspiration in case of clinical suspicion. Prepare laboratories for intraoperative gram stain, frozen section and cultures.
- Check previous incision and assess the skin condition. Decide the length and shape of new incision accordingly. Avoid parallel or anterior incisions.

## Radiological Assessment

- Ensure that adequate anteroposterior (AP) and lateral radiographs are available.
- Low AP radiograph of the pelvis is useful for determining relative limb length by comparing the inter-ischial line with a fixed point on the lesser trochanter.
- A cross-table lateral radiograph of the acetabulum is useful for evaluating acetabular version.
- Long films of the femur should be obtained.
- Special Judet views and CT scan can be useful to assess acetabular and femoral bone stock.
- MRI of the hip, using metal artifact reduction sequences (MARS) can be used to reveal occult causes of THA failure (Fig. 9.1).
- Preoperative templating is important to achieve leg length equality and to determine the appropriate size of the femoral and acetabular components to use. Pay attention to the magnification of the X-rays. Use the special markers to adjust measurements (Fig. 9.2).

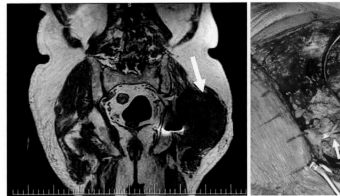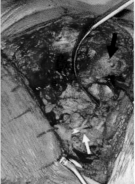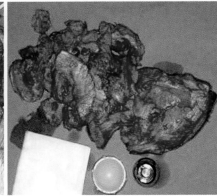

**Fig. 9.1** *Left*: MRI using metal artifact reduction sequences (MARS) of a patient with painful THA. Plain X-rays were inconclusive. MRI revealed a large soft tissue mass at the posterior and posterolateral aspect of the greater trochanter (*arrow*). *Middle*: patient underwent revision surgery and revision of the acetabular implant (*white arrow*: femur, *black arrow*: acetabulum). *Right*: the removed pseudotumor, with the revised acetabular liner and femoral head

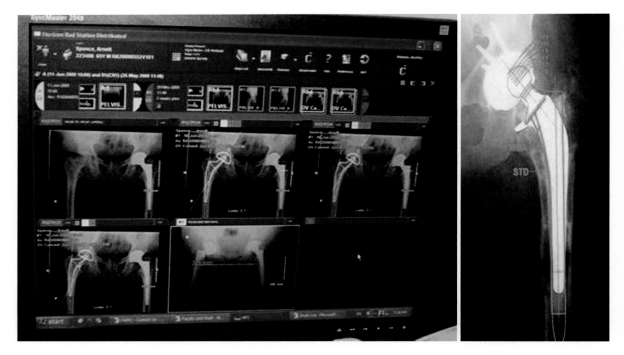

**Fig. 9.2** Preoperative templating is important in revision THA. Modern computerized templating can more accurately assist the appropriate implant selection

## Available Resources and Instrumentation

- Make sure that all equipments needed for previous implants removal are available (Stem extraction tools, head disassembly instruments, cement removal sets, flexible intramedullary reamers, trephine reamers, flexible osteotomes, reconstruction plates, and cages, cerclage wires, high speed burrs etc.) (Fig. 9.3).
- Consider all different sizes and types of femoral and acetabular implants that you may need. Always have alternative solutions available.

**Fig. 9.3** Cement removal instruments for revision THA

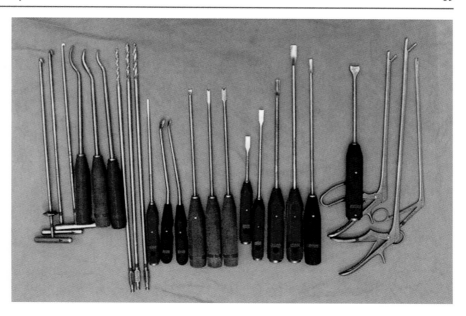

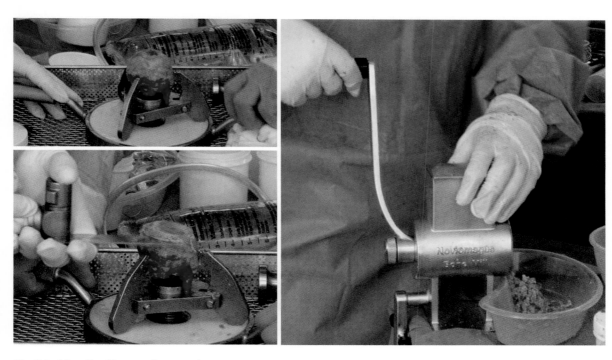

**Fig. 9.4** Morcelized bone graft preparation

- Plan carefully all the different types of grafts that might be needed (bulk grafts, strut grafts, morcelized bone (Fig. 9.4), etc.).
- Have C-arm and X-ray technician ready if needed.
- Have blood available for transfusion, and inform anaesthesia for possible prolonged operation. Consider having ICU/HDU bed booked.

## Operative Procedure

### Anesthesia

- Regional (spinal/epidural) or general anesthesia.
- At induction, administer prophylactic antibiotic as per local hospital protocol (e.g., second generation

cephalosporin). Consider a second dose if procedure is significantly prolonged. If infection is suspected, hold antibiotics until fluid and tissue cultures have been obtained.

## Patient Positioning

- Patient supine or lateral decubitus position (according to surgeon's experience and the desired approach) on a standard, preferably radiolucent, table.
- Patient prepped and draped in the usual fashion. Allow enough space to allow caudad or cephaland extension of the incision.

## Surgical Approach

- Surgical approach should: secure adequate exposure to remove previous implants, facilitate reconstruction of the bony defects of acetabulum or femur and allow new implant positioning.
- If possible, a previous incision should be followed. Skin problems are not as common as in revision total knee arthroplasties, however parallel or anterior incisions should be avoided.
- Usually direct lateral (Hardinge) or posterolateral approach is used for revision THA (Fig. 9.5). Each approach has strengths and weaknesses. Surgeon's experience, previous operations, and patient's anatomy, influence the choice of surgical approach.
- The trochanteric osteotomy can provide excellent exposure to both acetabulum and femur but carries the risk of trochanteric non-union and/or escape (Fig. 9.6).
- Trochanteric slide, as an alternative, reduces the risk of trochanteric non-union. Can be performed using lateral or posterolateral approach and it allows wide exposure to the acetabulum but also the femur.
- Extended trochanteric osteotomy (ETO) is used for more difficult revisions. In that case, the throchanter is removed along with a segment of the lateral femoral cortex. The length of the osteotomy is determined by the preoperative templating. ETO is useful to remove well-fixed uncemented femoral implants as well as cemented implants and remaining in the canal cement. Also, in cases of varus remodeling of the femur, ETO is mandatory in order to allow new straight stem positioning (Figs. 9.7 and 9.8).

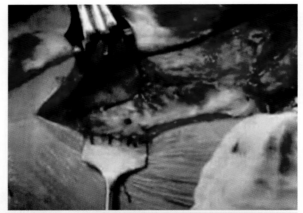

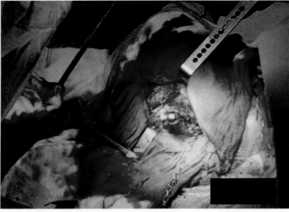

**Fig. 9.5** Posterolateral (*top*) or direct lateral approach (*bottom*) can be used, depending from the surgeon's experience and the previous operations and patient's anatomy

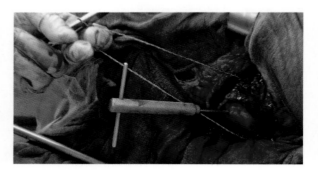

**Fig. 9.6** Trochanteric osteotomy

## Removal of Cemented Acetabular Components

- Exposing the rim of the acetabulum circumferential is crucial. When this is done, the cement – bone interface and the cement – cup interface is

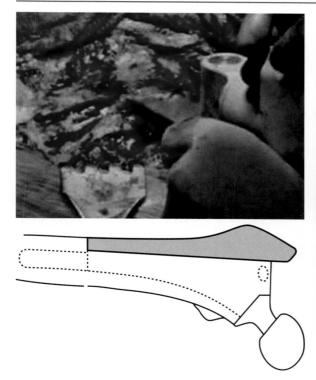

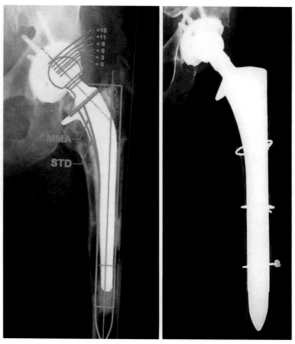

**Fig. 9.7** *Top*: taking in account the preoperative templating, extensive trochanteric osteotomy is performed using a saw. *Bottom*: diagram showing the osteotomized area

**Fig. 9.8** *Left*: ETO is useful to remove cemented implants, especially when a cement plug is difficult to be reached from the top of the femur. *Right*: cables or wires are used to reattach the osteotomized bone. Fixation of the new implant is achieved distally to the end of the ETO

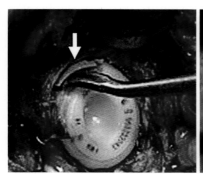

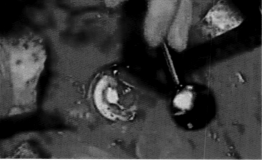

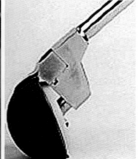

**Fig. 9.9** *Left*: removal of a well cemented liner. The rim of the acetabulum is exposed and curved osteotomes are used to disrupt the cement-implant interface (*arrow*). *Middle and right*: the

Explant (Zimmer) instrument has gained in popularity as it significantly facilitates removal of well fixed uncemented acetabular implants without compromising the acetabular bone stock

identified. Using curved thin osteotomes the cement-implant interface is disrupted. The implant is carefully removed. The remaining cement at the acetabulum is meticulously removed using thin osteotomes and cement splitters (Fig. 9.9).

- Start "breaking" the cement mantle from the "tear drop" area and proceed medially and superiorly.
- Alternatively, reaming of the cemented liner has been proposed up to the polyethylene cement interface and then removal of the cement as described above.

## Removal of Uncemented Acetabular Components

- Use the same approaches as described above.
- Expose meticulously the acetabular rim.
- Check the stability of the component. Consider liner exchange only, if possible, to avoid devastating bone loss.
- If screws are present the polyethylene liner has to be removed first. Use special liner extraction devises or osteotomes as appropriate to remove the liner. Alternatively, a screw can be used against the metal shell to pull out the polyethylene liner. Remove the screws carefully from the shell. If screws are broken, prefer to leave the broken parts in situ, rather than causing more bone loss.
- Use a high-speed burr to initiate exposure of the bone–implant interface. Then curved osteotomes can be used circumferential to disrupt the bone–implant interface. Alternatively, the Explant (Zimmer) instrument set can be used for easier and better results (Fig. 9.9).
- When cup is removed asses the degree of bone loss and plan the appropriate reconstruction technique.

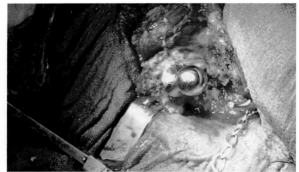

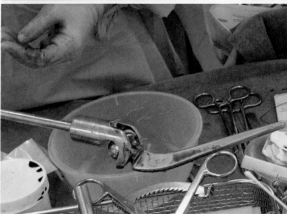

**Fig. 9.10** Removal of a cemented femoral stem

## Removal of Cemented Femoral Stem

- If implant is grossly loose, removal is relatively easy. Before removing the implant, it is very important to remove any bone from the implant's "shoulder," in order to avoid trochanteric fracture (Fig. 9.10).
- Sometimes, the implant can be easily separated from the well fixed cement mantle. Consider cement on cement technique if possible.
- If the implant is well fixed, then consider techniques that facilitate exposure, such as ETO (Fig. 9.11).
- Removal of well-fixed cement from the femur can be challenging. Proximal cement can be relatively easily removed using thin and flexible osteotomes and cement splitters. Be very careful to avoid fractures as proximal bone can be compromised due to osteolysis.
- Distal cement and cement plug can be very challenging to remove. Special instrumentation is usually needed, including fiberoptic light source, suction catheter, special long osteotomes, long pituitary rongeurs, hooked instruments, and different sized reamers. Ultrasound devices can also be very useful.

- Always consider ETO if reaching the distal cement is challenging. Controlled osteotomy is always better than devastating perforations and fractures. Always take in consideration varus remodeling, especially when you are trying to reach the distal cement plug or distal cement fragments, using straight tools.
- The cement plug is usually removed using the drill and tap technique. A long drill is centered in the distal plug, and a drill hole is made to it. C-arm can be used to confirm that there is no distal cortex penetration. Then a long tap is used to remove the plug. If removal of plug is very difficult and there is no sign of infection, then pushing the cement plug down to the distal femur is an acceptable option.

## Removal of Uncemented Stem

- Removal of loose uncemented stem can be very easy. Pay attention to release implant's "shoulder" before trying to remove it, as described above, to avoid trochanteric fractures.

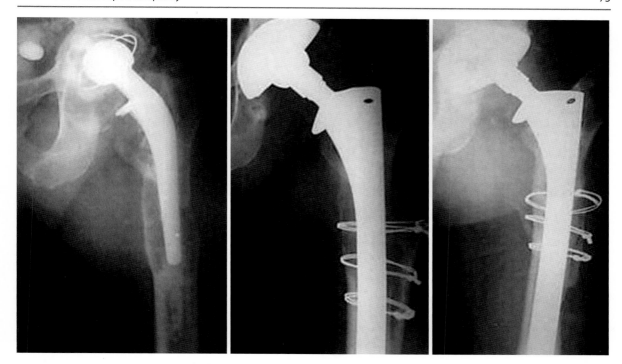

**Fig. 9.11** *Left*: cemented implant with still adequate cement mantle, that extends distally to the implant tip. *Middle*: the stem and cement was removed with an ETO successfully. A distal fit implant has been used. Osteotomy has been "closed" using three wires. *Left*: 7 years post-op, osteotomy has healed and the implant is stable

- Be sure that you know as much as possible regarding the implant's type and geometry. Have available implant-specific removal tools.
- Proximal coated uncemented stems can be removed using high-speed burrs and flexible thin osteotomes. Patiently detach the proximal part of the implant from the surrounding bone, making sure that no fracture is caused. If removal is difficult, then consider a short ETO.
- More distal porous coated, or fully porous coated stems can be very challenging to remove. Usually, ETO is required at least up to the beginning of the cylindrical part of the distal stem. The proximal part is then released from the bone using high-speed burr, flexible thin osteotomes, or a Gigli saw. An attempt can be made at that point to remove the stem using the extraction tools. If not successful, then a high-speed cutting burr is used to cut the metal stem at the junction of the cylindrical part. Appropriate-size trephines are then used to remove the distal part of the stem. This procedure can be hard and time consuming (Figs. 9.12 and 9.13). Be prepared and make sure that all instruments and at least five trephines are available.

## Reconstruction of the Femur and Acetabulum

- Implant removal in revision THA can be challenging, but it only represents the 50% of the whole procedure. The final goal in successful revision THA is to achieve stable fixation of the femoral and acetabular components resulting in pain free, functional total hip arthroplasty.

## Reconstruction of the Acetabulum

- Even though preoperative radiographic examination can give an estimation of the bone loss at the acetabular side, the remaining bone stock and the corresponding classification can be done only after removal of the acetabular component. Often, unpleasant surprises await the surgeon who has to be prepared.
- There are at least three classifications for assessment of acetabular bone loss: the AAOS Classification of Acetabular Deficiencies, the system described by Alan Gross, and the system described by Paprosky.

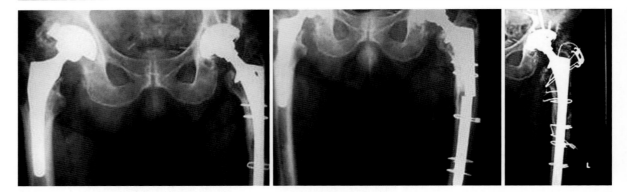

**Fig. 9.12** *Left*: this patient had a left hip revision 5 years ago. The short uncemented stem has been revised with a long fully porous coated stem, using an ETO. *Middle*: a fatigue fracture to the implant occurred. *Right*: the well fixed distal part of the implant was impossible to be removed without a new ETO. Trephines were used to release the distal fragment of the broken implant from the femur. Intraoperatively a trochanteric fracture occurred that was fixed with cables

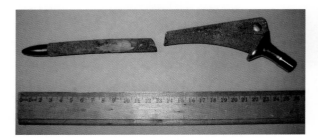

**Fig. 9.13** The removed broken implant

- According to Paprosky classification of acetabular bone defects (Table 9.1):
  - Type I and II defects can be usually treated with cemented or hemispheric uncemented cups, with or without screws, and with use of morcelized allograft where needed (Figs. 9.14–9.16).
  - Type III defects can be challenging even for the experienced arthroplasty surgeon.
  - For IIIA defects, large cups with screws can be used. Alternatively, superior figure of 7 distal femoral allograft with hemispherical cup, trabecular metal shell with superior augments, or high-hip center with hemispherical cup can be considered (Fig. 9.17).
  - For IIIB defects cage with cancellous allografts, custom triflange implants or trabecular metal implants with augments can be used (Fig. 9.18).
- For pelvic discontinuity, reconstruction acetabular plate can be used. Alternatively, acetabular

**Table 9.1** Paprosky classification of acetabular bone loss

| Type of defect | Acetabular rim | Columns | Remarks |
|---|---|---|---|
| I | Intact | Intact | No migration, no ischeal ostolysis, Kohler's line intact |
| II | Distorted but intact rim with adequate remaining bone to support a hemispherical implant | Intact | >50% host bone, A/P columns intact, hip center can be elevated <1.5 cm, Kohler line can be breached, some ischeal lysis is noted |
| III | Non-supportive rim | Severely compromised | Acetabular rim may not provide adequate stability. Ischeal lysis and Kohler's line disrupted. <br>– IIIA: 1.5–3 cm superior-lateral migration. 40–60% host bone. <br>– IIIB: >3 cm superior medial migration <40% host bone |

transplants or custom triflange implants have been proposed with good results. Lately, the "cup and cage" construct has been used with good midterm results.

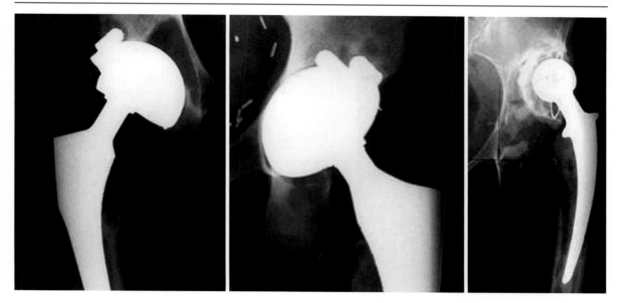

**Fig. 9.14** *Left*: type I acetabular bone defect according to Paprosky's classification. These defects can be easily managed with morcelized bone graft and uncemented or cemented acetabular shells. *Middle*: type II acetabular bone defect. *Right*: type III acetabular bone defect. These defects are difficult to be managed even from experienced arthroplasty surgeons

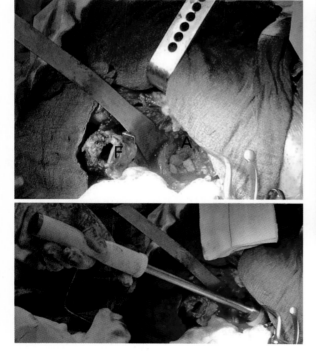

**Fig. 9.15** Impaction of morselized bone graft at the acetabulum (*F* femur, *A* acetabulum)

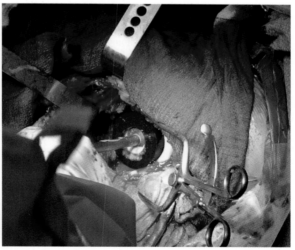

**Fig. 9.16** Introduction of a cemented cup

## Reconstruction of the Femur

- Similar with the acetabular bone loss, many classifications have been proposed for the femoral bone loss as well, that influence the decisions for femoral reconstruction techniques (Chandler and Penenberg, Endo-Klinik, Engh and Glassman, Paprosky et al.).

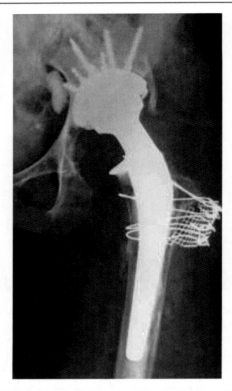

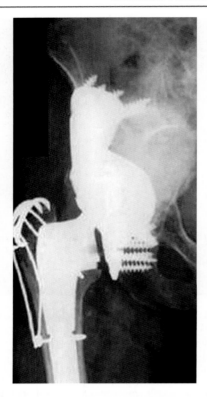

**Fig. 9.17** Severe type III acetabular bone defect that was treated with the "high hip center technique". In that case the stock deficiency and distorted acetabular anatomy preclude placement of the acetabular component at the true anatomic hip center

**Fig. 9.18** Severe type IIIB acetabular defect that was treated with morcelized bone graft and triflange implant successfully

- The Paprosky classification system evaluates the femoral diaphysis for its ability to support an uncemented fully porous coated prosthesis (Table 9.2).
  - For type I defects, femoral revision is straightforward and no additional bone graft is usually required. Defects are managed as a primary arthroplasty (Cemented or uncemented).
  - In type II defects, there is more extensive metaphyseal bone loss. For these defects a fully coated stem is preferred. Calcar replacement stems are often required to restore limb length (Fig. 9.19).
  - Type IIIA defects are characterized by extensive metaphyseal cancellous bone loss with some diaphyseal bone loss as well. There is adequate diaphyseal bone to support distal fixation. In these cases, fully coated bowed stem or, less commonly, a straight stem can be used.
  - Type IIIB <4 cm of intact diaphysis is remaining with extensive metaphyseal and diaphyseal bone

**Table 9.2** Paprosky et al. classification of femoral bone loss

| Type I | Minimal loss of metaphyseal cancellous bone. Intact diaphysis. |
|---|---|
| Type II | Extensive loss of metaphyseal cancellous bone. Intact diaphysis. |
| Type IIIA | The metaphysis is not supportive. There remains >4 cm of bone in the diaphysis to allow for a scratch fit. |
| Type IIIB | The metaphysis is not supportive. There remains <4 cm of bone in the diaphysis to allow for a scratch fit. |
| Type IV | Wide open canal without any appreciable isthmus to support an uncemented stem. |

loss. These defects are treated with modular tapered fluted stems or impaction grafting.
  - Type IV femurs have a widened femoral canal and no diaphyseal bone of sufficient quality for cementless fixation. These femurs are treated with impaction grafting, allograft prosthetic composite, modular revision stems or modular tumor megaprosthesis (Fig. 9.20).

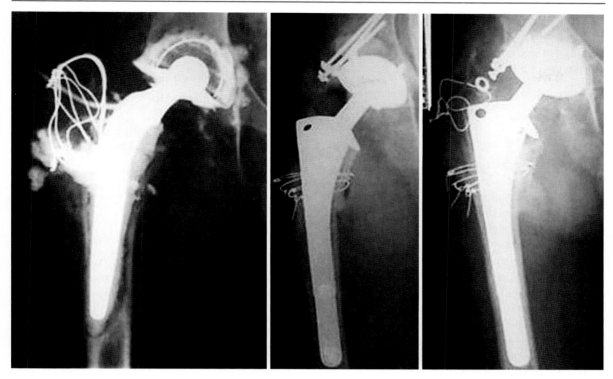

**Fig. 9.19** *Left*: type II femoral bone loss, according to Paparosky's classification in a patient with all cemented THA. *Middle*: successful reconstruction using a fully porous coated uncemented stem. *Right*: 10 years postoperative, no signs of revision failure

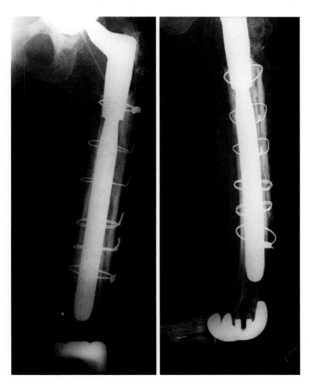

**Fig. 9.20** Severe type IV femoral bone defect that was treated with modular revision stem. Impaired femoral cortices were reinforced with strut grafts

## Wound Closure

- Irrigate the wound thoroughly.
- Use drain as per protocol.
- Identify and close fascia lata (PDS or Vicryl 2/0). Close subcutaneous fat with absorbable sutures.
- Skin closure with stainless steel surgical staples or non-absorbable sutures.

## Post-operative Care

- Position an abduction triangular pillow to maintain abduction of hip while patient is recovering from anesthesia.
- Continue antibiotics for 24 h post-op or according to culture results in case of infection.
- Start mechanical VTE prophylaxis at admission and continue until the patient no longer has significantly reduced mobility. Start pharmacological VTE prophylaxis after surgery and continue for 28–35 days.
- Routine bloods. Radiographs of pelvis (long films) on post-op day #2.

- Remove drain in 24 h.
- Begin physiotherapy on post-op day #1. Adjust program according the surgical exposure and the stability of the hip (Posterior, lateral precautions).

## Complications

- Infection.
- Intraoperative fractures.
- Non-unions of the osteotomies and also of the implanted bulk allografts.
- Dislocation (up to 20%). LLD, muscle atrophies and damage (especially abductors insufficiency), wrong implant positioning and implant fixation failure, all are some of the reasons leading to early or late dislocations.
- Nerve injuries. Extensive soft tissue strip and entrapment of nerves (especially sciatic nerve) to the scar tissue of previous operations can lead to reversible or not nerve injuries with devastating some times consequences for the patient.
- Heterotopic ossification.

- Vascular injuries.
- Deep venous thrombosis.
- Periprosthetic fractures.

## Outpatients Follow-Up

- Patients are assessed clinically and radiographically at 1, 3, 6, and 12 months, and every 5 years thereafter, unless GP's request.

## Further Reading

Gross AE, Goodman S. The current role of structural grafts and cages in revision arthroplasty of the hip. Clin Orthop Relat Res. 2004;429:193.

Paprosky WG, Magnus RE. Principles of bone grafting in revision total hip arthroplasty: acetabular technique. Clin Orthop Relat Res. 1994;298:147.

Younger TI, Bradford MS, Magnus RE, et al. Extended proximal femoral osteotomy: a new technique for femoral revision arthroplasty. J Arthroplasty. 1995;10:329.

Lieberman JR, Berry DJ, editors. Advanced reconstruction: hip. Rosemont: American Academy of Orthopaedic Surgeons; 2005.

# Trochanteric Osteotomy: Surgical Technique

# 10

Peter Bobak and Peter V. Giannoudis

## Introduction

- Advantages
  - Safest and easier hip dislocation
  - Best exposure to acetabulum and femur
  - Easier components' introduction
- Disadvantages
  - Rare limp to high detachment of trochanter after non-union

## Indications

- Disordered hip anatomy
- Shortening of femur is a prerequisite
- Primary and revision hip arthroplasty
- Obesity
- Intrapelvic protrusion of the acetabulum
- Trochanteric impingement

P. Bobak (✉)
Department of Trauma and Orthopaedic Surgery,
Leeds Teaching Hospitals NHS Trust,
Leeds, UK
e-mail: peter.bobak@leedsth.nhs.uk

P.V. Giannoudis
Academic Department of Trauma and Orthopaedic Surgery,
School of Medicine, University of Leeds,
Leeds, UK

## For Preoperative Planning (Clinical Assessment, Radiological Assessment), Anesthesia, Theater Preparations, Draping Look THA Chapter

### Patient Position

- Supine (should be done by the operating surgeon).

## Detachment

- Lateral skin incision over the mid-femur, curved posteriorly over the trochanter.
- Deep fascia incised in-line of skin incision.
- Landmarks: insertion of gluteus maximus, anterior edge of gluteus medius.
- Vastus lateralis ridge, trochanteric bursa (Fig. 10.1).
- Trochanteric bursa elevated in order to get access to the trochanter.
- Anterior edge of gluteus medius retracted.
- Using cutting diathermy soft tissue divided over the vastus lateralis ridge, moving anteriorly and over the neck of the femur the capsule opened.
- T-handle spike inserted to the neck-head (Fig. 10.2).
- Cholecystectomy forceps passed inside the capsule over the neck of the femur, between the notch of the trochanter and head of the femur, passed through the short rotators lateral (Fig. 10.3a).
- Gigli saw passed over the trochanter and neck.
- Diathermy used to check close proximity of the sciatic nerve.
- Hip positioned in flexion, slight adduction, internal rotation bringing the trochanter into the middle of the wound.

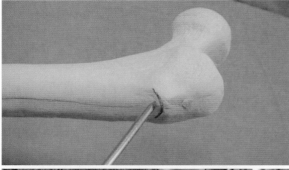

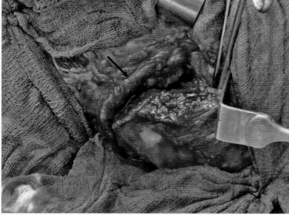

**Fig. 10.1** Vastus lateralis ridge is identified (*black arrow*)

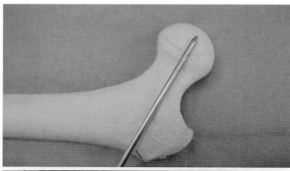

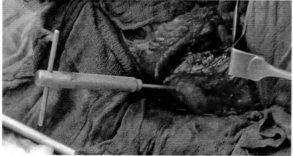

**Fig. 10.2** T-handle spike is delivered to the femoral neck-head

- Trochanter osteotomized by pulling the Gigli saw parallel to the shaft of the femur-cutting over the pin results dome shape osteotomy (Fig. 10.3b, c).
- Femoral neck resected. Direction of resection is to the edge of the trochanteric bed (Fig. 10.4).

## Reattachment

- The vertical double wire is passed through a drilled hole just distal to the edge of trochanteric bed in the middle of the trochanter /not the middle of the femur, there is more trochanter at the back (Fig. 10.5a).
- The strands are separated and secured in a small recess of the anterior and posterior neck of the femur (Fig. 10.5b, c).
- The spring wire is passed through a drilled hole in the proximal femur about 1–1.5 cm distal to the mid-point of the edge of the trochanteric bed, from front to back. The spring should sit on the anterior cortex of the upper femur (Fig. 10.6a–c).
- The trochanter is drilled from inside-out posterolaterally, just opposite the piriformis fossa. This is a double cortical part of the trochanter, outside the trochanteric bed. This hole will be for the posterior strand of the spring wire (Fig. 10.7).
- Wires pushed next to the cancellous surface of the medullary canal to facilitate cement delivery and stem insertion (Fig. 10.8).
- Stem cemented in place (Fig. 10.9). Hip is reduced.
- The anterior strand of the double wire is passed through the abductor muscles, staying close to the trochanter, front to back using the Charnley wire passer.
- The posterior strand is pulled through the same way, but back to front, the wires crossed over the trochanter (Fig. 10.10a).
- The double wires crossed again though the loop: posterior strand from back to front, anterior strand from front to back. The posterior strand of the spring wire is pulled through the hole of the trochanter posterolaterally/this wire can be used as a joystick to position the trochanter in to its anatomical bed (Fig. 10.10b).
- At first tighten the double wires to achieve near subperiosteal position (Fig. 10.11a).
- The anterior strand of the spring wire is passed through the abductor muscles, staying close to bone.

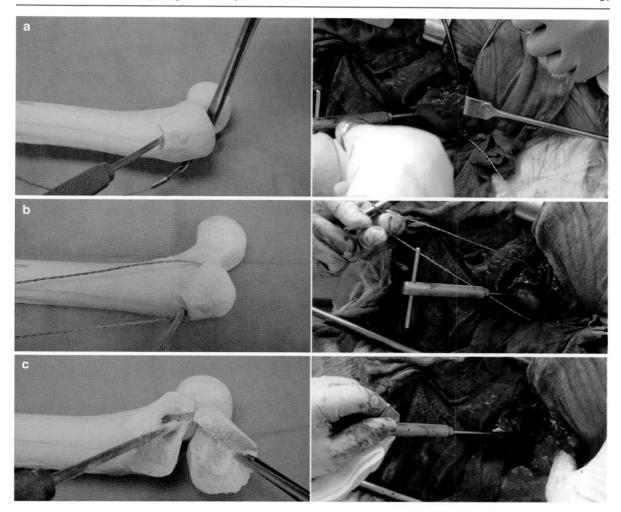

**Fig. 10.3** (**a**) Cholecystectomy forceps is passed over the neck and picks up the Gigli saw through the short rotators. (**b**) Trochanter is osteotomized by gentle pulling of the saw towards the knee and (**c**) cutting over the spike results chevron osteotomy

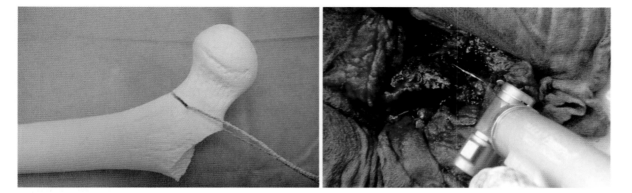

**Fig. 10.4** Neck resection aiming proximally to the edge of the trochanteric bed performed in-situ due to lost of adhesions

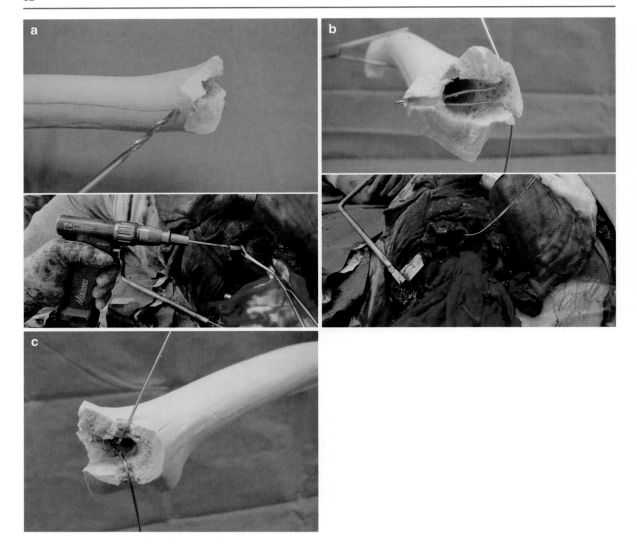

**Fig. 10.5** (**a**) First step of reattachment: drill hole to the double wire just distal to the vastus lateralis ridge, in the middle of the trochanter. (**b**) Position of the double wire and (**c**) the two strands of the double wire separated and secured in a small recess of the middle of the anterior and posterior neck of the femur

- Next tighten the spring wire until the spring is fully closed to deliver a 25-lb compression force (Fig. 10.11b).
- The wire tightener is twisted in a clockwise direction 90°, to lock the wire before further twisting and the wire is cut. It is important that the wire tightener is turned anticlockwise during further tensioning in order to avoid wire breakage.

- Tightening the spring wire could slacken the double wire. This will have to be tightening once more, the wire tightened is twisted just as before, and the wire is cut (Fig. 10.11c).
- The twisted end of the wires turned down and punched closed to the underlying bone (Fig. 10.12a–c).

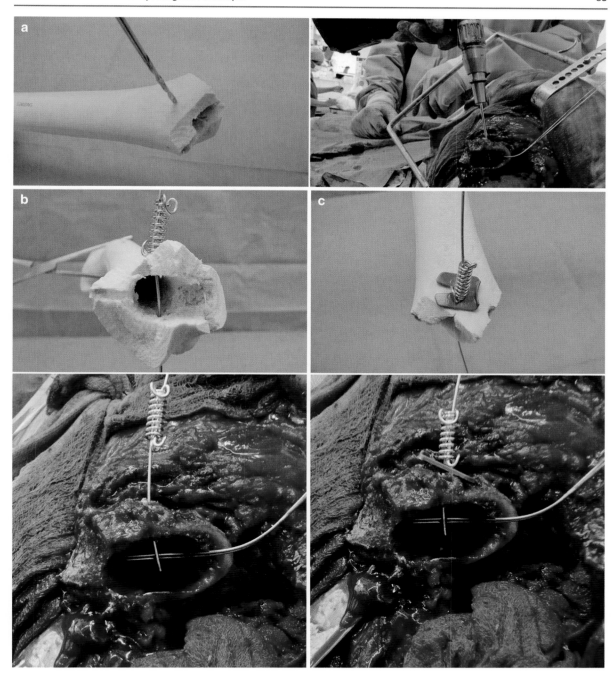

**Fig. 10.6** (**a**) Second drill hole for the single or spring wire, just 1–1.5 cm distal to the midpoint of trochanteric bed. (**b**) Position of the spring wire and (**c**) Small plastic inserted under the spring to prevent cement escaping

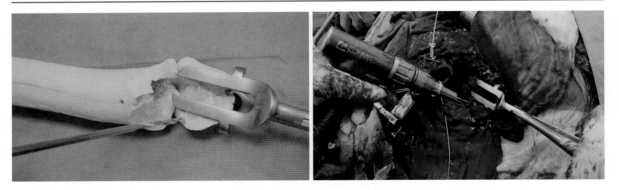

**Fig. 10.7** Third drill hole: for the posterior strand of the spring wire through the posterior lateral part of the trochanter

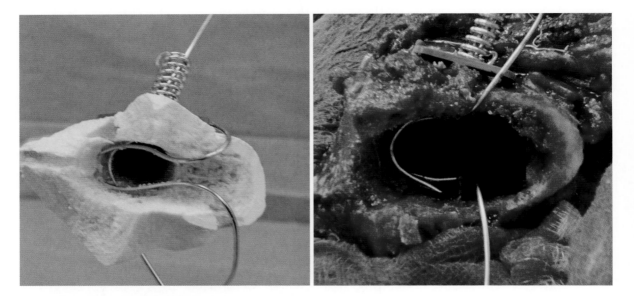

**Fig. 10.8** All the wires pushed to the inner surface of the canal

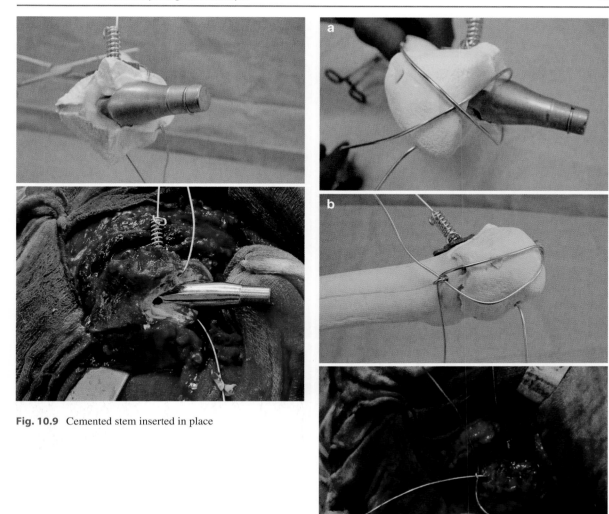

**Fig. 10.9** Cemented stem inserted in place

**Fig. 10.10** (**a**) The first cross of the double wire over the trochanter. (**b**) The second cross of the double wire is through the loop, note the posterior strand of the spring wire delivered through the posterolateral drill-hole of the trochanter

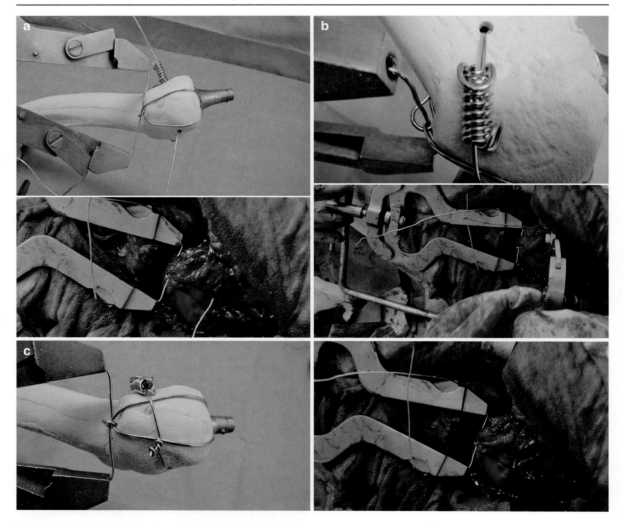

**Fig. 10.11** (**a**) The double wires tightened first. (**b**) The spring wire tightened next until full closure, twisted and cut and (**c**) the double wire tightened once more, twisted and cut

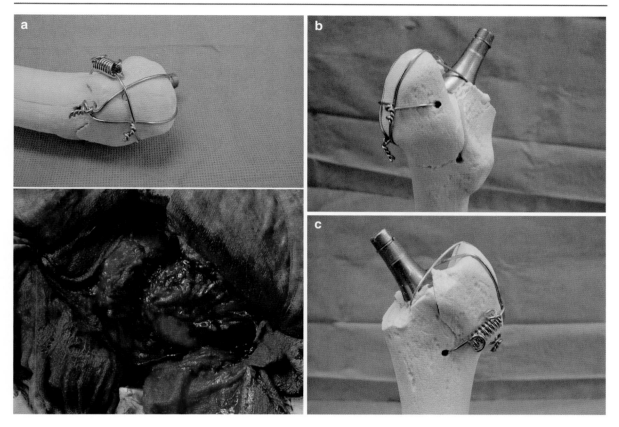

**Fig. 10.12** (**a**) Final configuration of trochanteric wires. Final configuration of stem (**b**) posterior view and (**c**) anterior view

## Further Reading

Jando VT, Greidanus NV, Masri BA, et al. Trochanteric osteotomies in revision total hip arthroplasty: contemporary techniques and results. Instr Course Lect. 2005;54:143–55.

Meek RM, Greidanus NV, Garbuz DS, et al. Extended trochanteric osteotomy: planning, surgical technique, and pitfalls. Instr Course Lect. 2004;53:119–30.

Archibeck MJ, Rosenberg AG, Berger RA, et al. Trochanteric osteotomy and fixation during total hip arthroplasty. J Am Acad Orthop Surg. 2003;11(3):163–73.

Parker MJ, Handoll HH. Osteotomy, compression and other modifications of surgical techniques for internal fixation of extracapsular hip fractures. Cochrane Database Syst Rev. 2009;2:CD000522.

# Excision of Heterotopic Ossification (HO) of the Hip

# 11

Peter V. Giannoudis, Fragkiskos N. Xypnitos, and Panayiotis N. Soucacos

## General Aspects

- Ectopic bone formation in the soft tissues.
- Etiology:
  - Brain injury (traumatic and non-traumatic).
  - Surgical interventions around the hip.
  - Local trauma.
- Pathophysiology:
  - The definitive causal factor is not yet clear.
  - Inappropriate differentiation of pluripotent mesenchymal stem cells.
  - Local and systemic factors.
- Clinical presentation:
  - Pain.
  - Limited range of motion.
  - Tenderness.
  - Limp.
  - Localized warmth.
  - Mild edema.
  - Erythema.
- Classification:
  - Most commonly with Brooker system (evaluation of ossification on a plain anteroposterior radiograph of the hip).

P.V. Giannoudis (✉)
Academic Department of Trauma and Orthopaedic Surgery,
School of Medicine, University of Leeds, Leeds, UK
e-mail: pgiannoudi@aol.com

F.N. Xypnitos
Department of Trauma and Orthopaedics Surgery,
Leeds Teaching Hospitals NHS Trust, Leeds, UK

P.N. Soucacos
Professor of Orthopaedic Surgery, University of Athens,
School of Medicine, Director, Orthopaedic Research &
Education Center (OREC), Athens, Greece
e-mail: psoukakos@ath.forthnet.gr

Grade 1: Islands of bone lie within the soft tissues about the hip.
Grade 2: Bony spurs protrude from either the femur or the pelvis, with a gap of more than 1 cm between opposing bony ends.
Grade 3: The gaps between the spurs are less than 1 cm.
Grade 4: Apparent ankylosis of the hip due to the heterotopic ossification.

## Indications

- Limited range of motion that interferes with the activities of daily living.
- Pain.
- Enhancement of bed to chair transfer.
- Easier perineal hygiene.
- Prevention of skin maceration.
- Enhancement of rehabilitation program in neurologically impaired individuals.
- Improvement of sitting balance by correction of malposition.

## Preoperative Planning

### Clinical Assessment

- History.
- Hip joint range of motion.
- Neurologic deficits.
- Any prior operations.
- Blood laboratory control for osteoclastic and osteoblastic markers (ALP, CTX-1 and P1NP).

P.V. Giannoudis (ed.), *Practical Procedures in Elective Orthopaedic Surgery*,
DOI 10.1007/978-0-85729-814-0_11, © Springer-Verlag London Limited 2012

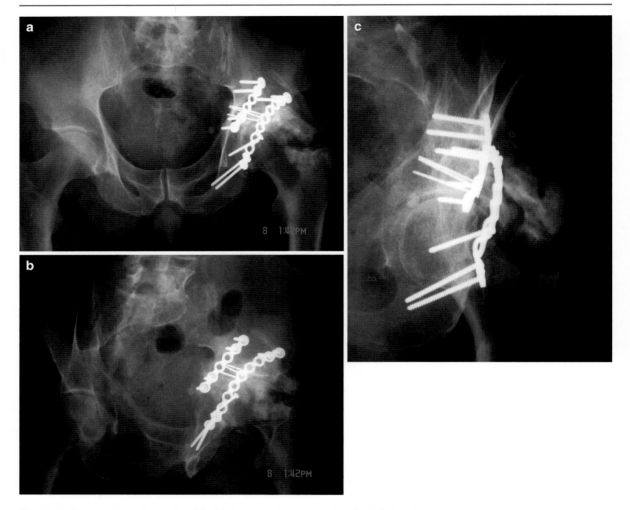

Fig. 11.1 Preoperative radiographs of the hip joint. (**a**) Anteroposterior, (**b, c**) Judet views

## Radiological Assessment

- Radiographs of the hip joint for staging (antero-posterior and Judet views) (Fig. 11.1a–c).
- CT for preoperative planning (Fig. 11.2).
- MRI can delineate the grade of HO as well as the presence of inflammatory phenomena.

## Operative Treatment

### Anesthesia

- Regional (spinal/epidural) or general anesthesia.
- Administration or prophylactic antibiotics as per local hospital protocol at induction.

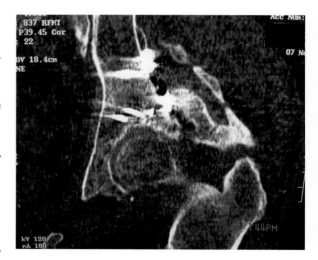

Fig. 11.2 Preoperative CT scan of same case

## Table Set Up

- The instrumentation is set up on the side of the operation.
- Position the table across the operating room so that the operating area lies in the clean air field.

## Patient Positioning

- In a lateral or prone position.
- Apply diathermy plate.
- Protect pressure areas.

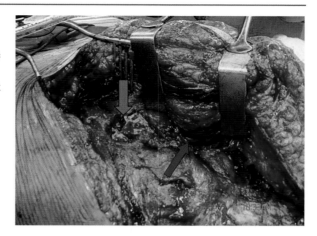

**Fig. 11.3** Identification of sciatic nerve (*blue arrow*) and of ectopic bone (*green arrow*)

## Draping and Surgical Approach

- Prepare the skin using antiseptic solutions (aqueous/alcoholic povidone-iodine) of the buttock and the lateral aspects of the thigh.
- The hip is re-exposed through the previous incision.
- In cases of no previous surgery, the surgical approach is modified according to the distribution of the ectopic bone.

## Kocher-Langenbeck Approach

- Utilize previous skin incision.
- The skin incision is carried through the subcutaneous tissue and superficial fascia onto the fascia lata of the lateral thigh and the thin deep fascia overlying the gluteus maximus muscle.
- Divide the fascia lata in line with the skin incision beginning at the distal aspect of the wound continuing approximately toward the greater tuberosity and ending at the first site of the gluteus maximus muscle fibers.
- Continue the proximal dissection by splitting the gluteus maximus muscle.
- The incision should be made between the upper one-third and lower two-thirds of the muscle as this is a relative avascular interval and in the desired plane of dissection.
- There is no internervous plain.
- Release of the gluteus maximus insertion to the femur allows adequate posteromedial retraction of the large mass of the gluteus maximus muscle without undue stretching on the inferior gluteal nerve.

- Whilst the tendon is released, care should be taken to avoid damage of the first perforating branch of the profunda femoris artery, which runs in close proximity.
- Locate the sciatic nerve (Fig. 11.3); the relationship between the sciatic nerve and quadratus femoris muscle should serve as a reference point.
- Identify the piriformis tendon running alongside the gluteus minimus muscle.
- It must be noted here that variability exists in relation to the sciatic nerve and the piriformis muscle. One therefore should be aware of the anatomic variability in this area, and prior identification of the sciatic nerve on the posterior surface of the quadratus femoris muscle will prevent intraoperative confusion and decrease the risk of iatrogenic sciatic nerve injury. Furthermore, scars from previous operations may alter normal anatomy of the area.
- After the identification of the piriformis tendon, it should be tagged with a suture and released from its insertion.
- Subsequently identify the obturator internus tendon with the superior and inferior gemeli muscles, which can be found just inferior and slightly deep to the piriformis.
- External rotation of the hip will relax the tendon allowing easier access to its deep surface. The obturator internus tendon is isolated, tugged with a suture and released from its insertion. Both the piriformis and obturator internus tendons should be incised approximately 1.5 cm from their insertion

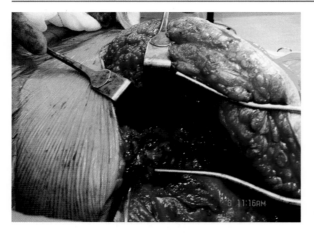

**Fig. 11.4** Use of a curved retractor (Langenbeck) superiorly to elevate the hip abductors from the external surface of the ilium

points into the greater trochanter to avoid injury to the blood supply of the femoral head.

- Elevate the obturator internus tendon away from the hip capsule along with the gemeli muscles.
- Access to the lesser sciatic notch is now possible, and a specially designed sciatic nerve retractor can be placed with its tip anchoring to the lesser sciatic notch.
- With the appropriate position of the sciatic nerve retractor, access is now possible to the posterior hip capsule and retroacetabular surface of the posterior column.
- Superiorly, the hip abductors are elevated from the external surface of the ilium with a curved retractor (Langenbeck) (Fig. 11.4).
- Care should be taken in the region of the greater sciatic notch not only to avoid injury to the sciatic

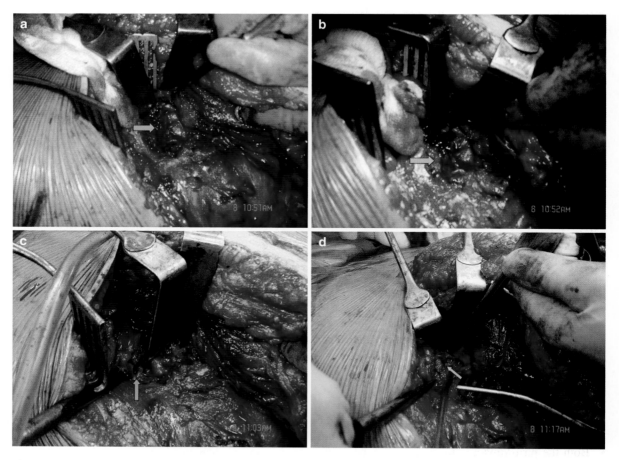

**Fig. 11.5** (**a**, **b**) Sharp dissection of ectopic bone from surrounding soft tissues, (**c**) removal of ectopic bone with a chisel, and (**d**) with a kerrison

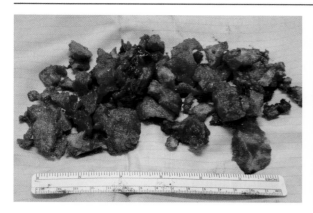

**Fig. 11.6**   The removed ectopic bone

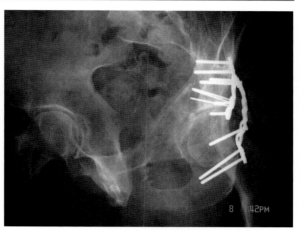

**Fig. 11.8** Postoperative obturator oblique view of the case shown in Fig. 11.1

- After the placement of a deep closed suction drain, the fascia lata gluteal fascia and subcutaneous tissues are closed in layers with 1.0 and 2.0 Vicryl absorbable sutures.
- The skin can be closed either with stainless steel surgical staples or monofilament nylon sutures in an interrupted manner.

## Pitfalls to Avoid and Tips

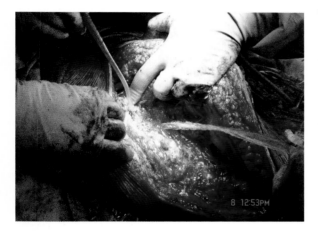

**Fig. 11.7**   Irrigation of the wound

nerve but also to the superior gluteal neurovascular bundle.
- The extent of the HO pattern dictates the extent of the surgical approach.
- Ectopic bone should be removed from surrounding soft tissues with sharp dissection, staying on bone wherever possible (Fig. 11.5a–d).
- The excised bony specimen (Fig. 11.6) is sent for histological examination.

## Closure

- The wound is irrigated thoroughly and hemostasis is achieved (Fig. 11.7).
- Both the piriformis and the obturator internus are reattached by using nonabsorbable sutures.

- Adequate exposure is paramount.
- The Kocher-Langenbeck approach to the soft tissues described above will not always be possible to follow due to the extent of the HO usually formed. In cases where complete distortion of the anatomical landmarks is present, removal of the ectopic bone formation should be initiated and performed in situ with the simultaneous protection of the sciatic nerve.
- Identification of the neurovascular structures is mandatory.
- The sciatic nerve should be isolated and protected throughout dissection of the HO about the hip.
- Timing for surgery:
  - After TBI.
    3–6 months from injury.
    Evidence of bone maturation at radiologic assessment.
  - After surgical intervention.
    >6 months.

- Recurrence prevention after surgical resection:
  - A single postoperative dose of 700 rad (within 72 h of surgery – best within the first 48 h).
- Measures to prevent HO formation after surgical interventions:
  - Pre/postoperative radiation.
  - Postoperatively indomethacin 75 mg per day for 6 weeks.

## Postoperative Rehabilitation

- Two further doses of prophylactic antibiotics.
- Routine bloods and radiographs of the hip in 24 h including Judet views (Fig. 11.8).
- The drain is removed in 24 h.
- Start mechanical VTE prophylaxis at admission and continue until the patient no longer has significantly reduced mobility, based on an assessment of risks. Start pharmacological VTE prophylaxis after surgery and continue until the patient no longer has significantly reduced mobility.
- Early passive and active physiotherapy.
- One session of low-dose (7 Gy) radiation on the first postoperative day.
- Discharged on indometacin 75 mg per day combined with a proton-pump inhibitor (omeprazole) for 6 weeks.

## Outpatients Follow Up

- Review at 3 weeks, 6 weeks, 3 months, 6 months, and 12 months with both clinical and radiographic assessment of the hip joint.
- Discharge from follow up after clinical and radiological evidence off non-recurrence of HO.
- Review again at the request of the GP.

## Further Reading

Board TN, Karva A, Board RE, Gambhir AK, Porter ML. The prophylaxis and treatment of heterotopic ossification following lower limb arthroplasty. J Bone Joint Surg (Br). 2007; 89-B:434–40.

Chao ST, Lee S-Y, Borden LS, Joyce MJ, Krebs VE, Suh JH. External beam radiation helps prevent heterotopic bone formation in patients with a history of heterotopic ossification. J Arthroplasty. 2006;21(5):731–6.

Manidakis N, Kanakaris NK, Nikolaou VS, Giannoudis PV. Early palsy of the sciatic nerve due to heterotopic ossification after surgery for fracture of the posterior wall of the acetabulum. A case report. J Bone Joint Surg (Br). 2009;91-B:253–7.

# Dunn's Procedure

**12**

Peter V. Giannoudis and Peter Templeton

## Indications

- The majority of cases of slipped upper femoral epiphysis can be managed with in situ cannulated screw fixation perpendicular to the epiphysis.
- Severe slips pose a problem for fixation as slips over 50° degrees or 50% are extremely difficult to fix with an in situ cannulated screw.
- Even if successful, the range of movement of the hip is often severely restricted due to impingement of the neck on the acetabulum.
- Complete slips are impossible to fix with an in situ screw.
- The Dunn's procedure is a cuneiform-shaped osteotomy of the proximal femoral neck which shortens the neck and allows reduction of the epiphysis onto the neck without tension on the posterior retinacular vessels. Thus, a relative indication for a Dunn's procedure is a slip more than 50°, especially if the neck is impinging on the acetabulum and an absolute indication is a complete slip. The acute component of the slip should be less than 1 month in duration.

P.V. Giannoudis (✉)
Academic Department of Trauma and Orthopaedic Surgery,
School of Medicine, University of Leeds, Leeds, UK
e-mail: pgiannoudi@aol.com

P. Templeton
Department of Trauma and Orthopaedic Surgery,
Leeds Teaching Hospitals NHS Trust, Leeds, UK

## Preoperative Planning

### Clinical Assessment

- Acute slips have a history of 3 weeks or less. The procedure is not recommended after 4 weeks of the onset of the acute slip.
- The leg is usually short and lies in external rotation.
- Movement of the hip is extremely painful and should be avoided.
- Plan for 2.5 h of theater time.

### Radiological Assessment

- AP view of the pelvis shows proximal femoral neck lying proximal to the epiphysis and may even appear to touch the acetabulum. Klein's line along the superior margin of the neck does not pass through the capital epiphysis.
- Cross table lateral or (unforced) frog leg lateral view demonstrates more clearly the severity of the slip which measures more than 50° in severe cases.

## Operative Treatment

### Anesthesia

- General anesthesia.
- Prophylactic intravenous antibiotics administered at the time of induction.
- Patient-controlled analgesia device postoperatively and femoral nerve block.

## Equipment

- Travers self retaining retractors.
- 2.5-mm-diameter drill.
- Osteotomes and mallet.
- 6.5-, 7.1-, or 8.0-mm-diameter cannulated screws. Using a cannulated screw that requires a 3.2-mm-diameter guide wire makes accurate placement much easier.
- Image intensifier.

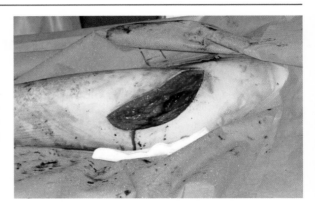

**Fig. 12.1** Posterolateral approach

## Table Setup

- Radiolucent table allowing unobstructed AP view of the pelvis.

## Patient Positioning

- Patient supine, sandbag, or "jelly" under lumbar region of affected side.
- Check that it is possible to perform AP view of pelvis with image intensifier.

## Fracture Reduction

- Do not attempt any form of reduction until the osteotomy has been performed.

## Draping and Surgical Approach

- Place a "U"-shaped isolation drape before preparing the skin with aqueous betadine or chlorhexidine.
- Then drape as per hip operation leaving thigh, buttock, and iliac crest freely accessible.
- Use a waterproof "sock" for the leg up to the knee.

## Incision

- Either posterolateral approach from just posterior to the anterior superior iliac spine extending laterally and distally to the lateral aspect of the upper thigh (Fig. 12.1).
- The interval between tensor fascia lata and gluteus medius is explored. Identify and coagulate veins at

the proximal extent of the wound. Try to preserve nerve to tensor fascia lata muscle.

- Clear fat from capsule and release gluteus minimus tendon from the greater trochanter.
- Do not place any retractors posterior to the neck of femur at any time to prevent damage to the blood supply to the head of the femur (Fig. 12.2a).
- Or use an anterior oblique incision centerd on a point 2 cm distal to the anterior superior iliac spine.
- Explore the interval between sartorius and tensor fascia lata muscles, protecting the lateral cutaneous nerve of the thigh which should be retracted medially.
- Divide conjoint tendon of rectus and reflect distally with stay suture of 1 Vicryl.
- Split iliac crest with knife and reflect lateral half to improve access.
- Expose capsule and divide in "L" shape along margin of acetabulum and then along superior border of neck of femur (Fig. 12.2b).
- If the anterior oblique incision is used, then a second incision will be required for the insertion of the cannulated screw from the lateral aspect of the femur.

## Procedure

- Expose the anterior aspect of the femoral neck which is displaced anteriorly relative to the proximal femoral epiphysis.
- Position the leg in adduction and external rotation to present the femoral neck.

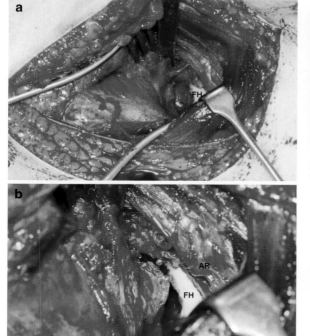

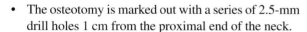

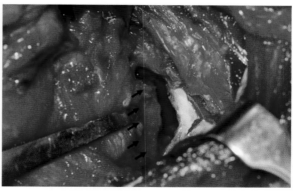

**Fig. 12.3** Osteotomy performed avoiding damaging the epiphysis (*arrows* showing osteotomy plane)

**Fig. 12.2** (**a**) Retractor must be positioned with extra care, avoiding any further disturbance on femoral head (FH) blood supply. (**b**) Capsular incision along the margin of acetabulum (*FH* femoral head, *AR* acetabular rim)

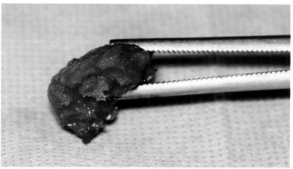

**Fig. 12.4** The bone chip removed after the osteotomy

- The osteotomy is marked out with a series of 2.5-mm drill holes 1 cm from the proximal end of the neck.
- Use an osteotome to complete the osteotomy taking care not to damage the periosteum on the posterior aspect of the neck (Fig. 12.3).
- Take your time to very carefully remove 1 cm of the neck with alternating use of the osteotomes and bone nibblers. Try to remove any prominent callus formed on the posterior aspect of the neck (Fig. 12.4). Do not remove anything, i.e., the growth plate, from the undersurface of the epiphysis.
- Once the neck is shortened enough to allow movement between the neck and epiphysis, gently apply traction, abduction, and internal rotation to reduce the neck onto the epiphysis. Further resection of the neck may be required to achieve an easy reduction without tension.
- The epiphysis should sit on the neck with an equal amount of overhang anteriorly, posteriorly, inferiorly, and superiorly.

## Implant Positioning

- Hold the position with a cannulated screw guide wire inserted from the lateral cortex of the proximal femur up the center of the neck into the middle of the epiphysis keeping 5 mm away from the articular surface. This procedure is technically very difficult and requires patience, spatial awareness, and a good image intensifier. The position of the guide wire must be checked on AP and lateral views by flexing the hip gently up to 90° taking care not to bend the guide wire.
- Ideally, the screw should be in the middle of the head, perpendicular to the epiphysis, or the epiphysis should lie in slight valgus.
- Use a single 7.1-mm or 8.0-mm-diameter screw (Fig. 12.5). In very obese children consider using 2×6.5-mm-diameter screws.

**Fig. 12.5** X-ray presenting the reduced slipped upper femoral epiphysis, stabilized with a cannulated screw

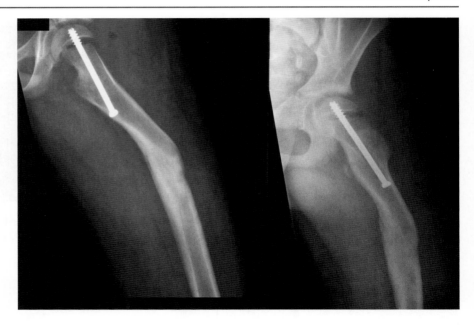

## Closure

- 1 Vicryl for the capsule, iliac crest, and rectus conjoint tendon
- 2.0 Vicryl for subcutaneous fat and fascia
- 3.0 Vicryl or PDS for subcuticular skin
- Dressing (no cast)

## Postoperative Rehabilitation

- Start mechanical VTE prophylaxis at admission and continue until the patient no longer has significantly reduced mobility, based on an assessment of risks. Start pharmacological VTE prophylaxis after surgery and continue until the patient no longer has significantly reduced mobility.
- Bed rest up to 7 days keeping leg on a pillow.
- Gently mobilize leg in bed with physiotherapist.
- Once comfortable, mobilize toe touching for 6 weeks.
- Then mobilize partial weight-bearing for 6 weeks further.

## Outpatient Follow-Up

- Review wound by outreach nurse at 2 weeks.
- Review at 6 weeks for an X-ray AP pelvis and progress to partial weight-bearing if no concerns.
- Review at 3 months for an X-ray AP pelvis and progress to full weight-bearing if osteotomy united (Fig. 12.6a, b).
- Arrange for cannulated screw fixation of opposite hip if not already performed. I prefer to perform once there is evidence that the osteotomy is healing due to the positioning required on a fracture table.

## Implant Removal

- I do not recommend routine removal of the implant unless there is a complication or the screw head is causing irritation.
- If screw removal is required, then it must be performed after the osteotomy has soundly united, i.e., several years later in which case it will be difficult to remove and broken screw removal set should be available.

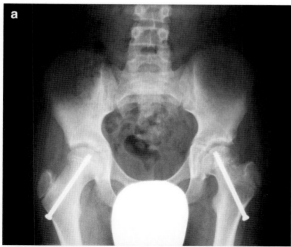

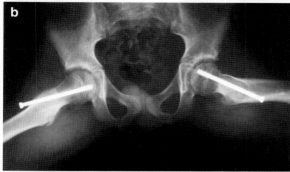

**Fig. 12.6** (**a**) AP and (**b**) lateral X-rays with the well reduced slipped epiphysis in a Risser 5 patient

## Further Reading

Dunn DM. The treatment of adolescent slipping of upper femoral epiphysis. J Bone Joint Surg Br. 1964;46:621–9.

Pelillo F, De Sanctis N, Benazzo F, et al. Slipped Upper Femoral Epiphysis (SUFE): to do or not to do in sufe. Hip Int. 2009;19 Suppl 6:S13–7.

Tins B, Cassar-Pullicino V, McCall I. Slipped upper femoral epiphysis: imaging of complications after treatment. Clin Radiol. 2008;63(1):27–40.

Uglow MG, Clarke NM. The management of slipped capital femoral epiphysis. J Bone Joint Surg Br. 2004;86(5):631–5.

# Treatment of Avascular Femoral Head Necrosis with Bone Morphogenetic Protein, a Collagen Scaffold and Filtered Autologous Mesenchymal Stem Cells

**13**

Georgio Maria Calori and Peter V. Giannoudis

## Indications

- Osteonecrosis of the femoral head (up to Stage IIIC of the Steinberg classification system).
- Patients under 55 years of age.
- No presence of radiological-documented arthritis of the hip.
- Nom BMP hypersensitivity.
- No underlying pregnancy.

## Preoperative Planning

### Clinical Assessment

- Pain is the first symptom. It is localized in the affected hip site with possible radiation of pain to the knee, often without related radiographical signs. Causes of early pain are: tissue ischemia, pressure increase inside the bone, microfractures in the avascular zone.

- Investigate any concomitant systemic disease (obesity, smoke, alcohol abuse, rheumatic disease, cancer, acute and chronic leukemia, sickle-cell disease).

### Radiological Assessment

- Anteroposterior (AP) and lateral X-rays of the affected hip (Fig. 13.1).
- Magnetic Resonance Imaging (MRI) to determine the exact size and position of the lesion in early stages. It allows to find the early trasformation of the hematopoietic marrow in fat marrow individuating those patients with higher risk before the lesion of the femoral head takes place (Fig. 13.2).

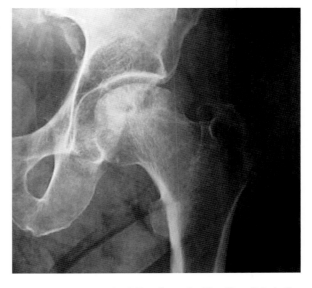

**Fig. 13.1** Anteroposterior (AP) radiograph of the affected hip (radiographic changes can appear even up to 6 months after pain onset)

G.M. Calori (✉)
Academic Department of Trauma and Orthopaedic Surgery,
Instituto Ortopedico Gaetano Pini,
Milan University, Milan, Italy
e-mail: gmc@studiocalori.it

P.V. Giannoudis
Academic Department of Trauma and Orthopaedic Surgery,
School of Medicine, University of Leeds, Leeds, UK

P.V. Giannoudis (ed.), *Practical Procedures in Elective Orthopaedic Surgery*,
DOI 10.1007/978-0-85729-814-0_13, © Springer-Verlag London Limited 2012

**Fig. 13.2** Magnetic Resonance Imaging (MRI) showing the exact size and position of the AVN lesion in the left hip

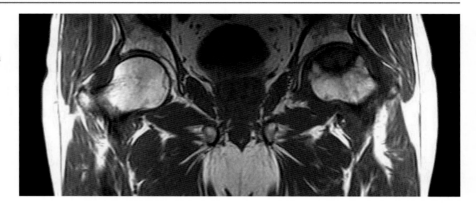

**Fig. 13.3** (**a**) 14-mm-diameter cannulated reamer and cannulated guide designed for the reamer. (**b**, **c**) Cannula with reservoir for BMP-7 with pushing device

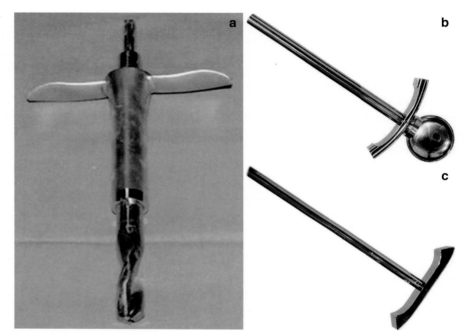

## Operative Treatment

### Anesthesia

- Regional (spinal/epidural) and/or general anesthesia.
- At induction, administer short-therapy prophylactic antibiotic as per hospital protocol (e.g., first generation cephalosporin).

### Table and Equipment

- Instrumentation set including guide wire, 14-mm diameter cannulated reamer, cannulated guide designed for the reamer (Fig. 13.3a), cannula with reservoir for BMP-7 with pushing device (Fig. 13.3b, c).
- A radiolucent table or a fracture table with the appropriate traction devices.
- An image intensifier or CT equipment.
- Bone marrow aspiration trocar for harvesting Mesenchymal Stem Cells (MSC's).
- A bone marrow concentration device.
- A collagen scaffold.

### Table Setup

- The instrumentation is set up on the side of the operation.
- Image intensifier is from the contralateral side.

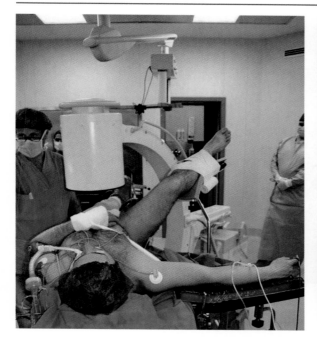

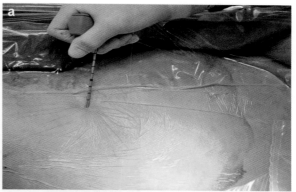

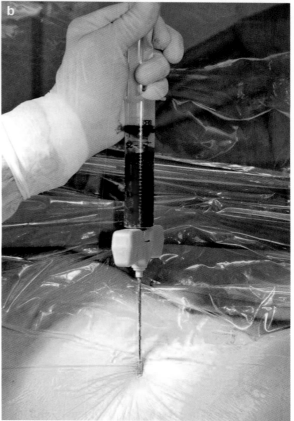

**Fig. 13.4** Patient supine with the injured leg positioned in a footplate attached to the leg extensions of the fracture table. Uninjured leg in a leg holder in wide abduction with adequate padding over the peroneal nerve

## Patient Positioning

- Supine with the affected leg positioned in a foot-plate attached to the leg extensions of the fracture table (Fig. 13.4).
- Position the opposite leg in a leg holder in wide abduction with adequate padding over the peroneal nerve.

## Iliac Crest Harvesting

- Clean the skin around the iliac crest with the usual antiseptic solutions (10% povidone-iodine solution, chlorhexidine gluconate, 4%).
- Identify the Anterior Iliac Crest (AIC) by locating the center of prominence of anterior superior iliac spine, just under lip of crest chosen site.
- Highlight the procedure site with an indelible pen.
- Place a sterile drape with a fenestrated opening over the AIC.
- Fill the necessary number of 30-mL syringes (added with heparin solution or other anticoagulant). Usually at least 60 mL of bone marrow aspirate is required.

**Fig. 13.5** (a) Punctioning of the skin vertically over the Anterior Iliac Crest. (b) Attaching the syringe to the needle and aspiration of the marrow into the syringe until is filled

- Hold aspiration needle vertically to puncture the skin. Press the needle with a slight twisting motion through the cortical bone and advance it about 1 cm into the marrow cavity. Unlock and remove the obturator (Fig. 13.5a, b).

**Fig. 13.6** Application of a transparent, plastic, adherent isolation drape directly over the proposed incision site

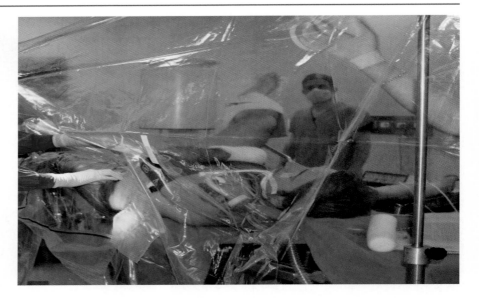

- Attach a 30-mL syringe to the needle and aspirate marrow into the syringe until it is fullfilled. Repeat the procedure until all two syringes are filled. Give the material collected to the technical assistant to process them.
- If not enough harvest can be obtained from the procedure site, then reposition needle changing depth, angle, or location until harvesting is successfull. Try the contralateral side if necessary.
- Remove aspiration needle and achieve hemostasis. Suture skin if necessary and cover with a sterile dressing.
- Concentrate the bone marrow aspirate as per instructions of the bone marrow concentration device (usually a volume between 6-8mls is obtained).

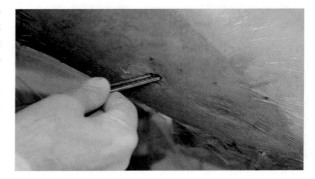

**Fig. 13.7** Mid-lateral longitudinal incision, extending distally from the great trochanter for 1.5–2 cm

## Draping and Surgical Approach

- Prepare the skin over the proximal femur with antiseptic solution.
- Apply a transparent, plastic, adherent isolation drape directly over the proposed incision site (Fig. 13.6).
- Perform a mid-lateral longitudinal incision, extending distally from the great trochanter for 1.5–2 cm (Fig. 13.7). Divide the fascia lata and the vastus lateralis muscle in line with the skin incision.

## Core Decompression

- Place the guide wire into the center of the necrotic area of the femoral head under fluoroscopic or CT

control (Fig. 13.8a, b). Check the position of the wire in the AP and lateral planes.
- Determine the reaming distance using the measuring device.
- Ream coaxially the femur with 14-mm-diameter cannulated reamer under image intensifier control to confirm that the guide wire is not advancing into the pelvis up to 1 cm from the chondral surface (Fig. 13.9a, b).
- Remove bone up to the subchondral level in order to achieve core decompression (Fig. 13.10).

## Graft Positioning

- Prepare a scaffold of cancellous bone permeated with autogenous filtered bone marrow cells. The scaffold is a decalcified, flexible, and mouldable equine bone

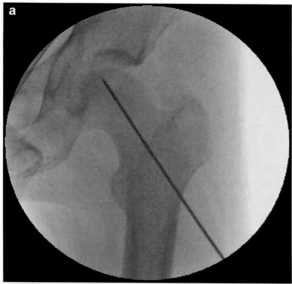

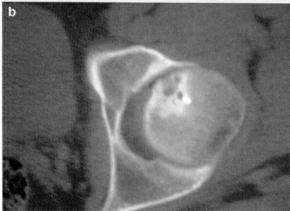

**Fig. 13.8** (**a, b**) Placing of the guide wire into the center of the necrotic area of the femoral head under fluoroscopic or CT control

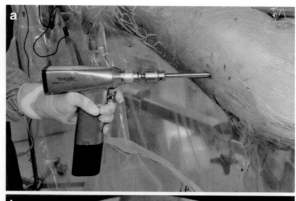

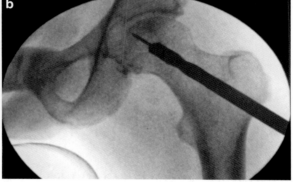

**Fig. 13.9** (**a, b**) Reaming coaxially the femur with a 14-mm cannulated reamer under image intensifier control to confirm that the guide wire is not advancing into the pelvis

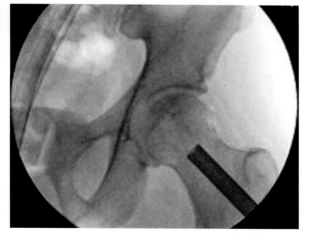

**Fig. 13.10** Removing of bone up to the subchondral level in order to achieve core decompression

tissue with collagen, which expands after loading with filtrated bone marrow cells (Fig. 13.11a).

- Apply BMP-7 following preparation (dilution of active substance with 2.5 ml of normal saline) on the reservoir of the cannula. Advance BMP-7 at least 2 cm from the reservoir inside the tunnel of the cannula.
- Insert the scaffold using the appropriate instrumentation under fluoroscopic guidance until the implant reaches the subchondral plate (this advancement of the scaffold ensures delivery of the BMP into the affected AVN area and at the same time the scaffold contains the protein within the femoral head) (Fig. 13.11c).
- Obtain final fluoroscopic or CT imaging in both the AP and lateral views (Fig. 13.11d, e).

## Closure

- Irrigate the wound thoroughly and achieve hemostasis.

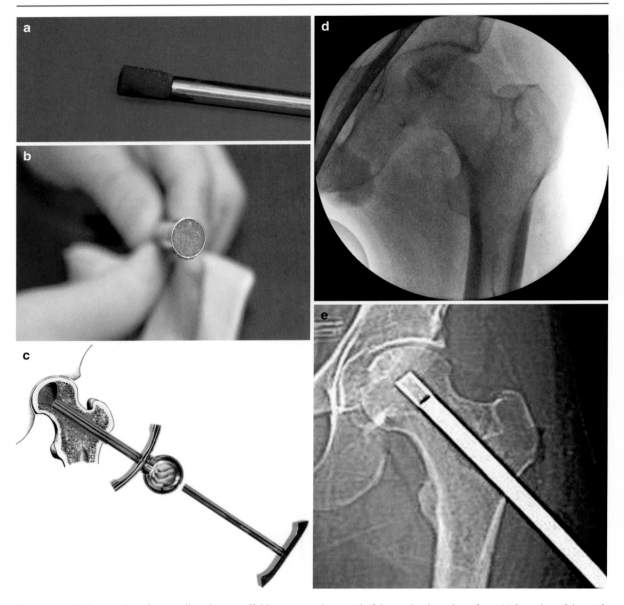

**Fig. 13.11** (**a**) Preparation of a cancellous bone scaffold permeated with autogenous filtered bone marrow cells. (**b**) Application of BMP-7 onto the reservoir and advancement of BMP-7 inside the tunnel of the trochar by at least 2cm. (**c**) Insertion of the scaffold using the appropriate instrumentation under fluoroscopic guidance. (**d**, **e**) Final control with fluoroscopic or CT imaging

- Close the fascia lata and the subcutaneous fat with adsorbable sutures.
- Skin closure and covering with sterile dressing.

## Postoperative Rehabilitation

- Obtain Postoperative radiographs.
- Routine blood examination.

- Two more doses of antibiotics.
- Prescribe thromboprophylaxis for a period of 6 weeks as per local department protocol.
- Non-weight-bearing with use of crutches for 3 weeks, then mobilize partial weight-bearing (20–25% of the overall weight) for 3 weeks, and then progressive weightbearing for 6 weeks with physiotherapy assistance.

**Fig. 13.12** (**a**) CT control 6 months after operation, documenting partial bone formation in the former necrotic area. (**b**) Radiographic control 12 months after surgery documenting absence of head deformation with complete bone formation

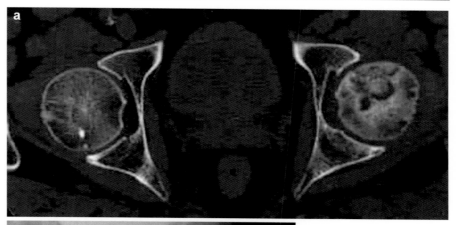

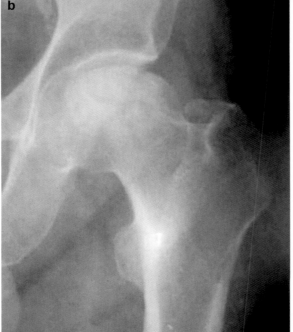

## Outpatient Follow-Up

- Review after 1 month with radiographs of the hip and then every 3 months for the first year, then every 6 month for the second year, then once a year (Fig. 13.12a, b).
- Evaluate at the 6-months and 12-months follow-up by using Harris Hip Score.

## Further Reading

Garrigues GE, Aldridge 3rd JM, Friend JK, et al. Free vascularized fibular grafting for treatment of osteonecrosis of the femoral head secondary to hip dislocation. Microsurgery. 2009;29(5):342–5.

Aldridge 3rd JM, Urbaniak JR. Avascular necrosis of the femoral head: role of vascularized bone grafts. Orthop Clin North Am. 2007;38(1):13–22.

Yen CY, Tu YK, Ma CH, et al. Osteonecrosis of the femoral head: comparison of clinical results for vascularized iliac and fibula bone grafting. J Reconstr Microsurg. 2006;22(1):21–4.

Tang CL, Mahoney JL, McKee MD, et al. Donor site morbidity following vascularized fibular grafting. Microsurgery. 1998;18(6):383–6.

# Femoral Neck Non-union (Intracapsular)

**14**

Peter V. Giannoudis and Rozalia I. Dimitriou

## Indications

- Previously stabilized femoral neck fracture that failed to progress to union within 6 months of fixation.
- Usually young individual below the age of 60.
- Above the age of 60, hip replacement is the procedure of choice.
- Non-union associated with pain and impaired hip function.

## Pre-operative Planning

### Clinical Assessment

- Obtain detailed previous history.
- Document comorbidities.
- Document pain killer intake and smoking habits.
- Assess leg length discrepancy and presence of rotational deformity.
- Document range of hip motion.
- Assess neurovascular status of the limb.
- Request blood investigations (FRC, CRP, ESR) to exclude low grade infection.

P.V. Giannoudis (✉)
Academic Department of Trauma and Orthopaedic Surgery,
School of Medicine, University of Leeds, Leeds, UK
e-mail: pgiannoudi@aol.com

R.I. Dimitriou
Department of Trauma and Orthopaedic Surgery,
Leeds Teaching Hospitals NHS Trust, Leeds, UK

## Radiological Assessment

- Anteroposterior (AP) and lateral views (Fig. 14.1a, b) of the affected hip joint.
- AP pelvis X-ray will provide useful information of the opposite hip for comparison purposes.
- Investigate the state of the blood supply of the affected femoral head by requesting PET scan (If blood supply is compromised then consider total hip replacement rather than revision of fixation.).
- CT scan will provide useful information of the non-union site and the underlying type of non-union (atrophic or hypertrophic).

## Operative Treatment

### Anesthesia

- General or regional (spinal or epidural) anesthesia.
- Administration of prophylactic antibiotics is refrained until acquisition of intra-operative tissue cultures.

### Table and Equipment

- Availability of extraction kit for removal of the implant previously inserted.
- DHS instrumentation set – ensure the availability of the complete set of implants especially a 2-hole plate 135° (Fig. 14.2).
- A cannulated 6.5-mm instrumentation set.
- Osteotomes in case that open reduction will be necessary.

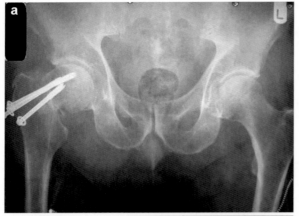

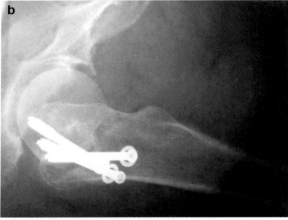

**Fig. 14.1** (**a**) AP pelvis radiograph illustrating non union (failure of previous fixation of an intra-capsular right neck of femur fracture stabilized with three cannulated screws). (**b**) Lateral radiograph of the hip illustrating the metal work failure

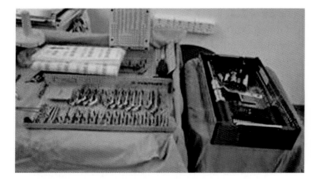

**Fig. 14.2** DHS instrumentation set is shown – ensure the availability of the complete set of implants

- Standard radiolucent operating table with the appropriate traction devices.
- Image intensifier.

## Table Set up

- The instrumentation is set up at the site of the operation.
- Image intensifier is from the contralateral side.
- Position the table diagonally across the operating room so that the operating area lies in the clean air field.

## Patient Positioning

- Supine with a well-padded radiolucent pudendal post.
- Uninjured leg positioned in a leg holder (i.e., Lloyd Davies with adequate padding over the peroneal nerve) or in wide abduction by a footplate attached to the leg extensions of the fracture table.
- A footplate attached to the other leg extension of the fracture table holds the injured leg (Fig. 14.3).

## Reduction of Non-union

- Restoration femoral neck's high and inclination is essential for optimum mechanical stability (Fig. 14.4a, b). A varus position of reduction must be avoided.
- If reduction is not possible by closed maneuvers and the traction applied, then open reduction is advisable. A valgus osteotomy may be necessary to achieve optimum reduction.

## Draping and Surgical Approach

- Prepare the skin over the proximal femur with the usual antiseptic solutions (aqueous/alcoholic povidone-iodine).
- Apply transparent, plastic, adherent "isolation" drape directly over the proposed incision site. This vertical drape is anchored above on a rail.
- A direct lateral approach is made to the proximal femur from the greater trochanter extending distally (Fig. 14.5).
- Divide the fascia lata in line with the skin incision (Fig. 14.6).
- Expose the proximal femur by splitting the vastus lateralis along its fibers or by elevating the vastus lateralis off the lateral intermuscular septum

**Fig. 14.3** A footplate attached to the other leg extension of the fracture table holds the injured leg

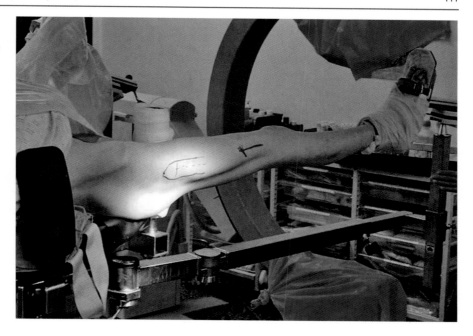

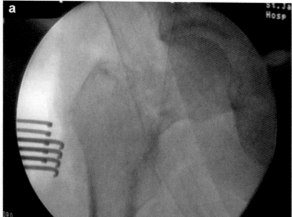

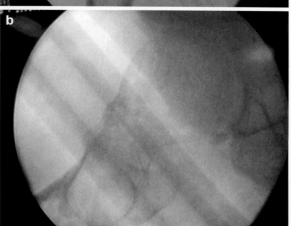

**Fig. 14.4** Application of traction – fluoroscopic images (**a**) AP and (**b**) lateral illustrating satisfactory reduction of the non-union

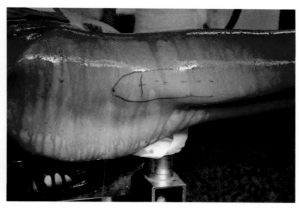

**Fig. 14.5** A direct lateral approach is made to the proximal femur from the greater trochanter extending distally

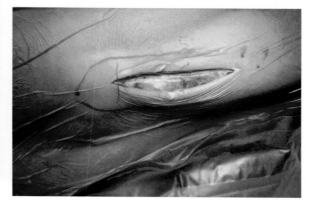

**Fig. 14.6** Divide the fascia lata in line with the skin incision

(beware of the perforators as they pierce the lateral intermuscular septum).

- At this stage, the previous cannulated screws can be removed with the appropriate screwdriver.

## Implant Insertion

- The lesser trochanter marks the level of entry of a 135° angle plate.
- Under fluoroscopic control insert a threaded 3.2-mm guide pin by power using the appropriate fixed angle guide.
- The body of the guide must be flush and parallel with the lateral cortex.
- Advance the guide pin toward the apex of the femoral head monitoring its position on the image intensifier.
- Place the tip in the subchondral bone. The guide pin must lie in the center of the femoral head in the anteroposterior and lateral views.
- Determine the lag screw length and reaming distance using the measuring device.
- Set the reamer 5 mm shorter than the length measured. Ream the femur by using the "triple reamer" (Fig. 14.7a, b).
- Ream coaxially, and use image intensification views to confirm that the guide pin is not advancing into the pelvis or being withdrawn at the conclusion of the reaming.
- Tap the bone in young patients and when dealing with hard sclerotic bones.
- Insert the lag screw over the centering sleeve after assembling it on the insertion device. Advance the tip of the screw up to the non-union level using the image intensifier for guidance (Fig. 14.8).
- On this occasion a diluted dose of a growth factor (BMP-7) was injected via the DHS screw into the site of the non-union in order to optimize the biological substrate of the local environment (this treatment represents the author's chosen option on this occasion, other surgeons may prefer to proceed with an open approach and to graft with autologous bone graft harvested from the iliac crest of the non-union site).
- For the injection of the growth factor, incline the fracture table towards the healthy hip site so that the injection material will not escape backwards out of the screw (Fig. 14.9).

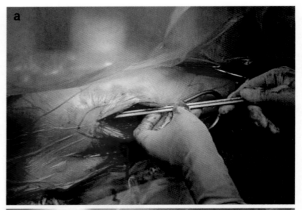
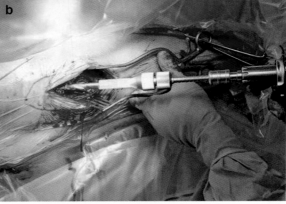

Fig. 14.7 (a) Set the reamer 5 mm shorter than the length measured. (b) Ream the femur by using the 'triple reamer

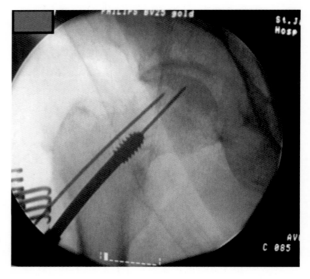

Fig. 14.8 Fluoroscopic image showing advancement of the tip of the screw up to the non-union level

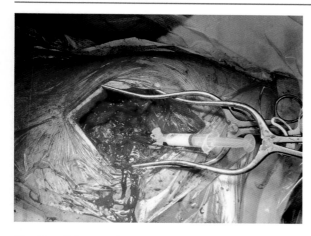

**Fig. 14.9** Injection of the growth factor is shown through the DHS screw

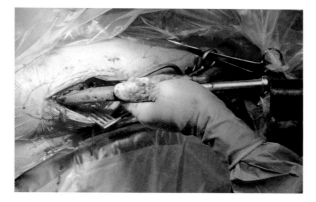

**Fig. 14.10** Advance the side plate over the lag screw shaft and use the plate tamper to fully seat the plate

- After injection of the growth factor, advance the tip of the screw beyond the non-union site. The tip-to-apex distance (TAD) (sum of the distances from the apex of the femoral head to the tip of the lag screw on both anteroposterior and lateral views, correcting for magnification) must ideally be less than 25 mm. Before the advancement of the DHS screw a 3.2-mm guide wire can be inserted into the femoral neck superiorly to control better the rotation (not to lose reduction).
- On completion of the screw insertion, the handle of the insertion device must be parallel to the axis of the femoral shaft (perpendicular if a Richards compression

screw is used) to allow the correct slotting of the lag screw to the plate barrel.
- Advance the 4-hole side plate (or 2 hole if indicated) over the leg screw shaft and use the plate tamper to fully seat the plate (Fig. 14.10)
- Unscrew the lag screw retaining rod and remove the guide pin.
- Remove also the second guide wire inserted to control rotation.
- Secure the plate to the femoral shaft using a plate clamp or a Haygroves clamp.
- Using the 3.5-mm twist drill through the neutral drill guide, make screw holes corresponding to the 4 holes in the plate.
- Determine the screw length using the measuring gauge. Use 4.5-mm screws after tapping to secure the plate (Fig. 14.11a–c).
- A compression screw through the lag screw to compress the fracture primarily (caution in osteoporotic bones) is optional and available for use.
- Insert a guide wire from the 6.5-mm cannulated set superiorly and in the midline of the femoral neck on the lateral view (if possible).
- Determine the lag screw length and reaming distance using the measuring device.
- Ream coaxially and use image intensification views to confirm that the guide pin is not advancing into the pelvis or being withdrawn at the conclusion of the reaming.
- Insert the appropriate-length 6.5-mm screw with a washer and remove the guide wire.
- Obtain final radiographs in both the anteroposterior and lateral planes (Fig. 14.12a, b).

## Closure

- Irrigate the wound thoroughly and achieve hemostasis.
- Close fascia lata (No1 PDS/Vicryl) and the subcutaneous fat with absorbable sutures (2/0 PDS/Vicryl).
- Skin closure – stainless steel surgical staples, monofilament non-absorbable suture or absorbable suture placed in the subcuticular layer.
- A drain has not been used on this occasion due to the implantation of the growth factor.

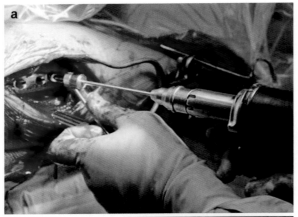

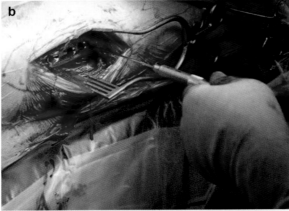

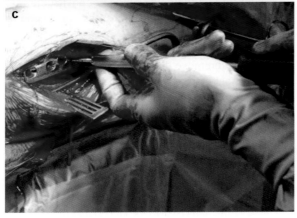

**Fig. 14.11** (**a**, **b**) and (**c**) Determine the screw length using the measuring gauge. Use 4.5 mm screws after tapping to secure the plate

## Postoperative Rehabilitation

- Two further doses of prophylactic antibiotics, if intraoperative cultures are negative.
- Start mechanical VTE prophylaxis at admission and continue until the patient no longer has significantly reduced mobility, based on an assessment of risks. Start pharmacological VTE prophylaxis after surgery and continue until the patient no longer has significantly reduced mobility.
- Routine bloods and radiographs of the pelvis in 24 h.
- Mobilize toe touch weight bearing at the earliest and tailor physiotherapy to meet individual needs and demands.
- Progress to full weight bearing at approximately 8 weeks following the revision surgery.

## Outpatient Follow up

- Review at 4, 8, and 12 weeks and at 6, 12, and 24 months with radiographs of the hip.
- Discharge from the follow up after clinical and radiological evidence of fracture healing (Fig. 14.13a, b).

## Postoperative Complications

- Superficial and deep Infection.
- Failure of metal work.
- Persistent non–union.
- Avascular necrosis of femoral head.

## Implant Removal

- No removal is indicated unless there is good evidence of soft tissue irritation.

**Fig. 14.12** (**a**) Postoperative xrays AP and (**b**) lateral illustrating the fixation of the femoral neck non-union

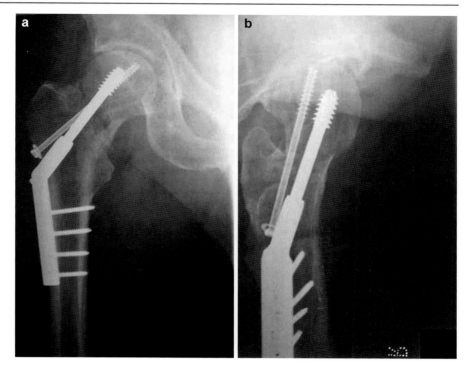

**Fig. 14.13** (**a**) Radiographs of the right hip AP and (**b**) lateral at 12 months follow up illustrating healing of the femoral neck non-union

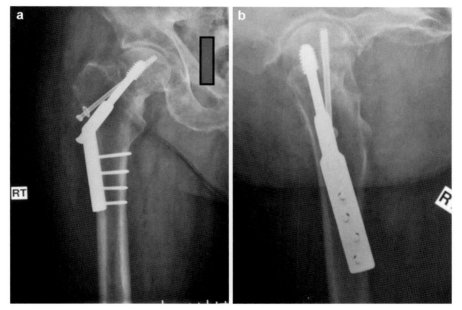

## Further Reading

Dhar SA, Gani NU, Butt MF, et al. Delayed union of an operated fracture of the femoral neck. J Orthop Traumatol. 2008;9(2): 97–9.

Van Must AB. Femoral neck non-unions: how do I do it? Injury. 2007;38 Suppl 2:S51–4.

Min BW, Bae KC, Kang CH, et al. Valgus intertrochanteric osteotomy for non-union of femoral neck fracture. Injury. 2006;37(8):786–90.

# Subtrochanteric Femoral Non-union

# 15

Peter V. Giannoudis and Nikolaos K. Kanakaris

## Indications

- Previous stabilized femoral subtrochanteric fracture that failed to progress to union.
- Early implant failure.
- Non-union associated with pain and impaired hip function.

## Preoperative Planning

### Clinical Assessment

- Obtain detailed previous history.
- Document comorbidities.
- Document painkiller intake and smoking habits.
- Assess leg length discrepancy and presence of rotational deformity.
- Document range of hip motion.

P.V. Giannoudis (✉)
Academic Department of Trauma and Orthopaedic Surgery,
School of Medicine, University of Leeds, Leeds, UK
e-mail: pgiannoudi@aol.com

N.K. Kanakaris
Department of Trauma and Orthopaedic Surgery, Leeds
Teaching Hospitals NHS Trust, Leeds, UK

- Assess neurovascular status of the limb.
- Request blood investigations (FRC, CRP, ESR) to exclude low-grade infection.

### Radiological Assessment

- Anteroposterior (AP) (Fig. 15.1) and lateral views of the affected hip joint.
- CT scan will provide useful information of the non-union site (type of non-union) and the presence of sequestrum in case of infected non-union.

## Operative Treatment

### Anaesthesia

- General or regional (spinal, epidural) anaesthesia.
- Administration of prophylactic antibiotics is refrained until acquisition of intraoperative tissue cultures.

### Table and Equipment

- Availability of extraction kit for the removal of the implant (IM nail) previously inserted.
- Blade plate (condylar plate) instrumentation set – ensure the availability of the complete set of implants (Fig. 15.2a, b).
- Osteotomes.
- Standard radiolucent operating table with the appropriate traction devices.
- Image intensifier.

**Fig. 15.1** AP pelvis radiograph illustrating right subtrochanteric non-union (failure of previous fixation with an intramedullary implant)

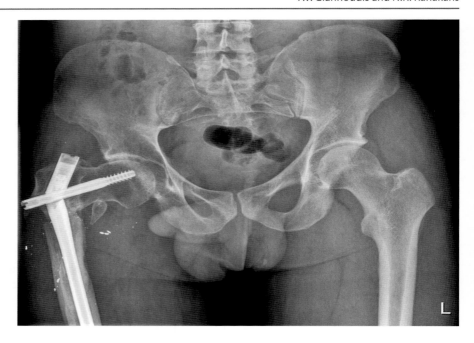

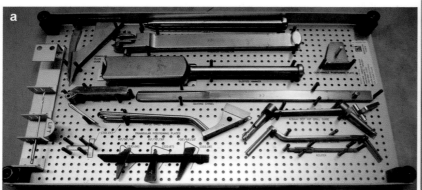
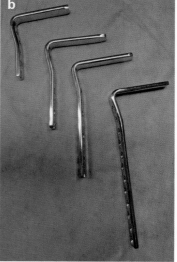

**Fig. 15.2** (**a**) Blade plate (condylar plate) instrumentation set is shown. (**b**). Ensure the availability of the complete set of implants

## Table Setup

- The instrumentation is set up at the site of the operation.
- Image intensifier is from the contralateral side.
- Position the table diagonally across the operating room so that the operating area lies in the clean air field.

## Patient Positioning

- Supine with a well-padded radiolucent pudendal post.
- Uninjured leg positioned in a leg holder (i.e., Lloyd Davies with adequate padding over the peroneal nerve) or in wide abduction by a footplate attached to the leg extensions of the fracture table.

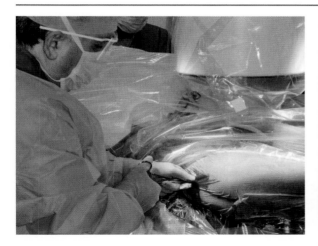

**Fig. 15.3** Opening of the proximal incision facilitates access to the great trochanter by splitting the fascia lata longitudinally and dividing the fibers of the gluteus maximus muscle

## Draping and Surgical Approach

- Prepare the skin over the proximal femur with the usual antiseptic solutions (aqueous/alcoholic povidone-iodine).
- Apply transparent, plastic, adherent "isolation" drape directly over the proposed incision site. This vertical drape is anchored above on a rail.

## Removal of Broken Implant (IM Nail)

- Utilize previous proximal and distal incisions.
- Opening of the proximal incision facilitates access to the great trochanter by splitting the fascia lata longitudinally and dividing the fibers of the gluteus maximus muscle (Fig. 15.3).
- Remove any ectopic bone formation with osteotomes and bone nibblers.
- Remove with a screw driver the cup of the nail.
- Open previous incision made over greater trochanter and remove lag screw of nail using the appropriate screw driver (Fig. 15.4a, b).
- Remove proximal locking screws and then the broken part of the proximal nail (if necessary use extraction rod inserted in the nail under image intensifier control).
- Remove distal locking screws.
- Remove the distal part of the broken nail by inserting an extraction hook (Fig. 15.5a, b).
- Take tissues for microbiology assessment (culture and sensitivities).

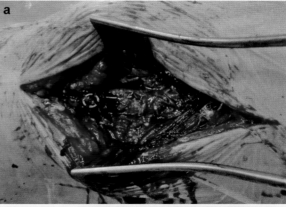

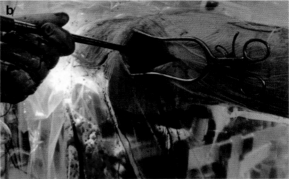

**Fig. 15.4** (**a**) Lag screw of nail is shown. (**b**) Removal of the lag screw with appropriate screw driver

- Ream the intramedullary canal at least 2 mm above the previous maximum reaming head size used.
- Send reamings to microbiology.
- Connect the proximal incision to the incision made to remove the proximal locking screws and extend incision distally 8–10 cm from the tip of the greater trochanter along the axis of the femoral shaft (Fig. 15.6).
- Split the fascia lata in the line of the femur along the entire length of the wound.
- Reveal the vastus lateralis and by using the index finger as a guide to the lateral aspect of the femoral shaft (using the cutting diathermy), cut down right on the bone.
- Using bone levers, retract the anterior and posterior parts of the vastus thus getting easy access to the proximal femur.
- Using osteotomes and bone nibblers, debride the non-union site (Fig. 15.7a–c).
- Send cultures again to microbiology.
- Make sure the bed of the non-union is vascular following the debridement.

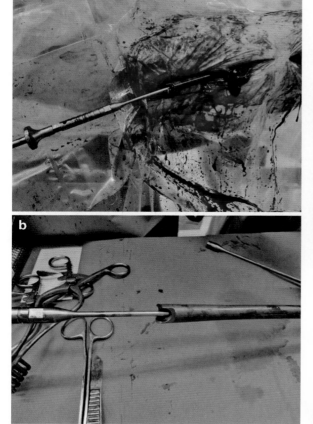

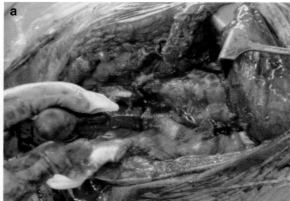

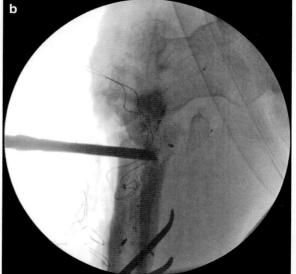

**Fig. 15.5** (**a**) Using an extraction hook, the distal part of the broken nail is removed. (**b**) Extracted piece of broken nail is shown with the hook attached

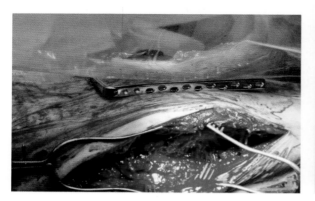

**Fig. 15.6** Incision is extended distally 8–10 cm from the tip of the greater trochanter along the axis of the femoral shaft. The blade plate implant to be used has been placed over the anterior aspect of the femur indicating the length of the incision required

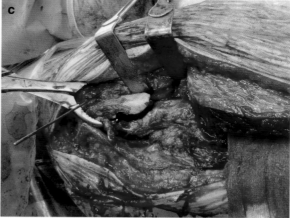

**Fig. 15.7** (**a**) Using osteotomes, the non-union site is refreshed down to healthy bleeding tissue. (**b**) Fluoroscopic image illustrating the use of the osteotome at the non-union site. (**c**) The non-union site is fully exposed, and the non-vital tissues were removed

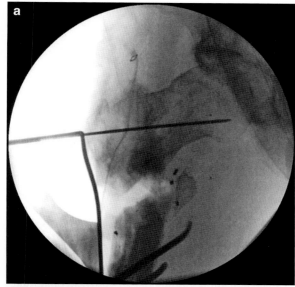

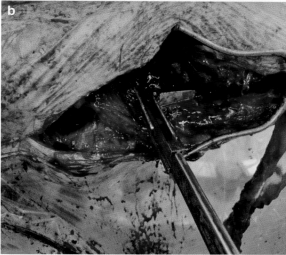

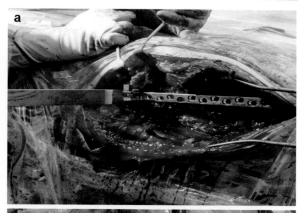

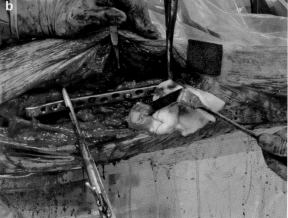

**Fig. 15.9** (**a**) Insertion of the chosen plate into the plate holder is shown. The blade is pushed by hand into the pre-cut channel. (**b**) The plate is inserted and initially is held in place with Hargroves reduction clumps until it is stabilized with the screws

**Fig. 15.8** (**a**) Fluoroscopic image showing the position of the guide wire in the femoral neck for choosing the appropriate level of the point of insertion of the seating chisel. (**b**) Intraoperative image illustrating the placement of the seating chisel on the lateral border of the greater trochanter

## Condylar Plate 95° Insertion

- Using the preoperative radiographs, template the healthy side for the length of the condylar blade as well as the length of the plate (number of holes) to be used.
- Condylar guide with an angle of 95° is used as a guide and is brought up to and along the lateral cortex of the femur.

- A Kirschner wire is inserted into the tip of the greater trochanter parallel to the top of the condylar guide.
- The position of the guide wire is checked under II control and is used for the insertion of the seating chisel (Fig. 15.8a, b).
- Make sure that the point of entry must be in the anterior part of the greater trochanter.
- The entry for the seating chisel is predrilled with a 4.5-mm drill bit, enlarged with a router.
- The position of the seating chisel is checked with image intensifier.
- This allows checking whether the length that was chosen preoperatively is still valid.
- The chosen plate is inserted into the plate holder, and the blade is pushed by hand into the pre-cut channel and with light hammer blows is advanced in the bone (Fig. 15.9a, b).

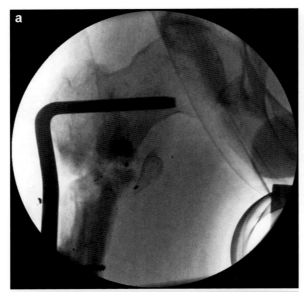

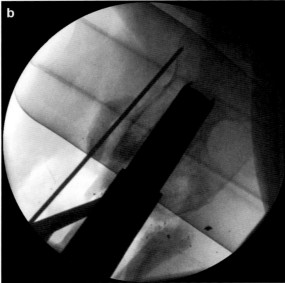

**Fig. 15.10** (**a**, **b**) Fluoroscopic image AP and lateral showing correction of the femoral neck-shaft angle

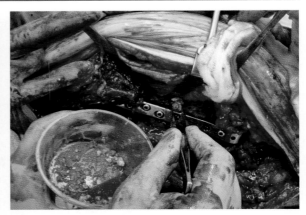

**Fig. 15.11** Cancellous bone chips are implanted in the non-union site

- Using the 3.2-mm drill sleeve in the holes of the plate will allow guiding the 3.2-mm drill bit through the two cortices.
- Having determined the screw length, insert the corresponding self-tapping cortex screws.
- The plate is fixed securely now on the bone.
- Implant the appropriate previous chosen bone graft in the non-union site for biological stimulation (this can be autologous iliac crest bone graft, BMP-7, or cancellous bone chips form the local hospital bone bank) (Fig. 15.11).
- Take intraoperative fluoroscopic images of the fixation.

## Closure

- Irrigate the wound thoroughly and achieve hemostasis.
- Close fascia lata (No.1 PDS/Vicryl) and the subcutaneous fat with absorbable sutures (2/0 PDS/Vicryl).
- Skin closure – stainless steel surgical staples, monofilament non-absorbable suture, or absorbable suture placed in the subcuticular layer.

## Postoperative Rehabilitation

- Two further doses of prophylactic antibiotics.
- Longer duration of antibiotics if the intraoperative samples taken are found to be positive for infection (duration of treatment minimum 6–8 weeks).

- Seat the plate with the impactor when the plate is about 5 mm from the bone having first removed the plate holder.
- The plate must come to lie in line with the femoral shaft and be held with a hay groves reduction forceps.
- This maneuver will correct the femoral neck-shaft angle (Fig. 15.10a, b).

**Fig. 15.12** (a) Radiographs AP and (b) lateral illustrating healing of the previous subtrochanteric non-union stabilized with the condylar blade plate implant (12 month follow-up)

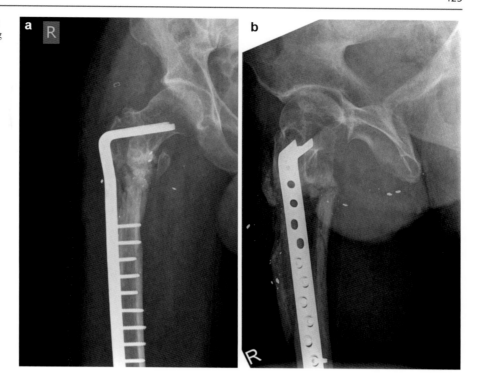

- Start mechanical VTE prophylaxis at admission and continue until the patient no longer has significantly reduced mobility based on an assessment of risks. Start pharmacological VTE prophylaxis after surgery and continue until the patient no longer has significantly reduced mobility.
- Routine bloods and radiographs of the pelvis in 24 h.
- Mobilize toe-touch weight-bearing at the earliest and tailor physiotherapy to meet individual needs and demands.
- Progress to full weight-bearing at approximately 8 weeks following the revision surgery.

## Outpatient Follow-up

- Review at 4, 8, 12 weeks and at 6, 12, 24 months with radiographs of the hip.
- Discharge from the follow-up after clinical and radiological evidence of fracture healing (Fig. 15.12a, b).

## Postoperative Complications

- Superficial and deep Infection.
- Failure of metal work.
- Persistent nonunion.
- Avascular necrosis of femoral head

## Implant Removal

- No removal is indicated unless there is good evidence of soft tissue irritation.

## Further Reading

Giannoudis PV, Atkins R. Management of long bone nonunions. Injury. 2007;38 Suppl 2:S1–2.

De Vries JS, Kloen P, Borens O, et al. Treatment of subtrochanteric nonunions. Injury. 2006;37(2):203–11.

Barquet A, Mayora G, Fregeiro J, et al. The treatment of subtrochanteric nonunions with the long gamma nail: twenty-six patients with a minimum 2-year follow-up. J Orthop Trauma. 2004;18(6):346–53.

# Femoral Shaft Non-unions: Exchange Nailing

# 16

Peter V. Giannoudis and Fragkiskos N. Xypnitos

## Indications

- Femoral shaft non-union following prior intramedullary nailing.
- Exchange nailing has been shown to be successful for the treatment of both atrophic and hypertrophic non-unions.

## Preoperative Planning

### Clinical Assessment

- Pain and disability.
- Occasionally a patient with a femoral shaft non-union will present without symptoms.
- Assess:
  - Patient's age.
  - Health status.
  - Activity level.
  - Osseous contact.
  - Deformity.
  - Infection.
  - Type of non-union.
  - The presence or absence of neuropathy.
  - The diameter of the nail in situ.

### Radiological Assessment

- Anteroposterior (AP) and lateral views (Fig. 16.1a, b) of the femoral shaft including the adjacent joints.
- Cable technique can be used to evaluate axial alignment, while for rotational alignment; lesser trochanter shape sign, cortical step sign, and diameter difference sign can be applied.
- In elusive cases perform a high resolution CT of the non-union site.

### Laboratory Tests

- Routine labs (FBC and biochemistry).
- In suspected infection, evaluate the ESR, CRP.

## Operative Treatment

### Anesthesia

- General or regional (spinal, epidural) anesthesia.
- Administration of prophylactic antibiotics is held before the acquisition of intra-operative cultures.

P.V. Giannoudis (✉)
Academic Department of Trauma and Orthopaedic Surgery,
School of Medicine, University of Leeds,
Leeds, UK
e-mail: pgiannoudi@aol.com

F.N. Xypnitos
Department of Trauma and Orthopaedics Surgery,
Leeds Teaching Hospitals NHS Trust,
Leeds, UK

P.V. Giannoudis (ed.), *Practical Procedures in Elective Orthopaedic Surgery*,
DOI 10.1007/978-0-85729-814-0_16, © Springer-Verlag London Limited 2012

**Fig. 16.1** Preoperative
radiographs demonstrating
femoral shaft nonunion.
(**a**) AP and (**b**) lateral views

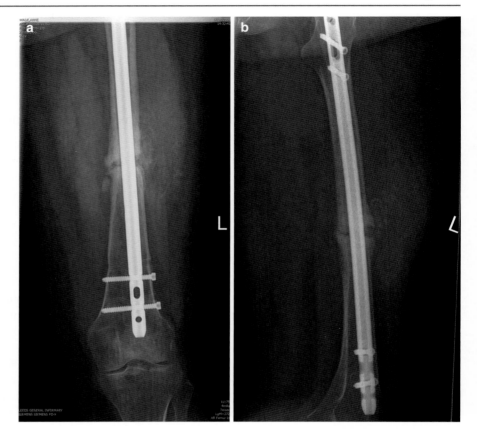

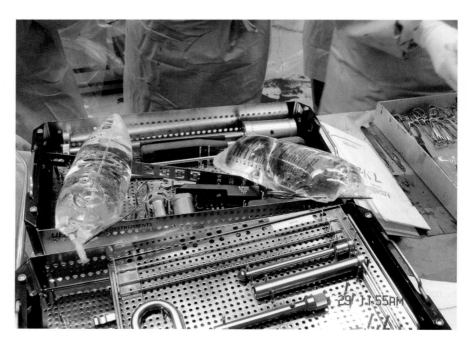

**Fig. 16.2** Nail instrumentation
set

## Table and Equipment

- Nail instrumentation set including a complete set of implants (Fig. 16.2).
- Standard radiolucent operating table.
- Image intensifier.

## Table Set Up

- The instrumentation is set up at the site of the operation.
- Image intensifier is from the contralateral site.

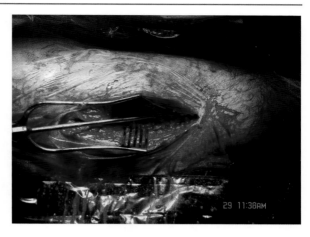

**Fig. 16.3** Utilization of previous skin incision

## Patient Positioning

- Supine position:
  - Allows the best control of the alignment. An adequate approach to the piriformis fossa and medullary canal is facilitated by adduction, flexion, and internal rotation of the hip joint.
  - The contralateral leg is positioned on a gyneco- logical leg holder with the hip and knee joint flexed, in order to facilitate easy access of the image intensifier in a lateral direction. Alter- natively, the contralateral leg can be positioned on the operating table, in order to provide intra- operative comparison of leg length, rotation, and alignment.
- Lateral position:
  - Provides comfortable access to the piriformis fossa, but control of alignment is more difficult.
- The tip of the greater trochanter must be visible in two directions under the image intensifier.

## Draping and Surgical Approach

- Prepare the skin from the gluteal area down to the foot using antiseptic solutions (aqueous/alcoholic povidone-iodine).
- Use previous incision (Fig. 16.3).
- Split the fascia lata longitudinally and divide the fibers of the gluteus maximus muscle.
- In the case that the non-union can be manually reduced, the previously placed nail should be removed, the femoral shaft should be realigned, and an exchange nailing should then be performed.

## Implant Removal

- Under image intensifier's control, the interlocking screws and existing nail should be removed.
- Obtain multiple intraoperative cultures from the retrieved nail and reaming (Fig. 16.4a, b).
- Meticulous wash of the intramedullary canal (Fig. 16.5).

## Implant Selection

- The exchange nail should be at least 1 mm larger in diameter (ideally 2–4 mm).
- In unstable patterns, we can improve mechanical stability by increasing the length of the nail, and the number of interlocking screws.
- In stable patterns with good cortical contact, unlocked or dynamically locked nails allow gradual compres- sion at the non-union site during weight-bearing.
- Statically locked exchange nail with slotted inter- locking holes can be used for gradual axial com- pression at the non-union site.
- Some recently developed nails allow the surgeon to apply compression acutely across the site of injury.

## Implant Positioning

- Use the previous entry point.
- In case of previous entry point malposition, identify the interval between the trochanter major and the piriformis fossa.

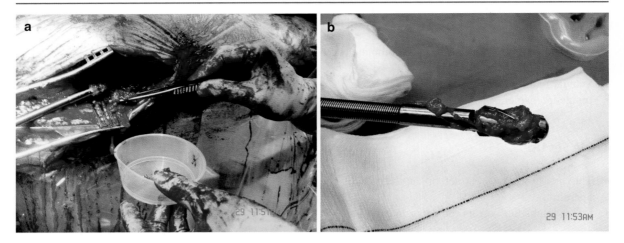

**Fig. 16.4** Intra-operative cultures from (**a**) reaming, (**b**) tip of reamer

**Fig. 16.5** Intramedullary
washing after nail removal

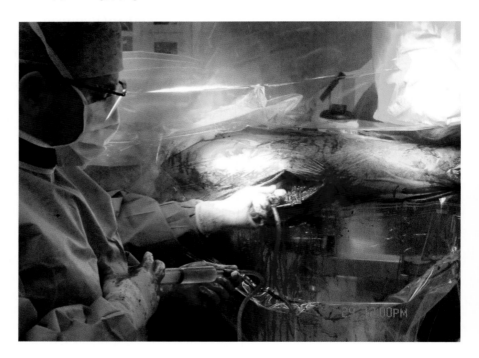

- The entry point:
  - For reamed femoral nails is slightly more lateral at the anterior aspect of the greater trochanter.
  - In nails with greater curvature has to be more posterior.
  - In nails with a proximal angulation can be the tip of the greater trochanter.
- The entry point can be opened with a 3.5 mm guide pin. Drive the pin into the center or the medullary canal.
- Insert a second pin using the initial wire as a reference if the position of the guide wire is not perfect.
- In case of a cannulated nail, insert a long central guide wire and drive it through the non-union into the distal fragment at the center of the intercondylar notch.
- The guide wire is not extracted during the change of the reamer heads.
- The intramedullary canal should be over-reamed to at least 1 mm larger than the diameter of the new nail, with the intention to reach the maximal canal

**Fig. 16.6** Nail-insertion handle assembly. Nail introduction

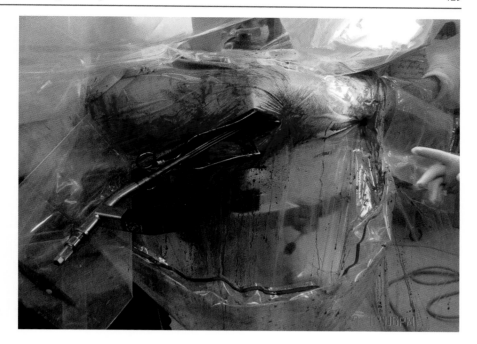

diameter possible while using fluoroscopy to avoid cortical breaching.

- The optimal length of the nail can be determined intra-operatively under image intensifier control by a central guide wire, a metal ruler or a nail.
- The implant is assembled with the insertion handle and the connection screw (Fig. 16.6).
- Insert the nail manually into the medullary canal by twisting movements or with slight blows of a hammer.
- Solid nails are introduced without a central guide wire. Use the proximal part of the nail as a "joy-stick" to manipulate the proximal fragment in order to introduce the nail.
- Drive the nail through the non-union (Fig. 16.7a), and place the tip of the nail directly into the center of the intercondylar notch (Fig. 16.7b).
- Control alignment rotation and bone length.
- By the insertion of the nail, distraction of the non-union site may be produced. Therefore, before proximal interlocking, reverse impaction can be performed after the distal interlocking screws are placed.
- For femoral distal locking screw insertion, use the free hand technique.
- With a measuring gauge, determine the bolt length.
- The locking screws have to pass both cortices.

- Check bone length and rotation before you proceed to lock the nail proximally.
- For insertion of the proximal locking screws use the aiming device and drill the holes for the screws.
- Remove the aiming device. An end cap maybe inserted into the internal thread.
- Exchange nailing is often combined with bone grafting:
  - Open bone-grafting (Fig. 16.8a, b).
  - Intramedullary grafting.
  - Delivery of autogenous iliac crest bone graft to the site of non-union through the medullary canal by means of a chest tube.
- In case of open bone-grafting, debridement of non-union site has to proceed (Fig. 16.9).

## Closure

- Irrigate the wound thoroughly and achieve haemostasis.
- Subfascial drainage is usually not necessary.
- Close fascia lata and the subcutaneous fat with absorbable sutures.
- Skin is closed with stainless steel surgical staples or monofilament nylon sutures in an interrupted manner.

**Fig. 16.7** (**a**) Control of nail's drive through the non-union site with fluoroscopy. (**b**) Control of nail's tip placement at the center of intracondylar notch with fluoroscopy

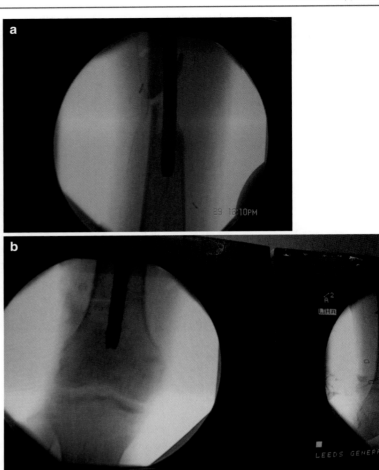

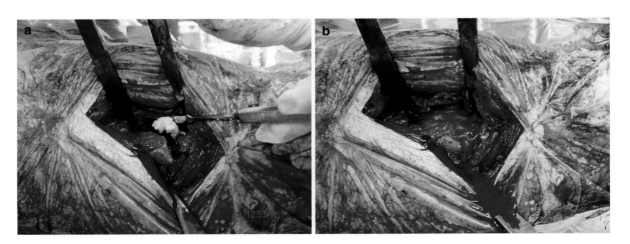

**Fig. 16.8** (**a**, **b**) Bone graft placement

## Pitfalls to Avoid and Tips

- Overream by an amount of 1–2 mm greater than the diameter of the new nail. Use sharp reamers with slow gradual reaming.
- Before proximal interlocking, reverse impaction can be performed after the distal interlocking screws are placed. Avoid excessive shortening.

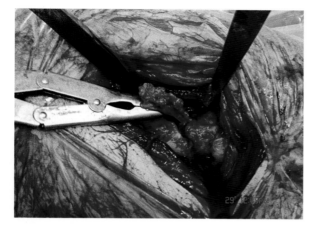

**Fig. 16.9** Non-union site debridement

- Following acute compression, the nail can be locked statically to provide added stability.
- Additional compression across the non-union site can be achieved by using a large femoral distractor in a compression mode.
- In cases where the nails are statically locked, care should be taken to avoid distraction of the non-union site.
- Non-unions, resultants of comminuted fractures do not respond to exchange nailing as favorably as non-unions following simple transverse or oblique fractures.

## Post-operative Rehabilitation

- Two further doses of prophylactic antibiotics. Chase the results of tissue samples taken intraoperatively and act accordingly.
- Routine bloods and radiographs of the femur at 24 h, including AP and lateral views.
- Start mechanical VTE prophylaxis at admission and continue until the patient no longer has significantly reduced mobility, based on an assessment of

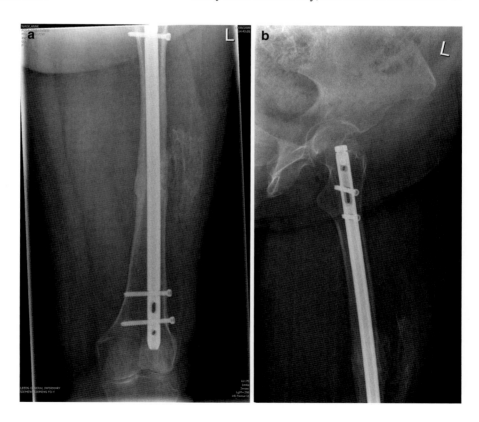

**Fig. 16.10** Radiographic assessment at 6 months postoperatively. (**a**) AP, (**b**) lateral

risks. Start pharmacological VTE prophylaxis after surgery and continue until the patient no longer has significantly reduced mobility.

- Postoperatively, watch for DTV, PE, and infection.
- Postoperatively, patients are encouraged to weight bear as tolerated.
- Physiotherapy on the first postoperative day with free active and passive range of motion exercises.
- To prevent postoperative soft tissue contraction or in case of soft tissue contraction, the patient is positioned in the bed with 90° flexed hip and knee joint for the first 3 days.

## Outpatients Follow Up

- Review at 3 weeks, 6 weeks, 3 months, 6 months and 12 months with both clinical and radiographic assessment (Fig. 16.10a, b) of the nonunion.
- Further radiological evaluation is performed only in patients that report continuing symptoms or in patients where there is no radiological sign of

healing. In such cases, a CT scan evaluation should take place.

- Discharge from follow up after clinical and radiological evidence of a healed non-union.
- Review again at the request of the GP.

## Implant Removal

- No removal is indicated unless there is good evidence of soft tissue irritation, and usually not before 1.5 years after implantation.

## Further Reading

Brinker MR, O'Connor DP. Exchange nailing of ununited fractures. J Bone Joint Surg Am. 2007;89:177–88.
Shroeder JE, Mosheiff R, Khoury A, Liebergall M, Weil YA. The outcome of closed, intramedullary exchange nailing with reamed insertion in the treatment of femoral shaft nonunions. J Orthop Trauma. 2009;23(9):653–7.
Wu CC. Exchange nailing for aseptic nonunion of femoral shaft: a retrospective cohort study for effect of reaming size. J Trauma. 2007;63:859–65.

# Distal Femoral Non-union

# 17

Peter V. Giannoudis and Nikolaos K. Kanakaris

## Indications

- Previous stabilized distal femoral fracture that failed to progress to union.
- Early implant failure.
- Non-union associated with pain and impaired knee function.

## Preoperative Planning

### Clinical Assessment

- Obtain detailed previous history of fracture fixation and any associated comorbidities.
- Document smoking habits and intake of pain killers.
- Evaluate mechanical axis, the presence of rotational deformity, and leg length discrepancy.
- Document the range of motion of the affected knee.
- Assess neurovascular status of the limb.
- Request blood investigations (FRC, CRP, and ESR) to exclude low-grade infection.

P.V. Giannoudis (✉)
Academic Department of Trauma and Orthopaedic Surgery,
School of Medicine, University of Leeds,
Leeds, UK
e-mail: pgiannoudi@aol.com

N.K. Kanakaris
Department of Trauma and Orthopaedic Surgery,
Leeds Teaching Hospitals NHS Trust,
Leeds, UK

## Radiological Assessment

- Anteroposterior (AP) and lateral views of the femur and knee (Fig. 17.1a, b).
- CT scan will provide useful information of the non-union site (type of non-union) and the presence of sequestrum in case of infected non-union (Fig. 17.1c).

## Operative Treatment

### Anesthesia

- General or regional (spinal or epidural) anesthesia.
- Administration of prophylactic antibiotics is refrained until acquisition of intraoperative tissue cultures.

### Table and Equipment

- Availability of extraction kit for removal of the implant (locking plate-LISS) previously inserted.
- Blade plate (condylar plate) instrumentation set – ensure the availability of the complete set of implants (Fig. 17.2a, b).
- Osteotomes.
- Standard radiolucent operating table (OSI).
- Image intensifier.

### Table Setup

- The instrumentation is set up at the site of the operation.
- Image intensifier is from the contralateral side.

**Fig. 17.1** (**a**) Antero-posterior (AP) and (**b**) lateral views of right distal femur illustrating non-union. (**c**) CT scan (coronal view) revealing distal femoral non-union

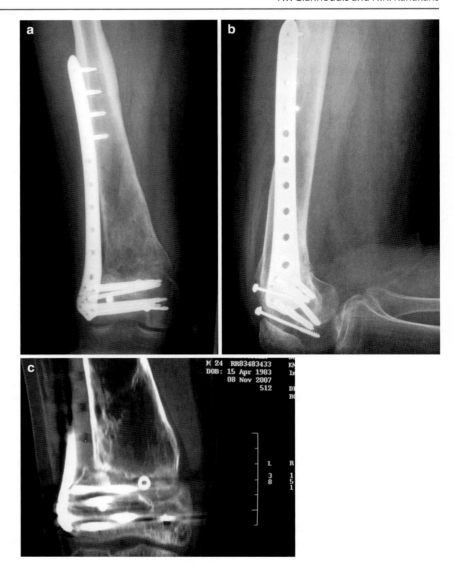

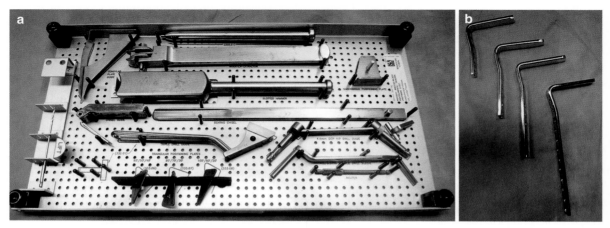

**Fig. 17.2** (**a**) Blade plate (condylar plate) instrumentation set is shown. (**b**) Ensure availability of the complete set of implants

**Fig. 17.3** Patient is supine on a radiolucent table. Image intensifier is positioned on the contralateral side

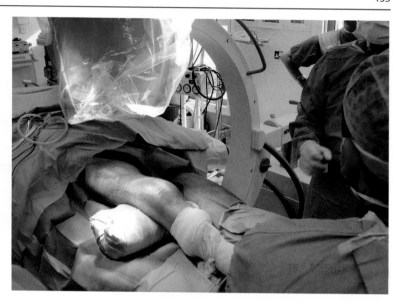

- Position the table diagonally across the operating room so that the operating area lies in the clean air field.

## Patient Positioning

- Supine position.
- Put towels under the distal part of the femur to bring the knee in slight flexion. Gastrocnemius which tends to bring the distal femur in recurvatum is relaxed, and the distal main fragment is supported (Fig. 17.3).

## Draping and Surgical Approach

- Prepare the skin around the knee joint extending to proximal femur with the usual antiseptic solutions (aqueous/alcoholic povidone-iodine).
- Apply transparent, plastic, adherent "isolation" drape directly over the proposed incision site.

## Removal of Implant (LISS Plate)

- Utilize previous incision made through the skin and subcutaneous fat exposing the fascia lata layer (Fig. 17.4a).

- Incise fascia lata layer longitudinally and expose the vastus lateralis fascia (Fig. 17.4b).
- Reveal the vastus lateralis using the index finger as a guide to the lateral aspect of the femoral shaft (using the cutting diathermy), cut down right on the plate moving in the line of the femur from the lateral supracondylar area proximally towards the subtrochanteric area (Fig. 17.5).
- Following adequate exposure, remove the screws and the LISS plate.
- Using the image intensifier, mark the margins of the non-union.
- Debride the scar tissue from the non-union site using osteotomes and bone nibblers.
- Send tissues to microbiology for culture and sensitivities.
- Make sure the bed of the non-union is vascular following the debridement.

## Condylar Plate 95° Insertion

- Using the preoperative radiographs, template for the length of the condylar blade as well as the length of the plate (number of holes) to be used.
- Condylar guide with an angle of 95° is used as a guide and is brought up to and along the lateral supracondylar cortex of the femur.

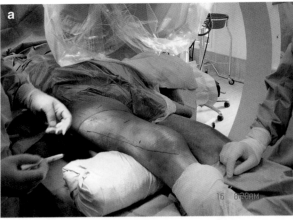
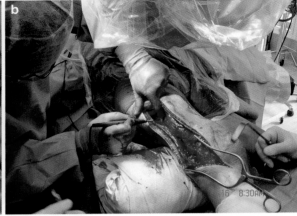

**Fig. 17.4** (**a**) Previous incision is utilized (dissect skin and subcutaneous fat exposing the fascia lata layer). (**b**) Fascia lata layer is incised longitudinally exposing the vastus lateralis fascia

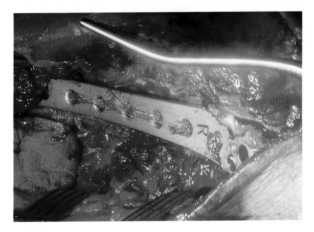

**Fig. 17.5** Fascia of vastus lateralis is incised exposing the plate

- A Kirschner wire is inserted parallel into the knee joint and another one over the femoral condyles.
- The position of the guide wire is checked under II control and is used for the insertion of the seating chisel.
- Make sure that the point of entry must be in the anterior part of the lateral femoral condyle.
- The entry for the seating chisel is predrilled with a 4.5-mm drill bit enlarged with a router.
- The position of the seating chisel is checked with image intensifier.
- This allows checking whether the length that was chosen preoperatively is still valid.
- The chosen plate is inserted into the plate holder and the blade is pushed by hand into the precut channel and with light hammer blows is advanced in the bone.

- Seat the plate with the impactor when the plate is about 5 mm from the bone having first removed the plate holder.
- The plate must come to lie in line with the femoral shaft and be held with a hey groves reduction forceps.
- Using the 3.2-mm drill sleeve in the holes of the plate will allow guiding the 3.2-mm drill bit through the two cortices.
- Having determined the screw length, insert the corresponding self-tapping cortex screws.
- The plate is fixed securely now on the bone (Fig. 17.6a).
- Implant the appropriate previous chosen bone graft in the non-union site for biological stimulation (this can be autologous iliac crest bone graft, BMP-7, or cancellous bone chips from the local hospital bone bank) (Fig. 17.6b).
- Take intraoperative fluoroscopic images of the fixation.

## Closure

- Irrigate the wound thoroughly and achieve hemostasis.
- Close vastus lateralis fascia and fascia lata (No.1 PDS/Vicryl) and the subcutaneous fat with absorbable sutures (2/0 PDS/Vicryl) (Fig. 17.7a, b).
- Skin closure – stainless steel surgical staples, monofilament non-absorbable suture or absorbable suture placed in the subcuticular layer.

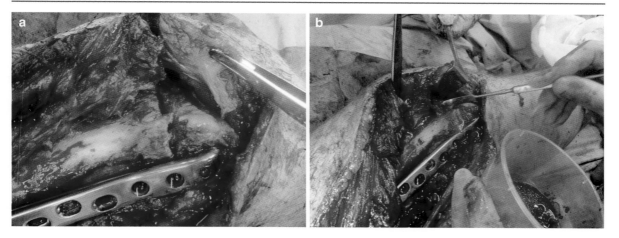

**Fig. 17.6** (**a**) Blade plate is fixed securely on the bone as shown. (**b**) Autologous bone graft is implanted at the non-union site

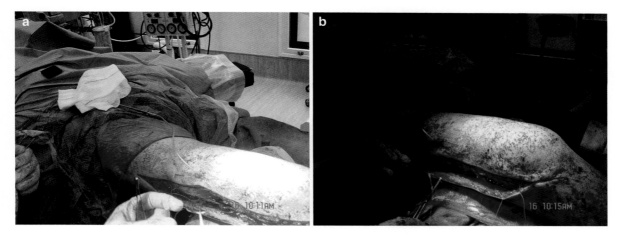

**Fig. 17.7** (**a**) Fascia lata layer is shown to be sutured with (1/0 Vicryl) suture. (**b**) Fat layer is shown to be sutured with absorbable (2/0/Vicryl) suture

## Postoperative Rehabilitation

- Two further doses of prophylactic antibiotics.
- Longer duration of antibiotics if the intraoperative samples taken are found to be positive for infection (minimum duration of treatment is 6–8 weeks).
- Routine bloods and radiographs of the knee (distal femur) (Fig. 17.8a, b) in 24 h.
- Start mechanical VTE prophylaxis at admission and continue until the patient no longer has significantly reduced mobility, based on an assessment of risks. Start pharmacological VTE prophylaxis after surgery and continue until the patient no longer has significantly reduced mobility.

- Mobilize toe-touch weight bearing at the earliest and tailor physiotherapy to meet individual needs and demands.
- Progress to full weight bearing at approximately 8 weeks following the revision surgery.

## Postoperative Complications

- Watch for compartment syndrome.
- Superficial and deep Infection.
- Failure of metal work.
- Persistent non-union.

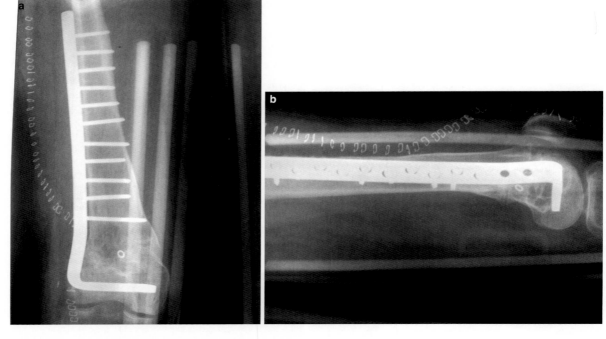

**Fig. 17.8** (**a**) AP and (**b**) lateral postoperative radiographs showing the right distal femoral non-union to have been stabilized with a blade plate

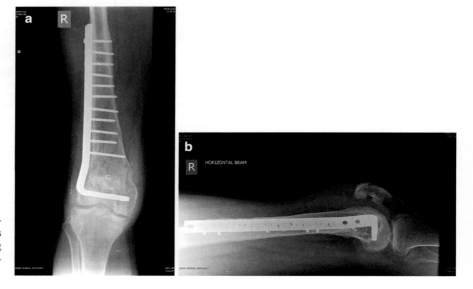

**Fig. 17.9** (**a**) AP and (**b**) lateral postoperative radiographs (6 months follow-up) showing union of the previous right distal femoral non-union

## Outpatient Follow-Up

- Review at 4, 8, and 12 weeks and at 6, 12, and 24 months with radiographs of the hip.
- Discharge from the follow-up after clinical and radiological evidence of fracture healing (Fig. 17.9a, b).

## Implant Removal

- No removal is indicated unless there is good evidence of soft tissue irritation.

## Further Reading

Kanakaris NK, Lasanianos N, Calori GM, Verdonk R, Blokhuis TJ, Cherubino P, et al. Application of bone morphogenetic proteins to femoral non-unions: a 4-year multicentre experience. Injury. 2009;40 Suppl 3:S54–61.

Schandelmaier P, Partenheimer A, Koenemann B, Grün OA, Krettek C. Distal femoral fractures and LISS stabilization. Injury. 2001;32 Suppl 3:SC55–63.

Calori GM, Tagliabue L, Gala L, D'Imporzano M, Peretti G, Albisetti W. Application of rhBMP-7 and platelet-rich plasma in the treatment of long bone non-unions: a prospective randomised clinical study on 120 patients. Injury. 2008;39(12):1391–402.

Giannoudis PV. Fracture healing and bone regeneration: autologous bone grafting or BMPs? Injury. 2009;40(12): 1243–4.

# Knee Arthroscopy

**18**

## Ram Venkatesh

## Indications

- Diagnosis and treatment of meniscus (Fig. 18.1a) and articular cartilage (Fig. 18.1b) problems
- Removal of loose bodies (Fig. 18.1c)
- Washout of septic arthritis
- Synovial biopsy
- Ligament reconstruction (Fig. 18.1d)

## Diagnosis and Investigations

- Diagnosis usually clinical
- Investigations
  - Radiographs
  - MRI

## Preoperative

- Consent and place mark on limb to be operated (Fig. 18.2)
- Safe surgery check list

## Anesthesia

- General or regional anesthesia

R. Venkatesh
Department of Trauma and Orthopaedic Surgery,
Leeds Teaching Hospitals NHS Trust, Leeds, UK
e-mail: ram.venkatesh@leedsth.nhs.uk

## Examination Under Anesthesia

- Important step prior to every arthroscopy
- Exam both knees
- Assess range of movement
- Ligament stability – collateral ligaments, Lachman test (Fig. 18.3a, b), Anterior drawer test (Fig. 18.4), and Pivot shift (Fig. 18.5a, b).
- Patella tracking

## Setup

- Patient supine
- Leg holder or side support to help control joint position (Fig. 18.6a)
- Bottom end of table removed if using leg holder
- Soft support underneath opposite thigh to flex the hip (Fig. 18.6b)
- Tourniquet applied high up in the thigh
- Surgeon on the opposite side of the arthroscopy cart (Fig. 18.7)

## Portals

- *Standard portals* (Fig. 18.8)
  - Anterolateral (vertical incision <1 cm made close to the patellar tendon at the soft spot above the Gerdy's tubercle) (Fig. 18.9).
  - Anteromedial (horizontal incision made arthroscopy guided after initial marking with a needle as a reference) (Fig. 18.10).

**Fig. 18.1** (**a**) Probing medial meniscus and demonstrating posterior horn tear (*arrows*) (picture obtained with permission from www. kneejointsurgery.com). (**b**) Femoral condyle's articular cartilage lesion (*arrow*) (picture obtained with permission from kneejointsurgery.com). (**c**) Loose body intra-articularly (*arrow*) (picture obtained with permission from kneejointsurgery.com). (**d**) ACL graft (hamstrings) in place (*arrow*) (picture obtained with permission from www.kneejointsurgery. com)

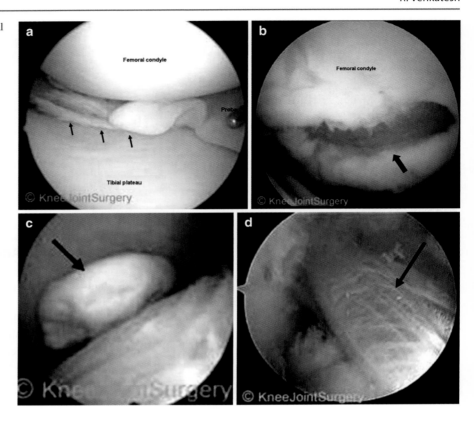

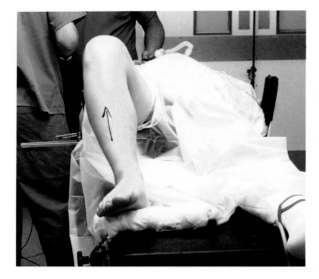

**Fig. 18.2** Mark on the limb to be operated

- *Accessory portals*
  - Superolateral portal as drainage portal.
  - Lateral portal to remove loose body from gutter.

- Posteromedial portal to visualize back of knee.
- Accessory anterior portal for bucket handle tears menisci.

## Diagnostic Arthroscopy

### Sequence of Examination of Joint

- Insert the sheath from the anterolateral portal (Fig. 18.11a–c).
- Introduce the camera in anterolateral portal.
- Visualize patellofemoral joint and then into medial compartment.
- Make anteromedial portal.
- Go back into patellofemoral joint and probe via anteromedial portal.
- Examine suprapatellar pouch and lateral and medial gutters.
- Examine medial compartment – meniscus and cartilage (Fig. 18.12).
- Then examine notch and transfer scope in to the lateral compartment.

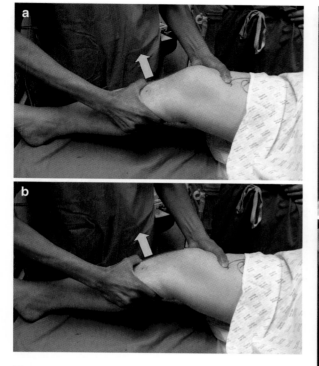

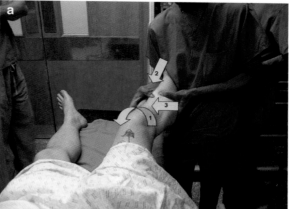

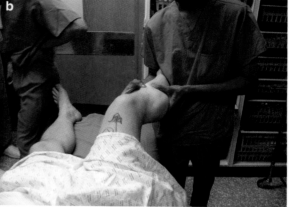

**Fig. 18.3** Lachman test. (**a**) Patient supine with knee at approximately 20° of flexion. Secure and stabilize with one hand the distal femur. Grasp proximal tibia with the other hand and apply anterior translation force (*arrow*). (**b**) Evaluate anterior translation of tibia [compare the modification in curvature depicted with the red line between (**a** and **b**)] and assess the end point (firm or soft)

**Fig. 18.5** Pivot shift. (**a**) Patient supine. Abduct hip to relax iliotibial band. Knee in full extension. Grasp leg with both hands and tuck patient's ankle under your arm. Apply internal rotation (*arrow 1*) with axial load (*arrow 2*) and valgus stress (*arrow 3*). (**b**) Flex the knee while maintaining these forces. The tibia will be anterolaterally subluxed on the distal femur and a clunk will be felt at 30° of knee flexion

- Assess ACL and PCL.
- Examine lateral compartment – meniscus and cartilage.

### Wound Closure

- Steristrips (Fig. 18.13) or simple suture
- Bulky bandage

### Local Anesthetic

- Infiltration to joint and/or around portals

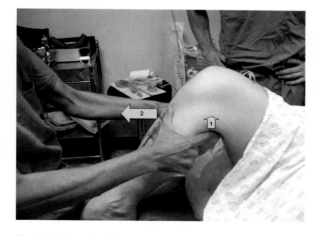

**Fig. 18.4** Anterior drawer test. Patient supine with hip at 45° of flexion and knee at 90° of flexion. Grasp tibia just below the joint line. Place the thumbs along the joint line and with the index fingers palpate hamstring tendons to ensure that they are relaxed (*arrow 1*). Apply anterior force to the tibia (*arrow 2*) and evaluate translation and end point

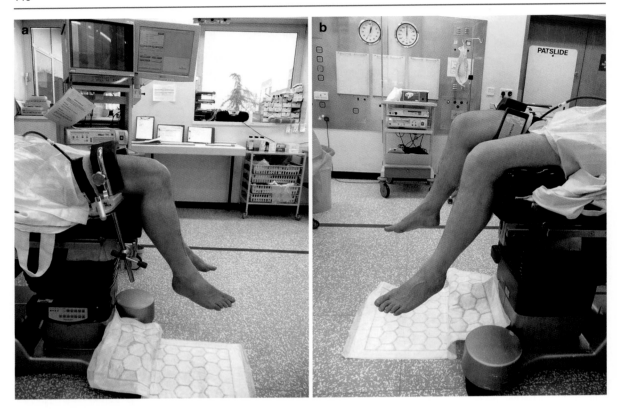

**Fig. 18.6** (**a**) Set up using a leg holder. (**b**) Flexion of the opposite thigh

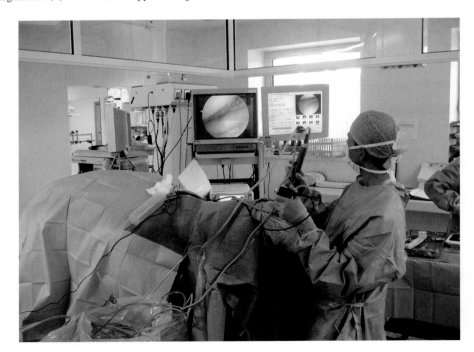

**Fig. 18.7** Patient – surgeon – equipment in the operating theater

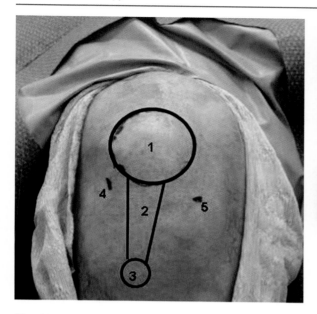

Fig. 18.8 Standard portals. (1) Patella, (2) patellar tendon, (3) tibial tubercle, (4) anterolateral portal, and (5) anteromedial portal

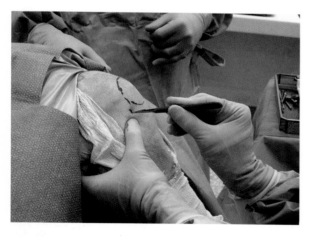

Fig. 18.9 A vertical incision is utilized for the anterolateral portal, close to the patellar tendon at the soft spot above the Gerdy's tubercle

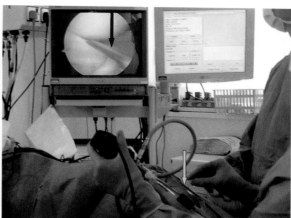

Fig. 18.10 Using a needle as a reference to make the anteromedial portal: The image of the needle at the monitor (*blue arrow*). The image of the needle penetrating the skin (*yellow arrow*).

risks. Start pharmacological VTE prophylaxis after surgery and continue until the patient no longer has significantly reduced mobility.

- Mobilize weight bearing as comfort allows.
- Remove bulky bandage at 24–48 h.
- Simple adhesive dressing.
- Increase range of movements.
- Physiotherapy.

## Complications

- Residual pain
- Stiffness
- Swelling
- Bleeding
- Painful portals
- Infection – rare (<0.1%)
- Thrombosis – <0.1%
- Nerve injury – 0.01%
- Complex regional pain syndrome

## Postoperative

- Start mechanical VTE prophylaxis at admission and continue until the patient no longer has significantly reduced mobility, based on an assessment of

**Fig. 18.11** (**a**) Insertion of the sheath, (**b**) sheath in place, and (**c**) sheath armed with a blunt obturator

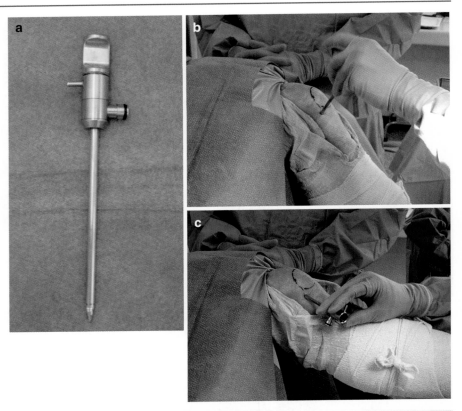

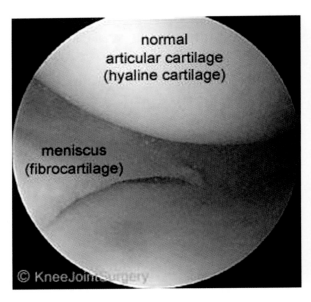

**Fig. 18.12** Normal meniscus and articular cartilage in the medial compartment of a knee (picture obtained with permission from www.kneejointsurgery.com)

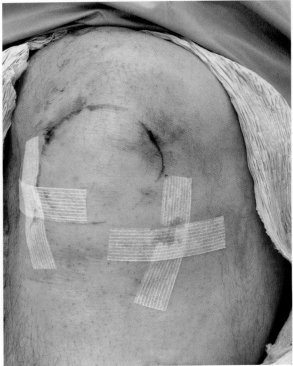

**Fig. 18.13** Wound closure with Steristrips

## Further Reading

Siparsky PN, Kocher MS. Current concepts in pediatric and adolescent arthroscopy. Arthroscopy. 2009;25(12):1453–69.

Levy BA, Dajani KA, Whelan DB, et al. Decision making in the
multiligament-injured knee: an evidence-based systematic
review. Arthroscopy. 2009;25(4):430–8.

Smith TO, Hing CB. A meta-analysis of tourniquet assisted
arthroscopic knee surgery. Knee. 2009;16(5):317–21, Epub
2009 Feb 23.

Rosenberg TD, Metcalf RW, Gurley WD. Arthroscopic meniscectomy. Instr Course Lect. 1988;37:203–8.

# Knee Arthroscopic Partial Meniscectomy

**19**

Ram Venkatesh

## Indication

- Diagnosis and treatment of meniscus tears

## Diagnosis and Investigations

- The diagnosis is mostly clinical. The diagnostic composite mentioned below would have a sensitivity to identify a meniscus tear with a positive predictive value of >90% if all five factors are present.
- *Diagnostic Composite*
  1. A history of "catching" or "locking" as reported by the patient
  2. Pain with forced hyperextension
  3. Pain with maximum flexion
  4. Pain or an audible click with McMurray's test
  5. Joint line tenderness to palpation
- Radiographs to rule out degenerative arthritis
- MRI useful if clinical diagnosis inconclusive (Fig. 19.1)

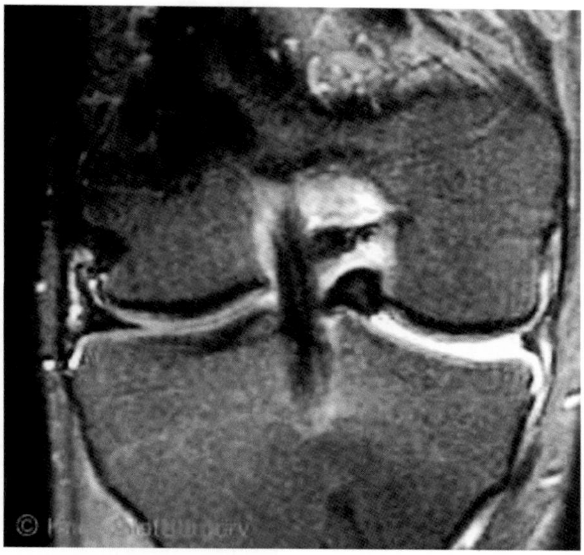

**Fig. 19.1** A bucket handle tear of the medial meniscus with the fragment displaced into the notch

## Preoperative

- Consent and place mark on limb to be operated
- Safe surgery check list

## Anesthesia

- General or regional anesthesia

## Examination Under Anesthesia

- Exam both knees
- Assess range of movement, especially full extension
- Ligament stability – collateral ligaments, Lachman test, Pivot shift

R. Venkatesh
Department of Trauma and Orthopaedic Surgery,
Leeds Teaching Hospitals NHS Trust, Leeds, UK
e-mail: ram.venkatesh@leedsth.nhs.uk

P.V. Giannoudis (ed.), *Practical Procedures in Elective Orthopaedic Surgery*,
DOI 10.1007/978-0-85729-814-0_19, © Springer-Verlag London Limited 2012

**Fig. 19.2** (**a**) Probing meniscus and (**b**) demonstrating posterior horn tear of medial meniscus

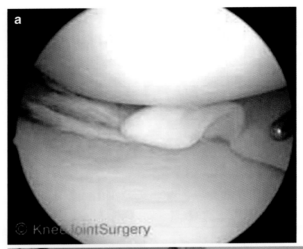

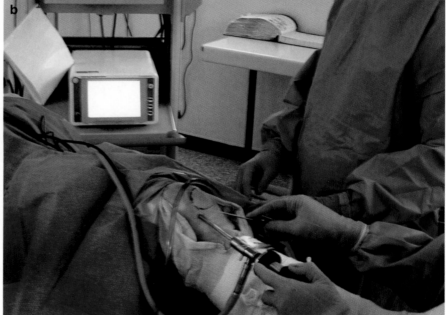

## Setup

- Patient supine
- Leg holder or side support to help control joint position
- Bottom end of table removed if using leg holder
- Soft support underneath opposite thigh to flex the hip
- Tourniquet applied high up in the thigh

## Portals

- Anterolateral and anteromedial.
- Accessory portals seldom required.
- Some surgeons use additional anterior portal to grasp bucket handle meniscal fragment.

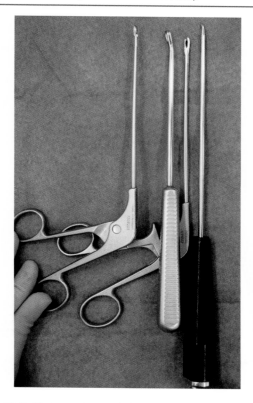

**Fig. 19.3** Various arthroscopic instruments

## Arthroscopic Technique

- Routine sequential examination of knee.
- Probe meniscus carefully (Fig. 19.2a, b).
- Get adequate visualization of posterior third of menisci.
- Adjust knee flexion angle and valgus/varus force to facilitate visualization.
- Use arthroscopic punches to perform meniscectomy (Fig. 19.3).
- Additional use of shavers to fashion meniscal edges if needed.
- Avoid sharp change in contours.

## Bucket Handle Tears

- Reduce meniscus fragment.
- Check if suitable for meniscus repair. The indications for meniscal repair are:
  1. Traumatic tear.
  2. Longitudinal unstable tear.

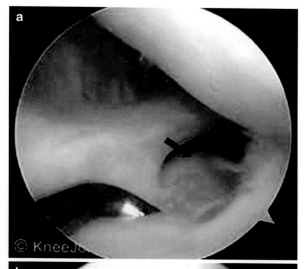

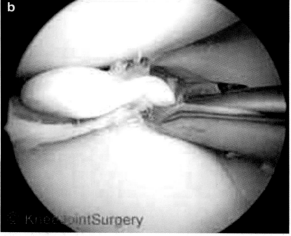

**Fig. 19.4** (**a**) Bucket handle meniscal tear not suitable for repair (*arrow*). (**b**) Use of an arthroscopic punch to perform partial menisectomy

  3. Tear in the peripheral third or vascular zone.
  4. The knee should be stable or else simultaneous ligament reconstruction should be performed.
- If repair is not indicated (Fig. 19.4a) then proceed to meniscectomy. The steps are as follows:
- Resect most of posterior attachment (Fig. 19.4b).
- Swap portals for camera (Fig. 19.5a, b).
- Resect anterior attachment fully (Fig. 19.6a, b).
- Grasp meniscus fragment, twist and remove (Fig. 19.6c, d).

**Fig. 19.5** (**a**, **b**) Swap
portals for camera in case of
a bucket handle meniscal tear

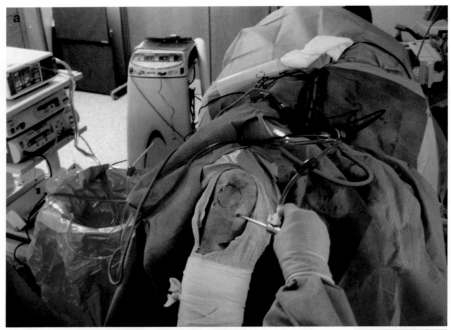

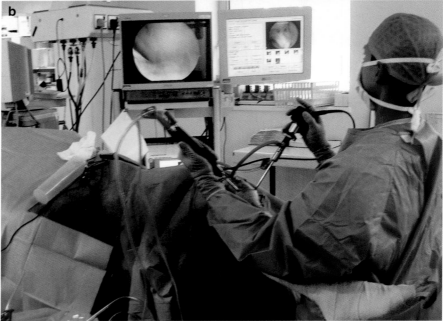

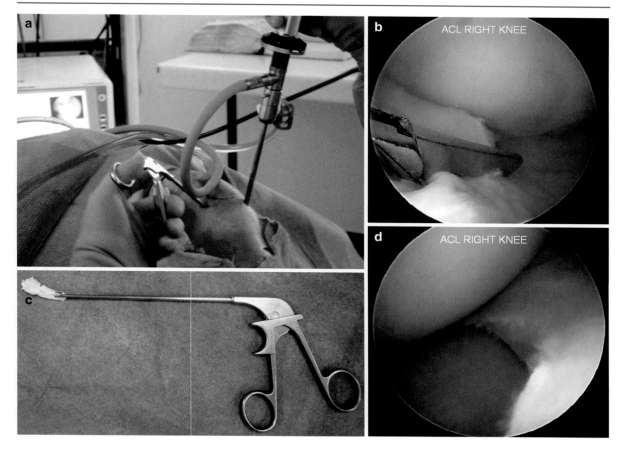

**Fig. 19.6** (**a**) Resect medial meniscus anterior attachment fully, (**b**) arthroscopic image of resection. (**c**) Meniscus fragment on the grasping forceps and (**d**) final result after meniscectomy

## Posterior Horn Tear Medial Meniscus

- Anteromedial portal has to be adequately low and closer to patellar tendon.
- Valgus force with knee in more extension.
- Avoid hip internal rotation.
- Knee flexion angle is more important than valgus force.
- Use low profile punches if needed.

## Wound Closure

- Steristrips or simple suture
- Bulky bandage

## Local Anesthetic

- Infiltration to joint and/or around portals

## Postoperative

- Start mechanical VTE prophylaxis at admission and continue until the patient no longer has significantly reduced mobility, based on an assessment of risks. Start pharmacological VTE prophylaxis after surgery and continue until the patient no longer has significantly reduced mobility.
- Mobilize fully weight bearing as comfort allows.
- Remove bulky bandage at 24–48 h.
- Simple adhesive dressing.

- Increase range of movements.
- Physiotherapy and resistance exercises.
- Return to sports training at 4–6 weeks.

## Complications

- Same as for routine knee diagnostic arthroscopy.
- Residual pain if there is additional chondral damage.
- Nerve injury risk is slightly higher for meniscus repair.
- Meniscectomy gives risk of secondary osteoarthritis.

## Further Reading

Fabricant PD, Jokl P. Surgical outcomes after arthroscopic partial meniscectomy. J Am Acad Orthop Surg. 2007;15(11): 647–53.

Meredith DS, Losina E, Mahomed NN. Factors predicting functional and radiographic outcomes after arthroscopic partial meniscectomy: a review of the literature. Arthroscopy. 2005; 21(2):211–23.

Bin SI, Kim JM, Shin SJ. Radial tears of the posterior horn of the medial meniscus. Arthroscopy. 2004;20(4):373–8.

# Arthroscopic Anterior Cruciate Ligament (ACL) Reconstruction

# 20

Ram Venkatesh and George Tselentakis

## Indication

- ACL rupture resulting in knee instability.

## Clinical Assessment

- History of pivoting injury.
- Symptoms of giving way.
- Positive Lachman test.
- Positive pivot shift.
- Absence of posterior sag of tibia.
- Assessment of other ligaments and also for meniscus tears.

## Radiological Assessment

### Investigations

- Radiographs
  - Look for Segond fracture (Fig. 20.1)

R. Venkatesh (✉)
Department of Trauma and Orthopaedic Surgery,
Leeds Teaching Hospitals NHS Trust,
Leeds, UK
e-mail: ram.venkatesh@leedsth.nhs.uk

G. Tselentakis
Department of Trauma and Orthopaedics,
East Surrey Hospital,
Surrey, UK

- MRI (Fig. 20.2)
  - It is not always mandatory, but is useful in doubtful cases and in combined injuries with meniscal and cartilage damage.

## Preoperative

- Prehabilitation.
- Treatment planning depends on coexisting meniscal and chondral injuries.

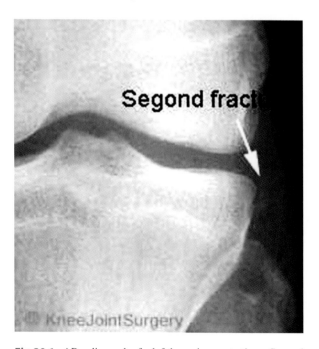

**Fig.20.1** AP radiograph of a left knee demonstrating a Segond fracture

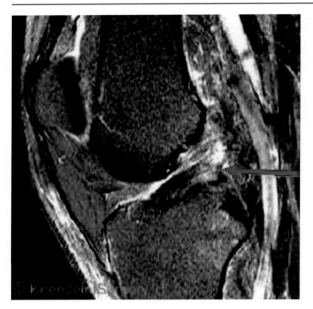

**Fig. 20.2** MRI sagittal scan demonstrating complete rupture of ACL

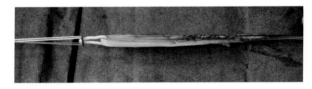

**Fig. 20.3** Autologous hamstring graft for ACL reconstruction

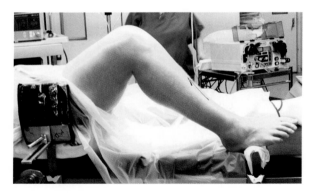

**Fig. 20.4** Leg holder and side support to help control joint position

- Consent and place mark on limb to be operated
- Safe surgery check list

## Anesthesia

- General or regional anesthesia.

## Timing of Surgery

- Minimal or no swelling.
- Minimal warmth.
- Good quadriceps muscle strength.
- Preferably symmetrical extension.

## Graft Choice

- Autologous – hamstring (Fig. 20.3), patellar tendon, and quadriceps tendon.
- Allograft – patellar tendon, hamstring, and achilles tendon.

## Equipment

### Setup

- Patient supine.
- Leg holder or side support to help control joint position (Fig. 20.4).
- Bottom end of table removed if using leg holder.
- Soft support underneath opposite thigh to flex the hip.
- Tourniquet applied high up in the thigh.
- To be able to drill femoral tunnel via low anteromedial portal at least 120° of flexion is necessary.

### Procedure

- Anterolateral portal close to patellar tendon (Fig. 20.5).
- Anteromedial portal preferably low (Fig. 20.5).
- Short vertical or transverse incision over hamstring insertion (usually 1 cm below level of tibial tuberosity) (Figs. 20.5 and 20.6).
- Gracilis and semitendinosus identified and bands divided (Fig. 20.7a–d).
- Use a tendon stripper to harvest hamstrings proximally (Fig. 20.8a–d).

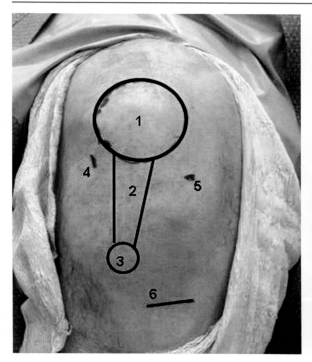

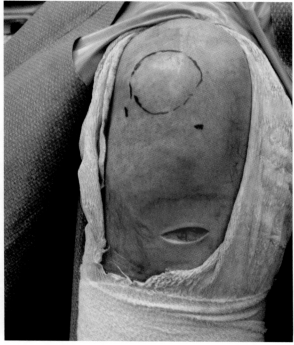

**Fig. 20.5** Standard portals. (1) Patella, (2) patellar tendon, (3) tibial tubercle, (4) anterolateral portal, and (5) anteromedial portal. (6) Incision for hamstring harvesting

**Fig. 20.6** Short horizontal incision over hamstring insertion (usually 1 cm below the level of the tibial tuberosity)

- Next, gracilis and semitendinosus are released from their tibial insertion.
- Grafts need to be prepared. For hamstring graft, the muscle needs to be removed from the tendon (Fig. 20.9). The edges of the tendon are whipstitched (Fig. 20.10a, b), and the tendon is pretensioned (Fig. 20.10c). Finally, the graft size is measured (Fig. 20.10d). For patellar tendon, graft sutures are placed through the bone plugs on either end.
- Appropriate surgery to meniscus tears and articular cartilage damage is performed.
- Remove ruptured ACL (Fig. 20.11) and identify middle of footprint of femoral and tibial attachments.
- Tunnels are made at the center of footprint (Figs 20.12a–e and 20.13a–c) for monobundle ACL reconstruction.
- Tunnel position single most crucial factor for success of ACL reconstruction (Figs. 20.14 and 20.15).
- Grafts passed through the tunnels (Fig. 20.16a–d) and fixed with aperture fixation (Fig. 20.17) using interference screws (Fig. 20.18) or using suspensory fixation.

- Tensioning of graft done at 20° flexion for single bundle ACL reconstruction (Fig. 20.19).

## Wound Closure

- Infiltrate appropriate volume of local anesthetic into graft harvest site (Fig. 20.20) and knee joint for postoperative pain relief.
- Steristrips or simple suture for the portals. Use 2/0 Vicryl for subcutaneous tissues and 3/0 Monocryl for skin (for the graft harvest site) (Fig. 20.21a).
- Bulky bandage (Fig. 20.21b).

## Postoperative

- Start mechanical VTE prophylaxis at admission and continue until the patient no longer has significantly reduced mobility, based on an assessment of risks. Start pharmacological VTE prophylaxis after

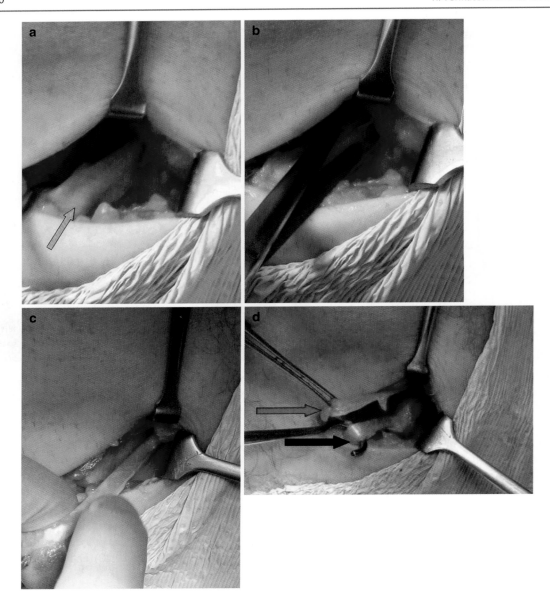

**Fig. 20.7** (**a**) Gracilis and semitendinosus identified and bands divided. (**c**) Identification of gracilis (*arrow*). (**b**) Release of attachments, (**c**) gracilis released and (**d**) gracilis (*red arrow*) and semitendinosus (*black arrow*)

surgery and continue until the patient no longer has significantly reduced mobility.
- Full weight bearing mobilization unless combined with meniscus repair or microfracture.
- Bracing not necessary.
- Early range of motion with an aim to regain early full extension and full flexion.
- Closed chain exercises.
- Staged program to regain motion, strength, and neuromuscular coordination.

- Frequency and rehabilitation program would depend upon individual needs and hospital setup.

## Complications

- Infection
- Stiffness
- Deep vein thrombosis
- Graft failure/re-rupture

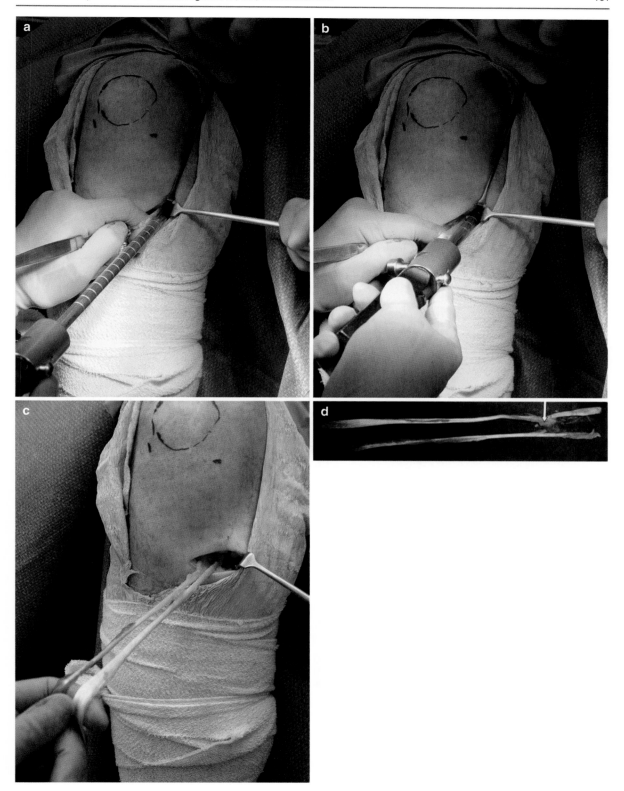

**Fig. 20.8** (**a**) Use a tendon stripper to harvest hamstring proximally. (**b**) Advancement of stripper. (**c**) Tendons released proximally and (**d**) tendons on the tendon board. The arrow shows the attachment of semitendinosus with the medial head of gastrocnemius muscle

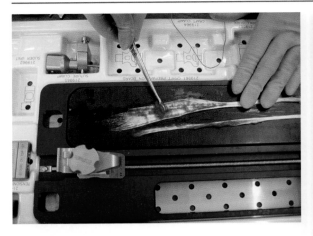

**Fig. 20.9** Removal of muscle from the tendon (hamstring graft)

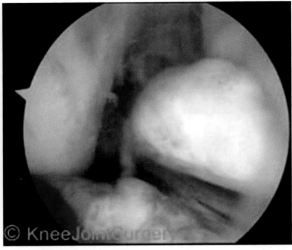

**Fig. 20.11** Remnants of a ruptured ACL

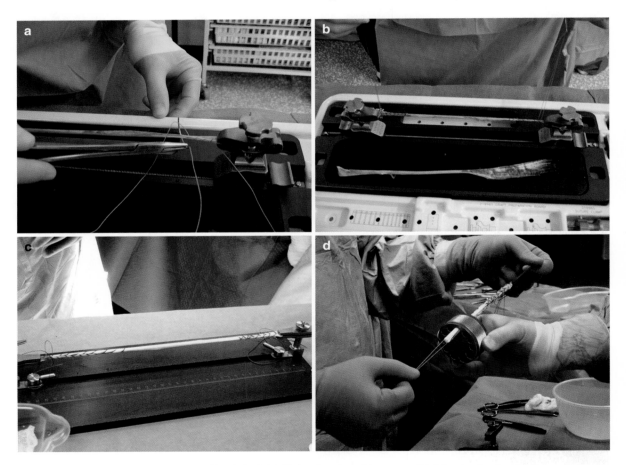

**Fig. 20.10** The edges of the tendon are whipstitched. (**a**) Fixing the edge with sutures. (**b**) After the fixation. (**c**) Pretensioning the graft on the tendon board and (**d**) measuring graft's diameter

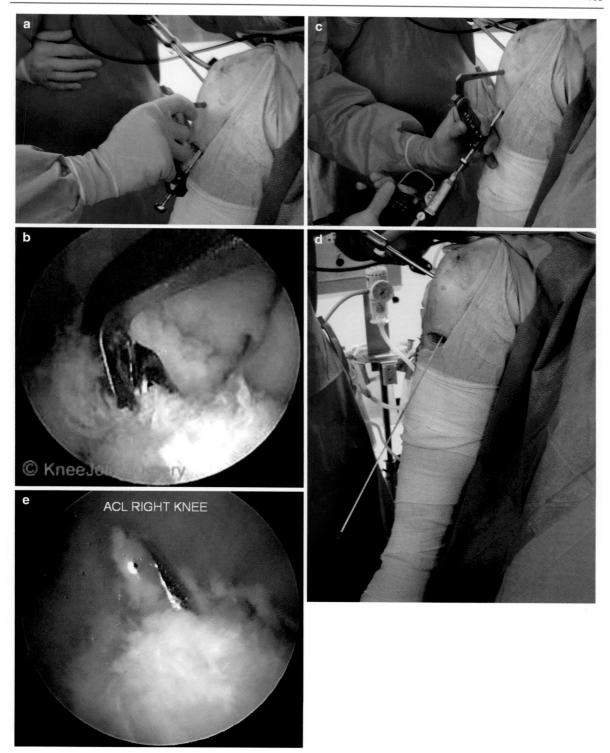

**Fig. 20.12** (**a**) Insertion of tibial drill guide. (**b**) Identify and place the tip of tibial drill guide on the middle of the footprint of tibia. (**c**) Insertion of guide wire, (**d**) guide wire in place, and (**e**) arthroscopic image of the tip of the wire

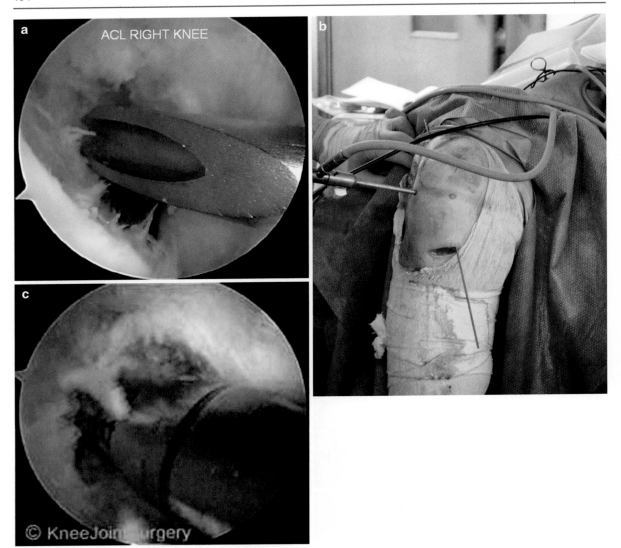

**Fig. 20.13** (**a**) Femoral drill guide at the correct position, (**b**) guide wire in place, and (**c**) drilling and measuring the femoral canal

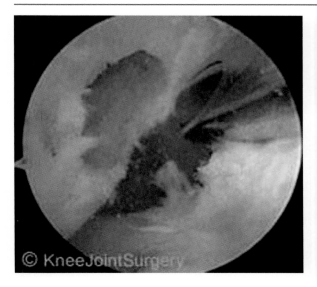

Fig. 20.14 Femoral tunnel is shown on the left at ten o'clock position

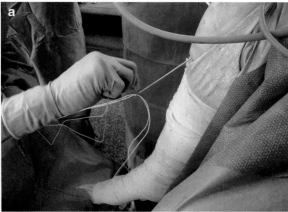

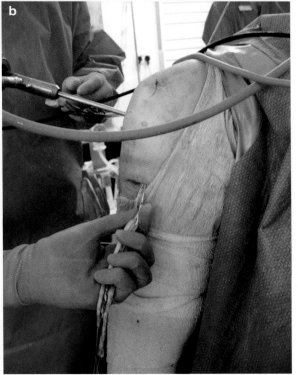

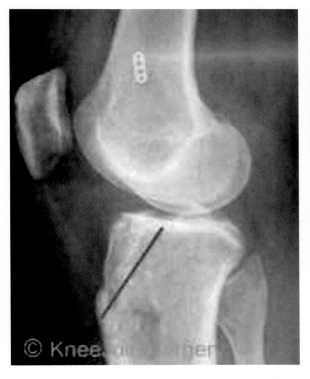

Fig. 20.15 Lateral radiograph showing tunnels with graft just behind Blumensaat's line

Fig. 20.16 Advancement of the graft through the tunnels (a) packing the sutures of the proximal part of the graft through the opening of the guide wire, (b) advancement of the graft, (c) the proximal part of the graft with the fixation button entering the femoral canal, and (d) graft in place

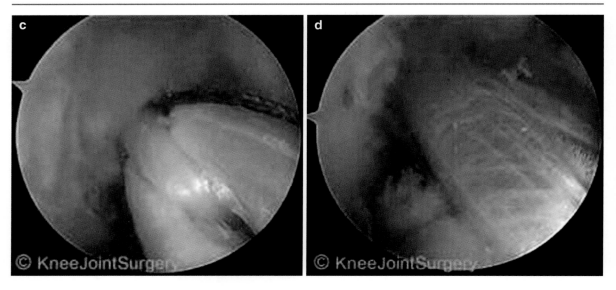

**Fig. 20.16** (continued)

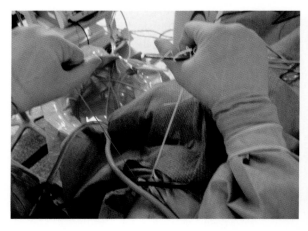

**Fig. 20.17** Flipping the fixation button maneuver

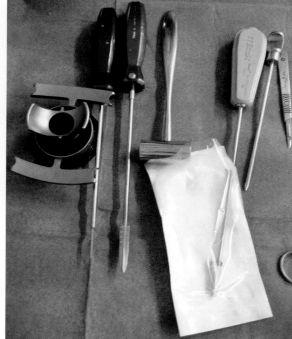

**Fig. 20.18** Instruments for tibial fixation

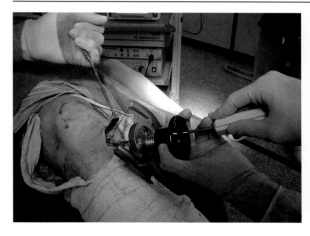

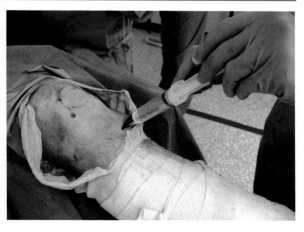

**Fig. 20.19**  Tensioning of graft at 20° flexion and fixation using interference screw

**Fig. 20.20**  Infiltration of local anesthetic into graft harvest site

**Fig. 20.21**  (**a**) Wound closure. (**b**) Bulky bandage

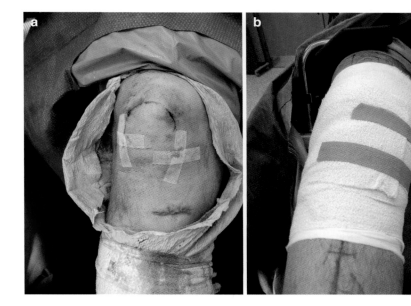

- Nerve or vascular injury
- Arthritis
- Anterior knee pain especially after patellar tendon graft

## Review

- At 2 weeks, 2 months, 6 months, and 1 year.
- Assess swelling and range of movements at early stages and muscle strength recovery and functional recovery at late follow-up.

## Further Reading

Hospodar SJ, Miller MD. Controversies in ACL reconstruction: bone-patellar tendon-bone anterior cruciate ligament reconstruction remains the gold standard. Sports Med Arthrosc. 2009;17(4):242–6.

Hapa O, Barber FA. ACL fixation devices. Sports Med Arthrosc. 2009;17(4):217–23.

Andersson D, Samuelsson K, Karlsson J. Treatment of anterior cruciate ligament injuries with special reference to surgical technique and rehabilitation: an assessment of randomized controlled trials. Arthroscopy. 2009;25(6): 653–85.

# Arthroscopic Posterior Cruciate Ligament (PCL) Reconstruction

# 21

Ram Venkatesh

## Indications

- PCL injury with combined ligament injuries.
- Symptomatic grade 2 or 3 PCL injuries – a significant proportion of grade 3 injuries have associated PLC or PMC injuries and need to carefully evaluate.

## Diagnosis

- Mechanism of injury gives the clue – posteriorly directed force to a flexed tibia.
- High velocity injuries and knee dislocations.
- Effusion less common.
- Examine knee at 90° flexion and observe normal step-off of tibia (Table 21.1).
- Assess posterior draw at 90° severe posterior draw suggests combined injuries (Fig. 21.1).
- Reverse pivot shift test.
- Dial test at 30° and 90° flexion (Fig. 21.2a, b).

## Investigations

- Stress X-rays at 90° flexion are extremely useful to assess posterior sag.
- MRI scans are useful in acute injuries but not so in chronic injuries (Fig. 21.3).

R. Venkatesh
Department of Trauma and Orthopaedic Surgery,
Leeds Teaching Hospitals NHS Trust, Leeds, UK
e-mail: ram.venkatesh@leedsth.nhs.uk

Table 21.1  Grades of tibial posterior sag

| Grade 1 | Tibial plateau is still anterior but can be posteriorly translated (<5 mm laxity) |
|---|---|
| Grade 2 | Flush with medial femoral condyle (5–10 mm laxity) |
| Grade 3 | Tibial plateau is posterior to the condyle (>10 mm laxity) |

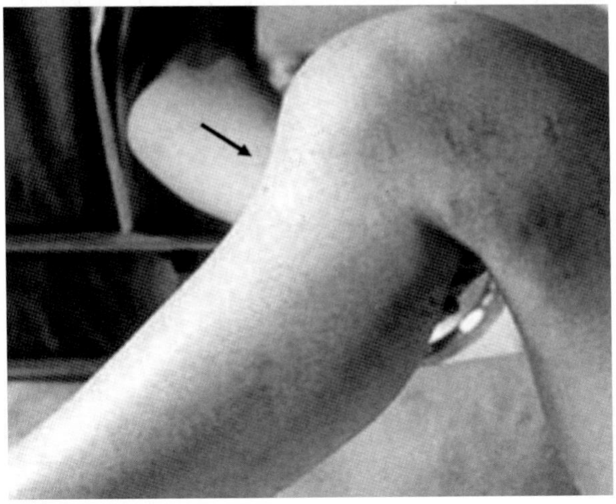

Fig. 21.1  Posterior tibial translation

## Preoperative

- Consent and place mark on limb to be operated
- Safe surgery check list

## Anesthesia

- General or regional anesthesia

P.V. Giannoudis (ed.), *Practical Procedures in Elective Orthopaedic Surgery*,
DOI 10.1007/978-0-85729-814-0_21, © Springer-Verlag London Limited 2012

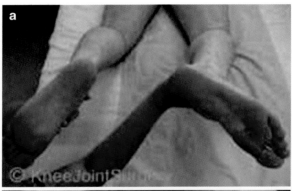

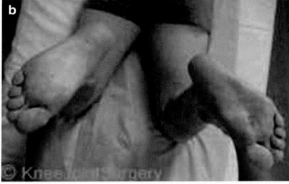

**Fig. 21.2** (**a**) Dial test at 30° with increased external rotation suggesting PCL and PLC injuries. (**b**) Dial test at 90° with increased external rotation suggesting PCL and PLC injuries (produced with permission from www.kneejointsurgery.com)

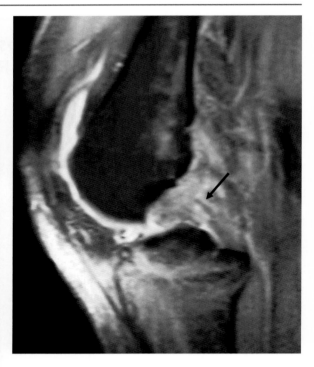

**Fig. 21.3** MRI scan presenting a PCL rupture (*arrow*)

## Timing of Surgery

- For acute knee dislocations, the ideal operative window is around 2 weeks post injury.
- Fluid extravasation can be a problem with earlier surgery (iatrogenic compartment syndrome).

## Graft Choice

- Autologous – hamstring, patellar tendon, quadriceps tendon.
- Allograft – Achilles tendon, hamstring.

## Setup

- Patient supine
- Leg holder or side support to help control joint position
- Bottom end of table removed if using leg holder

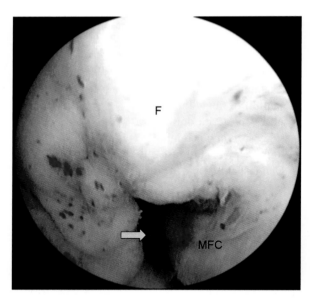

**Fig. 21.4** Arthroscopic image of a PCL rupture. Note the increased space (*arrow*) between the medial femoral condyle (*MFC*) and PCL (*F* fat pad)

- Soft support underneath opposite thigh to flex the hip
- Tourniquet applied high up in the thigh
- Ability to bring in the C Arm to take intraoperative imaging

**Fig. 21.5** (a) Drill guide for PCL surgery in place. (b) Fluoroscopic view during tibial tunnel preparation

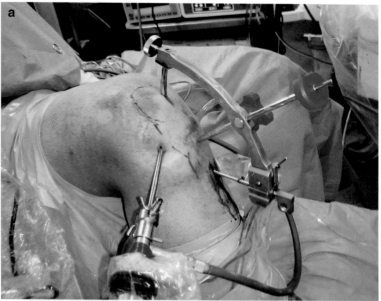

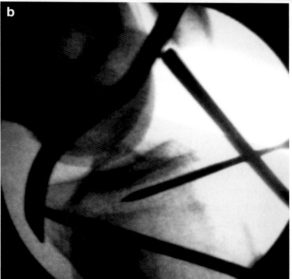

## Procedure

- Anterolateral portal close to patella tendon.
- Anteromedial portal and posteromedial portal.
- Short vertical or transverse incision over hamstring insertion (usually 1 cm below level of tibial tuberosity).
- In single-bundle reconstruction, it is the anterolateral bundle that is reconstructed.
- Conduct a diagnostic arthroscopy (Fig. 21.4) – check for other pathologies.

- Try to retain some of remnant PCL and sweep posterior capsule from posterior tibial ridge.
- Low entry point on anteromedial tibia to avoid killer turn at the back of tibia. The tunnel exits 10–14 mm below the joint line at the back of the tibia (Fig. 21.5a, b).
- Neurovascular structures need protection and guide wire and drill tip visualized and protected throughout.
- Femoral tunnel drilled inside out or outside in protecting trochlea cartilage.
- Graft fixation using interference screws (Fig. 21.6).

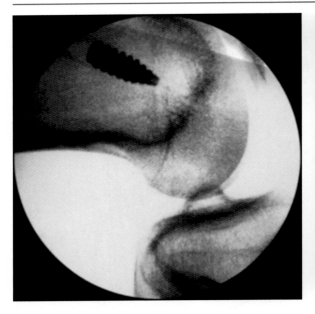

**Fig. 21.6** Fluoroscopic view of femoral interference screw

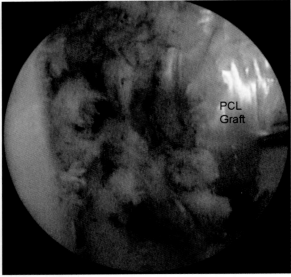

**Fig. 21.7** PCL graft in place

- In single-bundle reconstruction, the graft is tensioned at 70° knee flexion (Fig. 21.7).
- In multi-ligament surgery, ACL reconstruction performed next and then collateral ligament surgery.

## Postoperative Period

- Start mechanical VTE prophylaxis at admission and continue until the patient no longer has significantly reduced mobility, based on an assessment of risks. Start pharmacological VTE prophylaxis after surgery and continue until the patient no longer has significantly reduced mobility.
- Regain passive range of movements.
- Avoid open chain and also active hamstring exercises.
- Staged rehabilitation to regain motion, strength, and neuromuscular coordination.

## Complications

- Infection
- Stiffness

- Deep vein thrombosis
- Graft failure
- Re-rupture
- Nerve or vascular injury
- Arthritis
- Anterior knee pain

## Review

- At 2 weeks, 2 months, 6 months, and 1 year.
- Assess swelling and range of movements at early stages and muscle strength recovery and functional recovery at late follow-up.

## Further Reading

Matava MJ, Ellis E, Gruber B. Surgical treatment of posterior cruciate ligament tears: an evolving technique. J Am Acad Orthop Surg. 2009;17(7):435–46.

Petrigliano FA, McAllister DR. Isolated posterior cruciate ligament injuries of the knee. Sports Med Arthrosc. 2006;14(4):206–12.

Peccin MS, Almeida GJ, Amaro J, et al. Interventions for treating posterior cruciate ligament injuries of the knee in adults. Cochrane Database Syst Rev. 2005;(2):CD002939.

# Posterolateral Corner (PLC) Repair

# 22

Ram Venkatesh

## Indications

- Acute posterolateral corner injury either isolated or as combined injury.

## Clinical Assessment

- History of varus or twisting injury.
- Symptoms of giving way.
- Positive varus instability (Fig. 22.1).
- Positive dial test.
- Presence of posterolateral bruising.
- Assess neurovascular injury especially common peroneal nerve.

## Radiological Assessment

### Investigations

- Radiographs
  - Look for fibula neck fracture or increased lateral joint space.
- MRI
  - To assess integrity of lateral collateral ligament and popliteus.
  - Assess biceps femoris and common peroneal nerve integrity.
  - Look for multi ligament injury.

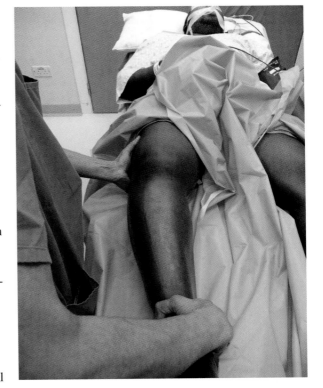

**Fig. 22.1** Varus instability

## Preoperative

- Assess neurovascular status.
- Angiogram may be necessary in some cases (knee dislocation).
- Consent and place mark on limb to be operated.
- Safe surgery check list.
- If associated nerve injury, plastic surgery input may be necessary for nerve repair.

R. Venkatesh
Department of Trauma and Orthopaedic Surgery,
Leeds Teaching Hospitals NHS Trust, Leeds, UK
e-mail: ram.venkatesh@leedsth.nhs.uk

P.V. Giannoudis (ed.), *Practical Procedures in Elective Orthopaedic Surgery*,
DOI 10.1007/978-0-85729-814-0_22, © Springer-Verlag London Limited 2012

**Fig. 22.2** Patient's position

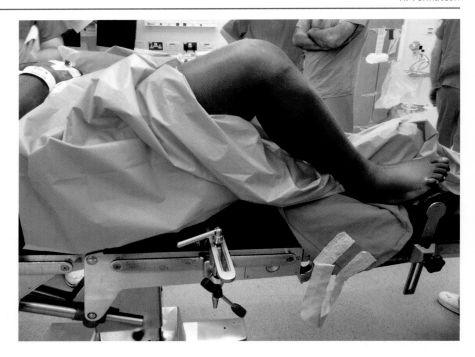

## Anesthesia

• General or regional anesthesia.

## Timing of Surgery

• Within 2 weeks of injury.

## Setup

• Patient supine.
• Leg holder or side support to help control joint position (Fig. 22.2).
• Bottom end of table removed if using leg holder.
• Soft support underneath opposite thigh to flex the hip.
• Tourniquet applied high up in the thigh.

## Procedure

• Check common peroneal nerve prior to surgery.
• MRI scans useful to assess structures involved. Check biceps femoris as it is an important landmark for dissection.
• Dry arthroscopy useful as mentioned above.

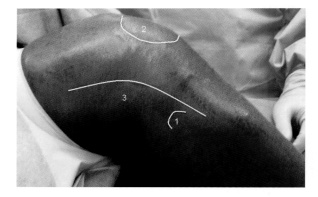

**Fig. 22.3** Anatomic landmarks: (1) fibular head, (2) patella, and (3) skin incision

• Lateral curvilinear incision (Fig. 22.3).
• Identify common peroneal nerve (Fig. 22.4a) through surgical window posteriorly to the iliotibial (IT) band.
• Fibular neck avulsion fracture fixed with anchors (Fig. 22.4b), screw with washer or tension band wiring.
• Inferior lateral geniculate artery may be encountered.
• Femoral attachment of LCL and popliteus identified through anterior window to IT band and reattached anatomically using anchors, suture, or recess technique.

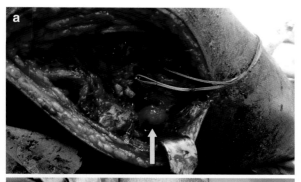

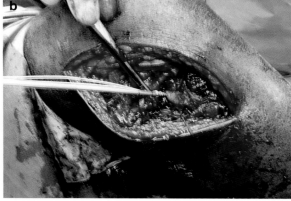

**Fig. 22.4** (**a**) Common peroneal nerve (*arrow*). (**b**) Fixation of fibular neck avulsion fracture with anchors

- LCL attachment on the femur is proximal and posterior to lateral epicondyle. The popliteus attachment is about 18 mm anterior and distal to this point.
- Popliteofibular ligament is present in most patients and identified close to musculotendinous junction and repaired.
- Direct repair of midlateral capsule (Fig. 22.5), IT band tear, meniscus tear, or biceps femoris tear may be needed.
- Occasionally, augmentation with hamstring graft or a slip of IT band or biceps femoris may be necessary.
- Tensioning is done at 30° knee flexion and slight internal rotation and valgus.

## Wound Closure

- Closure 1/0 vicryl for fascia and 2/0 vicryl for subcutaneous tissues and 3/0 monocryl continues for skin.

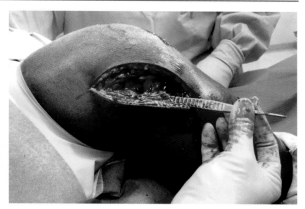

**Fig. 22.5** Rupture of midlateral capsule with forceps entering the articular space

## Postoperative Rehabilitation

- Start mechanical VTE prophylaxis at admission and continue until the patient no longer has significantly reduced mobility, based on an assessment of risks. Start pharmacological VTE prophylaxis after surgery and continue until the patient no longer has significantly reduced mobility.
- Aim to regain range of motion.
- Knee brace for 12 weeks.
- Avoid active hamstring exercises and external rotation of tibia for 3 months. Initial period of non-weight-bearing followed by closed chain quadriceps physiotherapy and gentle leg presses from 6 weeks to 3 months.
- Exercise bike at 6 weeks with mini squats and proprioceptive exercises. Treadmill and straight line activities at 4 months.
- Sports after 10–12 months.

## Complications

- Infection.
- Stiffness.
- Deep vein thrombosis.
- Failure of repair.
- Nerve or vascular injury.
- Persistent instability.

## Review

- At 2 weeks, 2 months, 6 months, and 1 year.
- Assess swelling and range of movements at early stages and muscle strength recovery and functional recovery at late follow-up.

## Further Reading

Hospodar SJ, Miller MD. Controversies in ACL reconstruction: bone-patellar tendon-bone anterior cruciate ligament reconstruction remains the gold standard. Sports Med Arthrosc. 2009;17(4):242–6.

Hapa O, Barber FA. ACL fixation devices. Sports Med Arthrosc. 2009;17(4):217–23.

Andersson D, Samuelsson K, Karlsson J. Treatment of anterior cruciate ligament injuries with special reference to surgical technique and rehabilitation: an assessment of randomized controlled trials. Arthroscopy. 2009;25(6):653–85.

# Unicompartmental Knee Arthroplasty

# 23

Panayotis N. Soucacos
and Athanasios E. Karamitros

## Indications

- Noninflammatory osteoarthritis or osteonecrosis affecting either one compartment of the knee.
- Initially indicated for elderly rather sedentary population; however its use in younger and more active patients (as an alternative to high tibial osteotomy or total knee replacement) has increased. Results in young patients have yet to be evaluated as they are derived from series with short and midterm follow-up.
- Osteoarthritic changes in the opposite compartment or the patellofemoral joint not greater than Outerbridge grade II or even asymptomatic grade III are not contraindications.

## Contraindications

- Inflammatory arthritis.
- Synovial chondromatosis, villonodular synovitis.
- Absent anterior cruciate ligament.
- Tibiofemoral translation or shift >5 mm.
- Recurvatum >5°.
- History of infection.
- Obesity (BMI > 45).

P.N. Soucacos (✉)
Professor of Orthopaedic Surgery, University of Athens, School of Medicine, Director, Orthopaedic Research & Education Center (OREC), Athens, Greece
e-mail: psoukakos@ath.forthnet.gr

A.E. Karamitros
Third Academic Department of Trauma and Orthopaedic Surgery, School of Medicine, University of Athens, Athens, Greece

## Preoperative Planning

### Clinical Assessment

- Thorough clinical examination of the knee should be performed. Symptoms such as severe night pain or pain at rest as well as symptomatic patellofemoral arthritis should preclude an unicompartmental knee arthroplasty (UKA).
- Examine the knee for any deformation, contractures, and stability.
- Mechanical axis of the affected knee should not deviate more than 5° from neutral for a valgus knee or 10° for a varus one. These deviations should be passively corrected.
- Any flexion contracture should not exceed 15°. Preoperatively, the knee should be able to flex up to 100°.
- The anterior cruciate ligament and menisci should be intact.
- Patient's weight up to 80 kg is acceptable, but concern is raised when weight exceeds 90 kg.

### Radiological Assessment

- Standard anteroposterior (weight-bearing) of both knees and lateral X-rays of the affected knee as well as tangential views of the patella should be obtained.
- Surgeon should be able to estimate the mechanical axis through the X-rays and evaluate the condition of the patellofemoral joint and the opposite compartment.
- Note that the final decision about performing a UKR is always taken after thorough intraoperative inspection (Fig. 23.1a, b).

P.V. Giannoudis (ed.), *Practical Procedures in Elective Orthopaedic Surgery*,
DOI 10.1007/978-0-85729-814-0_23, © Springer-Verlag London Limited 2012

**Fig. 23.1** (**a**) AP X-ray presenting the osteonecrosis of the medial femoral condyle. (**b**) Lateral X-ray of the affected knee

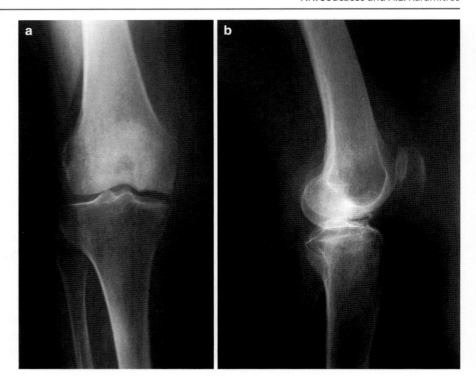

- MRI or scintigraphy should not be used routinely. Selectively, MRI can be used to exclude ligamentous or meniscal lesions when there is strong suspicion.

## Operative Treatment

### Anesthesia

- Preferably regional (spinal or epidural) and/or general anesthesia.
- Use of antibiotic prophylaxis.

### Table and Equipment

- Standard orthopedic operative table.
- Thigh tourniquet.

- Availability for intraoperative and final radiographs.
- Instrumentation, trial, and implants according to the implant selected.

### Patient Positioning

- Patient is placed supine on the operative table (soft supports under bony prominences), or with the leg in a leg holder at the level of the thigh, with 45° hip flexion and the knee allowed free to flex at least 120°.

### Draping

- Skin preparation of the entire leg including the foot (or below the tourniquet if placed) with use of local antiseptics.
- Standard draping of the entire leg provided that the knee is allowed to flex as noted previously.

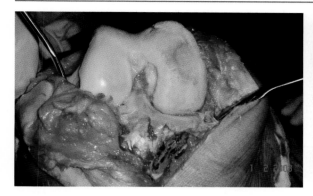

**Fig. 23.2** Intraoperative verification of osteonecrosis

## Surgical Approach and Technique

- Most surgeons use the standard medial parapatellar approach with eversion of the patella, which allows for thorough inspection of all three compartments.
- Alternatively, minimal procedures can be implemented. They are more technically demanding, highly depend on proper instrumentation but they certainly cause less damage and provide faster recovery.
- Proper implant positioning is crucial and appropriate instrumentation should always be used.
- Authors use the St Georg Sled (with Endo Model metal-backed tibial plateau) prosthesis (Waldemar/Link) and technique described corresponds to that implant.
- Tourniquet is used.
- A standard medial parapatellar approach is made. Patella is reverted and all three compartments are carefully inspected. According to the findings, a patient may not be a suitable candidate for UKA (Fig. 23.2).
- Meniscus and osteophytes are removed.
- Tibial cut is carried out with the tibial saw guide (available for medial and lateral compartment), which provides a posterior slope of 6°.
- The degree of correction of the preexisting deformity is a crucial issue in UKR. Overcorrection should be avoided and most authors agree on an undercorrection of 2–3° of the mechanical axis. Overcorrection leads to rapid progress of contralateral department disease.

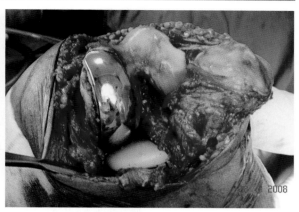

**Fig. 23.3** The prosthesis is implanted

- Templates are used for tibial sizing taking care to avoid overhanging.
- Preparation of the femoral size starts with cutting 3 mm of the posterior aspect of the femoral condyle.
- Using the appropriately sized femoral drill guide, anchoring holes are drilled. The borders of the drill guide are marked and cartilage inside the marked area is removed down to subchondral bone. A groove is made between the anchoring holes and the trial femoral prosthesis is placed.
- The leading edge of the femoral component should be "buried" into the trochlear cartilage. It is crucial to ascertain that the femoral component does not impinge on the patella. In such case, the part of the patella that makes the contact should be removed.
- Tibial trial components are inserted and trial reduction is made. Knee is tested for range of motion and stability. In a normal knee, there should be only a few millimeters' space between the components under valgus stress in a neutral position.
- The space for the keel of the metal-backed tibial prosthesis is prepared. Femoral prosthesis is cemented first followed by the tibial implant. Knee is extended allowing for the cement to harden.
- Before closure inspect carefully for remaining excess cement which has to be removed (Fig. 23.3).
- Tourniquet is released and hemostasis is carried out.
- Drains are not usually necessary.

**Fig. 23.4** Postoperative
(**a**) AP and (**b**) lateral
X-ray of the knee

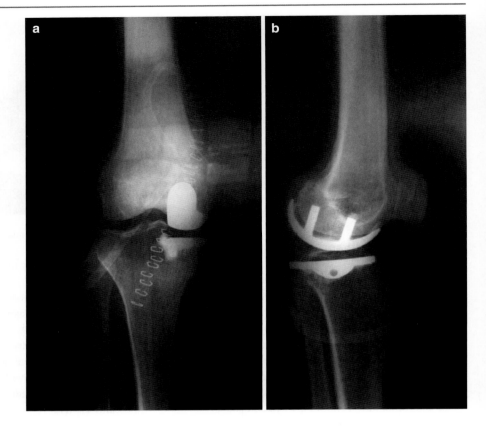

## Postoperative Treatment

- Routine antibiotic according to local protocols.
- Start mechanical VTE prophylaxis at admission. Continue mechanical VTE prophylaxis until the patient no longer has significantly reduced mobility. Start pharmacological VTE prophylaxis after surgery. Continue pharmacological VTE prophylaxis for 10–14 days.
- Patients sit on a chair and begin weight-bearing as tolerated with a walker or crutches the day after or even on the day of the surgery.
- Continuous passive motion device is used from the day of the surgery and throughout the hospitalization period.
- Muscle strengthening exercises begin on the day of the surgery.

## Complications

- Implant malposition.
- Retained cement.
- Intraoperative fracture (most frequently on the tibial side) or ligamentous injury medial collateral ligament avulsion.
- Hematoma formation.
- Deep vein thrombosis.
- Superficial wound infection or deep infection.
- Implant wear and/or loosening.
- Disease progress in the other compartments.
- When revision is necessary, it is usually straightforward. Almost always conversion is done to a primary TKR. Stemmed implants, augments, extended grafting, and custom-made implants are rarely required, especially in the lately described series.

## Follow-up

- Patients are assessed clinically and radiographically at 1, 3, 6, and 12 months and every 5 years thereafter, unless GP's request (Fig. 23.4a, b).

## Further Reading

Ackroyd CE, Whitehouse SL, Newman JH, Joslin CC. A comparative study of the medial St Georg Sled and Kinematic total knee arthroplasties. Ten-year survivorship. J Bone Joint Surg. 2002;84B:667–72.

Berger RA, Meneghini RM, Jacobs JJ, Sheinkop MB, Della Valle CJ, Rosenberg AG, et al. Results of unicompartmental knee arthroplasty at a minimum of 10 years of follow-up. J Bone Joint Surg. 2005;87A:999–1006.

Marmor L. Unicompartmental knee arthroplasty: 10 to 13 year follow-up study. Clin Orthop Relat Res. 1988;226:14–20.

O'Rourke MR, Gardner JJ, Callaghan JJ, Liu SS, Goetz DD, Vittetoe DA, et al. Unicompartmental knee replacement. A minimum twenty-one year follow-up, end-result study. Clin Orthop Relat Res. 2005;440:27–37.

Steele RG, Hutabarat S, Evans RL, Ackroyd CE, Newman JH. Survivorship of the St Georg Sled medial unicompartmental knee replacement beyond ten years. J Bone Joint Surg. 2006; 88B:1164–8.

Nice clinical guideline 92 – Venous thromboembolism: reducing the risk. Reducing the risk of venous thromboembolism (deep vein thrombosis and pulmonary embolism) in patients admitted to hospital. Jan 2010 (www.nice.org.uk/guidance/CG92)

# Total Knee Replacement (TKR)

# 24

Peter Bobak and Peter V. Giannoudis

## Indication

- Painful arthritis of the knee resulting decline in function, progressive deformity.

## Preoperative Planning

### Clinical Assessment

- In standing position from the front and the side, general assessment of:
  - Size
  - Muscle wasting
  - Alignment of the leg
  - Compare to the unaffected side:
    Valgus
    Varus
    Flexion deformity
- Record the posture of the affected leg and foot as it may suggest associated pathology above (hip) or below (foot and ankle) the knee.

P. Bobak (✉)
Department of Trauma and Orthopaedic Surgery,
Leeds Teaching Hospitals NHS Trust, Leeds, UK
e-mail: peter.bobak@leedsth.nhs.uk

P.V. Giannoudis
Academic Department of Trauma and Orthopaedic Surgery,
School of Medicine, University of Leeds,
Leeds, UK

- Look for changes of the skin:
  - Inflammation
  - Infection
  - Laceration
  - Swelling
  - Scars from previous surgery
- Feel the bony landmarks: femoral and tibial condyles, patella and the joint line, note range of movements (flexion, extension), and assess stability in both coronal and sagittal planes.
- Examine the distal vascular supply and neurological function of the limb.
- General preoperative medical assessment and routine blood tests – FBC, Electrolytes, Grp & Save, Cross-matched blood, ECG, MRSA screening.
- Thromboembolic risk should always be considered and prophylaxis used according to agreed protocol.

### Radiological Assessment

- Good quality and adequate X-rays – AP (fulllength) and lateral, ± patella views – are required for accurate preoperative planning (Fig. 24.1a, b) Some surgeons consider obtaining full-length x-rays.

## Operative Treatment

### Anesthesia

- Regional or general anesthesia ± nerve blocks.

**Fig. 24.1** (**a**) AP X-ray with full weight-bearing.
(**b**) Lateral X-ray of the knee

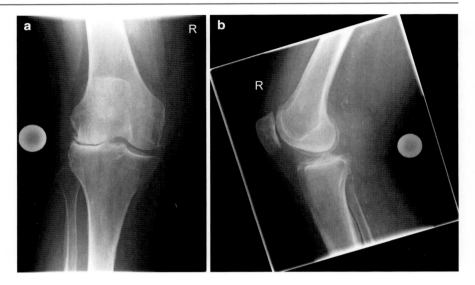

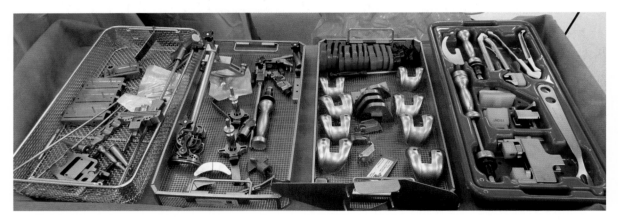

**Fig. 24.2** The tray for total knee replacement. Some small variations could be evident between the orthopedic industries

## Theater Preparations

- Confirm the correct patient and knee to be operated on.
- Operating theater should use ultra clean air systems for surgery.
- Implants and instruments specific to the operation must be available (Fig. 24.2).
- Antibiotic prophylaxis according to agreed protocol.
- The operative field should be free of hair.

## Patient Positioning

- Should be done by the operating surgeon.
- Supine position using upper thigh and foot supports to allow sufficient and stable flexion of the knee (Fig. 24.3).

- Check correct (proximal thigh) position of tourniquet, diathermy plate, flowtron, and pressure sore prevention gel pad to the contralateral leg.

## Draping and Surgical Approach

- Highest standard in antiseptic preparation is essential.
- The surgical site isolated with sterile drapes.
- Tourniquet inflated (300–350 mmHg) after elevation and flexion of the leg.
- *Varus knee*:
  - Midline skin incision terminates just at the medial aspect of tibial tuberosity (Fig. 24.4).
  - The incision through the superficial fascia to minimize undermining.

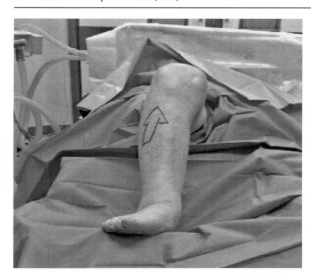

**Fig. 24.3** Supine position using upper thigh and foot supports to allow sufficient and stable flexion of the knee

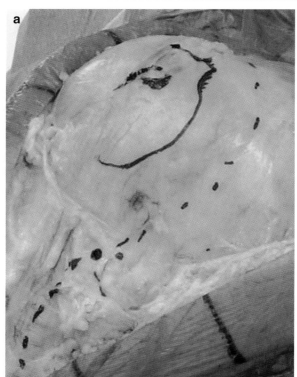

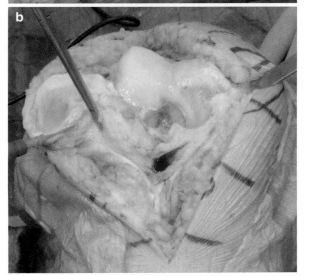

**Fig. 24.5** (**a**) Medial parapatellar arthrotomy preserving adequate volume of soft tissue to the patella for safe closure. (**b**) Infrapatellar fat pad excised to facilitate exposure

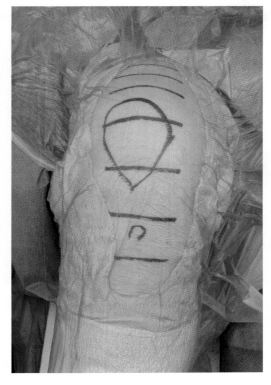

**Fig. 24.4** Patella and tibial tuberosity identified and marked, transverse lines aid closure

- Hemostasis of perforating vessels to the skin and deep fascia.
- Quadriceps tendon is freed up of soft tissues prior to arthrotomy.

- Medial parapatellar arthrotomy preserving adequate volume of soft tissue to the patella for safe closure (Fig. 24.5a).
- The patella is everted and part of the retropatellar fat pad excised to facilitate exposure (Fig. 24.5b).

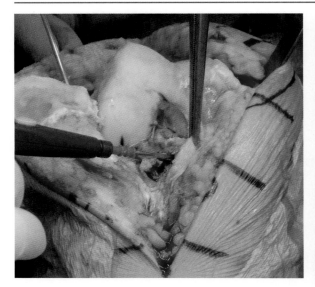

**Fig. 24.6** Soft tissue balancing releasing the medial soft tissue envelope

- Soft tissue balancing releasing the medial soft tissue envelope in a stepwise fashion until deformity is corrected/anterior synovium, deep MCL, posteromedial corner, superficial MCL in progression (Fig. 24.6).
- Remnants of menisci are removed to expose the tibial plateau.
- Retractors placed alongside the lateral and medial tibial plateau.
- Adequate visualization of the distal femur is essential prior to femoral cuts.
- Remove osteophytes and identify bony landmarks of the distal femur: condyles, anterior cortex, femoral intercondylar notch.
- Distal (at 4-6 degrees of valgus), anterior, and posterior femoral bone cuts in succession to achieve even flexion gap both laterally and medially (Fig. 24.7a, b).
- Assess trial femoral component.
- Tibia is brought forward with a PCL retractor.
- Remove marginal osteophytes from tibia to measure correct size.
- Tibial resection block positioned with external alignment guide to adjust rotation and tibial slope (Fig. 24.8a, b).
- Assess flexion-extension gap prior to tibial resection.

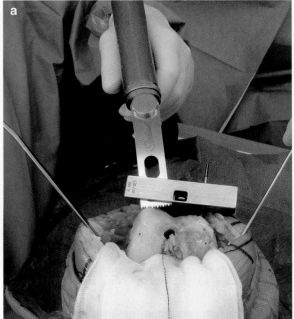

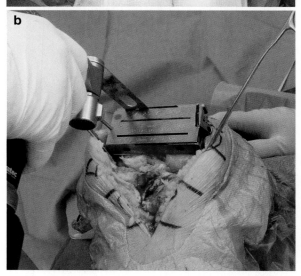

**Fig. 24.7** (**a**) Distal femoral cut. (**b**) Femoral cutting block for anterior and posterior preparation

- Final tibial preparation to accommodate the implant (Fig. 24.9).
- Laminar spreader used to access posterior aspect of the knee to remove femoral osteophytes and/or release any residual tightness if present – PCL may be excised (Fig. 24.10).

**Fig. 24.8** (**a**) Tibial resection block positioned with external alignment guide to adjust rotation and tibial slope, tibial marking stylus used to determine the amount of bone resected. (**b**) Tibial resection protecting soft tissue envelope and posterior structures with retractors

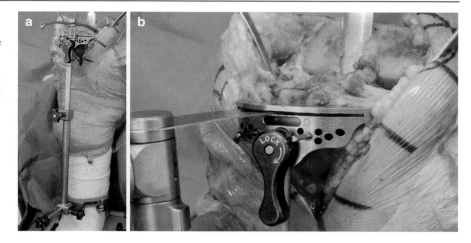

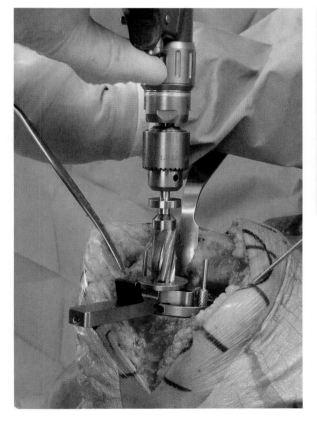

**Fig. 24.9** Final tibial preparation

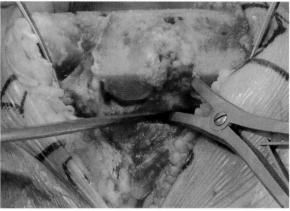

**Fig. 24.10** Laminar spreader used to access posterior aspect of the knee

- If patella is preserved, marginal osteophytes removed with circumferential soft tissue release.
- If patella is replaced, the bone cut should restore the patellar thickness.
- *Valgus knee:*
  - Skin incision is slightly to the lateral side of the midline.
  - Lateral arthrotomy extending through the medial edge of Gerdy's tubercle.
  - Incision of the synovium could be more postero-lateral to the incision of the retinaculum to facilitate closure.
  - Partial resection of fat pad, adhesions and removal of osteophytes to assist medial displacement of the patella.

- Trial reduction to assess stability, flexion-extension gap, patella tracking, and range of movements (Fig. 24.11a, b).

**Fig. 24.11** (**a**) Trial reduction. (**b**) Assessing stability

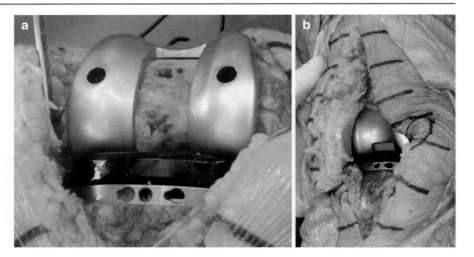

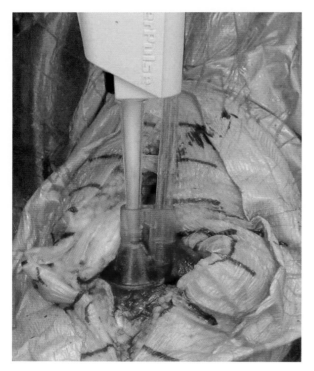

**Fig. 24.12** Pulse-lavage irrigation to remove fat and debris from the cut surfaces

- Soft tissue balancing in relation to the severity of deformity:
  Subperiosteal elevation of iliotibial band
  Release of LCL
  Popliteus in succession
- Bone cuts as above, but reduced valgus angle for distal femoral resection is recommended.
- Particular attention must be paid for correct tibial rotation.

- *Cemented components:*
  - Use pulse-lavage irrigation to remove fat and debris from the cut surfaces of the femur and tibia prior to cementation (Fig. 24.12).
  - Dry surface must be obtained to provide an optimal surface for cement injection.
  - The tibia is cemented first: cement is applied manually; pressurization of cement is achieved by use of thumb and digital pressure (Fig. 24.13a).
  - Cement is also placed evenly to the tibial component and it is then delivered on to the tibia (Fig. 24.13b).
  - Excess of cement released from the interfaces is removed.
  - Femoral component cemented in a similar fashion (Fig. 24.14). The femoral canal is sealed to minimize bleeding.
  - The knee is extended. One size bigger plastic trial may be used at this stage to maximize cement penetration. Excess of cement is removed (Fig. 24.15a).
  - Patella if replaced, cemented accordingly.
  - Appropriate polyethylene component is inserted (Fig. 24.15b).
  - If patella is preserved, marginal osteophytes removed with circumferential soft tissue release to facilitate adequate tracking (Fig. 24.16a, b).

## Closure

- Irrigation, infiltration with local anesthetic and epinephrine, drain.
- Closure in layers, deep fascia, subcutaneous tissues, and skin (Fig. 24.17a, b).

**Fig. 24.13** (**a**) Cement pressurization is achieved by digital pressure. (**b**) Bone cement is also placed evenly to the tibial component

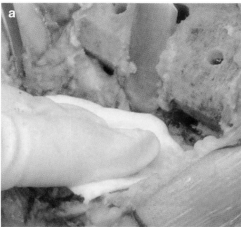
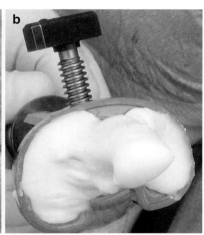

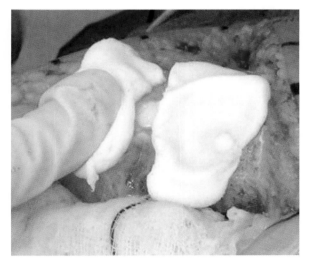

**Fig. 24.14** Femoral cementation. The femoral canal is sealed to minimize bleeding. Bone cement is placed on the femoral component

- Wound is covered with a bulky dressing (wool and crepe) that is reduced 24-48 hours after surgery (Fig. 24.18).
- Tourniquet is deflated and drain is opened.

## Postoperative Care

- Routine antibiotic according to local protocols.
- Start mechanical VTE prophylaxis at admission. Continue mechanical VTE prophylaxis until the patient no longer has significantly reduced mobility.

Start pharmacological VTE prophylaxis after surgery. Continue pharmacological VTE prophylaxis for 28 days.

- Observe blood loss and requirements for analgesia.
- Monitor vascular and neurological status of the leg.
- Mobilize weight-bearing and start ROM exercises with physiotherapist as early as possible, usually day 1 after surgery. Walking aids can be helpful and prescribed at this stage.
- Check X-ray and FBC (Fig. 24.19a, b).

## Complications

- Wound healing
- Fractures
- Patella clunk syndrome
- Stiffness
- Thromboembolic episode
- Extensor mechanism rupture
- Instability, flexion–extension inequality
- Neurovascular injury
- Infection
- Residual pain

## Follow-up

- Patients are assessed clinically and radiographically at 3/12 and 12/12 post surgery. Ideally indefinitive clinical and radiological follow-up is required. However, it's frequency is influenced by local and national guidelines.

**Fig. 24.15** (**a**) Knee is extended, one size bigger plastic trial may be used at this stage to maximize cement penetration. (**b**) Polyethylene component inserted

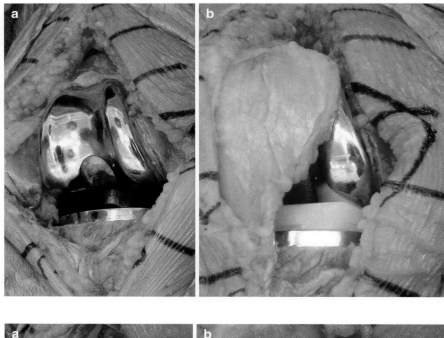

**Fig. 24.16** Final patellar preparation. (**a**) Circumferential soft tissue release. (**b**) Removal of marginal osteophytes

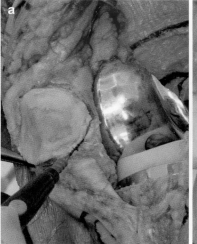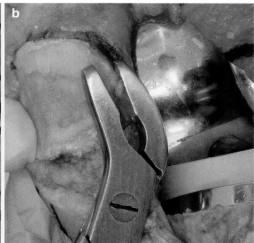

**Fig. 24.17** (**a**) Capsule is closed with uninterrupted sutures. (**b**) Skin clips

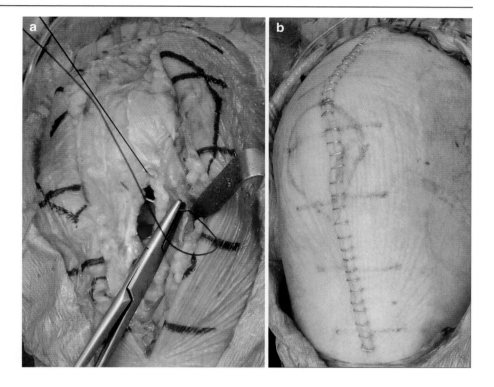

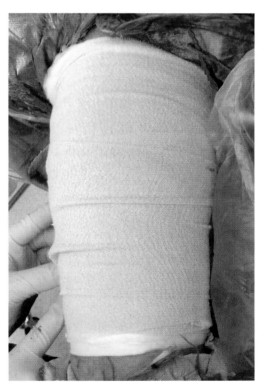

**Fig. 24.18** Wound covered with a bulky dressing

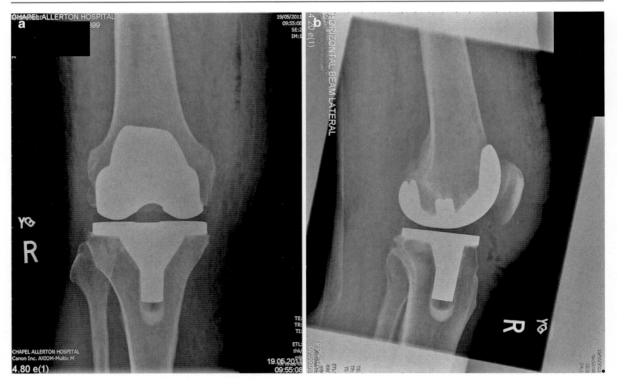

**Fig. 24.19** (**a**) Lateral and (**b**) AP postoperative radiographs

## Further Reading

Deirmengian CA, Lonner JH. What's new in adult reconstructive knee surgery. J Bone Joint Surg Am. 2009;91(12): 3008–18.

Brooks P. Orthopedics. 2011:9;34(9):e476–8. doi:10.3928/014774 47-20110714-32.

Schiavone Panni A, Cerciello S, et al. Stiffness in total knee arthroplasty. J Orthop Traumatol. 2009;10(3):111–8.

Gandhi R, Tsvetkov D, Davey JR, et al. Survival and clinical function of cemented and uncemented prostheses in total knee replacement: a meta-analysis. J Bone Joint Surg Br. 2009;91(7):889–95.

Nice clinical guideline 92 – Venous thromboembolism: reducing the risk. Reducing the risk of venous thromboembolism (deep vein thrombosis and pulmonary embolism) in patients admitted to hospital. Jan 2010 (www.nice.org.uk/guidance/ CG92).

# Revision Total Knee Arthroplasty

# 25

Peter V. Giannoudis, Fragkiskos N. Xypnitos, and Peter Bobak

## Indications

- Causes:
  - Loose femoral and/or tibial components (and/or patellar component in case of patellar resurfacing)
  - Osteolysis
  - Polyethylene wear
  - Implant fracture
  - Component malposition
  - Infection
  - Arthrofibrosis
  - Soft tissue impingement
  - Dysfunction of the extensor mechanism
  - Instability – subluxation – dislocation
  - Lack of motion
- Main indications:
  - Loosening
    Fracture-impending fracture
    Instability
    Pain
    Stiffness
- As soon as mechanical failure is apparent.
- Any delay will result in progressive bone loss and increased wear products with subsequent

creation of larger bone defects and metal-induced reactive synovitis.
- Challenging Procedure due to:
  - Extensive bone loss
  - Instability
  - Extensor mechanism dysfunction
  - Periarticular arthrofibrosis
- Before doing a revision, you should know the cause of the failure.

## Preoperative Planning

### Clinical Assessment

- History:
  - Primary symptom (pain, swelling, instability, or stiffness)
  - Time of onset
  - Duration and frequency of the symptoms
  - Activities that are associated with them
  - Comorbid conditions (e.g., diabetes, lumbar stenosis, etc.)
  - Notes from the previous procedure
  - Every patient who presents with a failure of a total knee arthroplasty must be evaluated for an infection, since the treatment of an infection-related failure of a total knee replacement is fundamentally different from the treatment of aseptic failure
- Clinical examination:
  - Knee
    Examine patient in three positions: non-weight-bearing, standing, and walking.

P. Bobak• F.N. Xypnitos
Department of Trauma and Orthopaedic Surgery,
Leeds Teaching Hospitals NHS Trust,
Leeds, UK

P.V. Giannoudis (✉)
Academic Department of Trauma and Orthopaedic Surgery,
School of Medicine, University of Leeds, Leeds, UK
e-mail: pgiannoudi@aol.com

P.V. Giannoudis (ed.), *Practical Procedures in Elective Orthopaedic Surgery*,
DOI 10.1007/978-0-85729-814-0_25, © Springer-Verlag London Limited 2012

Visual inspection, palpation, and stability testing:
  Knee joint range of motion
  Stability
  Patella tracking
– Neurovascular examination
– Adjacent joints
• Exclude symptoms from:
– Adjacent joints (ipsilateral hip and lumbar spine)
– Surrounding soft tissues (pes anserinus bursitis or iliotibial, patellar, or quadriceps tendinitis)
– Complex regional pain syndrome
– Neuroma
– Vascular claudication
– Fracture

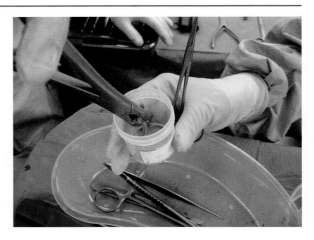

**Fig. 25.1** Periprosthetic tissues sent for histopathologic examination

## Laboratory Assessment

• Blood laboratory control:
– Inflammation markers: peripheral white blood count, CRP, and ESR
• Aspiration of the knee joint:
– Examine the aspirate for cells, organisms, and debris
– Send for cultures
– Check protein and glucose levels
– WBC count of between 1,100 and 3,000 cell/mm$^3$ is strongly suggestive of an infection
– When neutrophils are between 60% and 80%, infection is likely
– When the white blood cell count is <1,100 cells/mm$^3$ and the percentage of neutrophils is <64%, the negative predictive value is 98.2%
– When both are greater than these values, the positive predictive value for infection is 98.6%
• Intraoperatively:
– Gram stains (low sensitivity)
– Histopathologic examination of periprosthetic tissues (Fig. 25.1)
An average of more than ten polymorphonuclear cells per high-power field is diagnostic for infection
The periprosthetic tissues should not be fibrin to evaluate the results

## Imaging Assessment

• Radiographs
– Of the knee (hip-to-ankle weight-bearing)
Anteroposterior (Fig. 25.2a)

Lateral (Fig. 25.2b)
  Merchant views
– Of the ipsilateral hip
• Computed Tomography or Magnetic Resonance Imaging
– Assess:
The rotation of the femoral and tibial components
The extent of osteolytic lesions (requires metal artifact suppression)
• Radionuclide Scans
– Investigate:
Aseptic loosening
Infection
Complex regional pain syndrome
Periprosthetic stress fractures

## Operative Treatment

### Anesthesia

• Regional (spinal/epidural) or general anesthesia.
• At induction, administer prophylactic antibiotic as per local hospital protocol. If infection is suspected, hold antibiotics until fluid and tissue cultures have been obtained.

### Table and Equipment

• Standard orthopedic operative table.
• Thigh tourniquet.
• Availability for intraoperative and final radiographs.

**Fig. 25.2** (**a**) Anteroposterior and (**b**) lateral preoperative X-rays

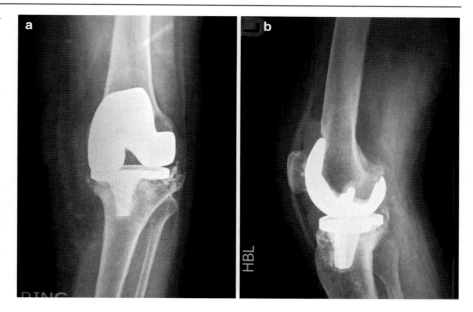

- Instrumentation, trial, and implants according to the implant selected (Fig. 25.3a, b).
- Availability for wedges, blocks (Fig. 25.3c), and allografts.

## Patient Positioning

- Should be performed by the operating surgeon.
- Supine position using upper thigh and foot supports to allow sufficient and stable flexion of the knee (Fig. 25.4a, b).
- Check correct (proximal thigh) position of tourniquet, diathermy plate, flowtron, and pressure sore prevention gel pad to the contralateral leg.

## Draping

- Highest standard in antiseptic preparation is essential.
- The surgical site is isolated with sterile drapes.
- Tourniquet is inflated (300–350 mmHg) after elevation of the leg and knee flexion.

## Surgical Approach

- Utilize previous incision whenever is possible (Fig. 25.5a).

- If all incisions were made more than 2 years previously and did not involve a surrounding soft tissue flap, the surgeon should choose the one that is most advantageous for the revision surgery. A minimum 6-cm skin bridge should be maintained if previous incisions cannot be utilized.
- The medial parapatellar arthrotomy is the workhorse of revision total knee arthroplasty (Fig. 25.5b).
- Remove previously placed sutures as part of the debridement.
- Suprapatellar and parapatellar regions debridement: Perform synovectomy in cases of hypertrophic synovitis (Fig. 25.6a, b).
- A medial release to the posteromedial corner of the tibia should then be performed.
- The patella is everted, and retractors are placed alongside the lateral and medial tibial plateau (Fig. 25.7).
- Remove the polyethylene insert to improve the ability to mobilize the soft tissues (Fig. 25.8).
- When the exposure is inadequate, consider a quadriceps snip or additionally a tibial tubercle osteotomy.
- If improved exposure of the components is still required, perform a medial femoral peel.
- Protect the extensor mechanism throughout the procedure (Fig. 25.9a, b).
- In fixed varus deformity, proceed in succession to subperiosteal release of medial collateral ligament (deep and superficial portions), pes anserine, semimembranosus, and posterior capsule.

**Fig. 25.3** (**a**, **b**) Trays of instruments and (**c**) tray with trial wedges and blocks

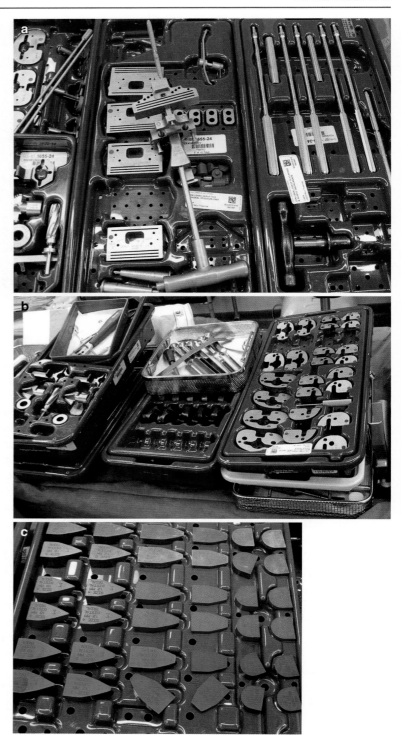

**Fig. 25.6** (**a**) Synovectomy. (**b**) The excised hypertrophic synovium

**Fig. 25.4** (**a**, **b**) Patient position

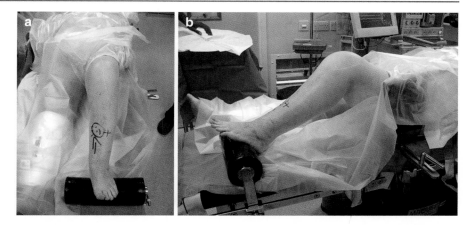

**Fig. 25.5** (**a**) Previous incisions for TKR (black arrow) and for tibial plateau fracture fixation (yellow arrow). (**b**) Patella and tibial tuberosity identified and marked. Transverse lines aid closure

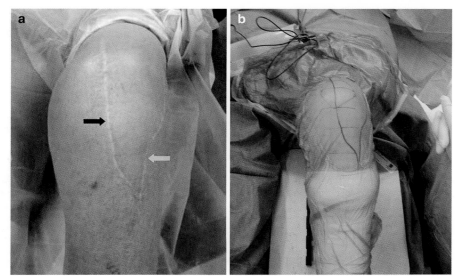

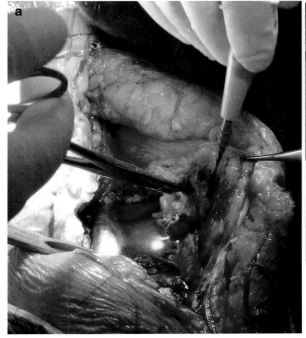

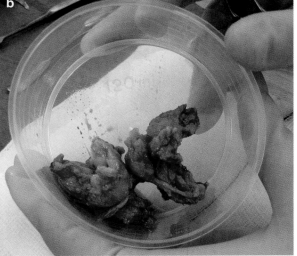

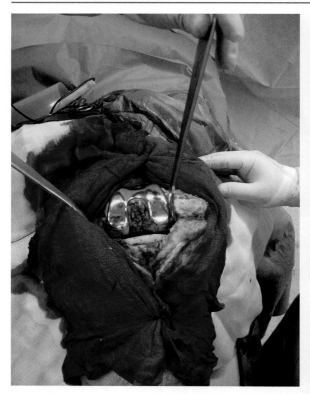

**Fig. 25.7** Eversion of the patella and retractor placement alongside the lateral and medial tibial plateau

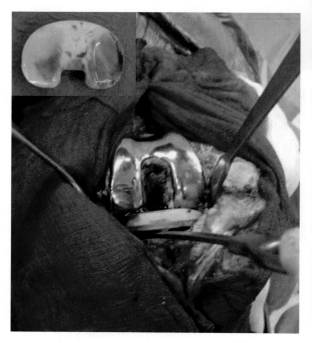

**Fig. 25.8** Removal of the polyethylene insert

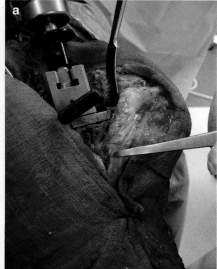

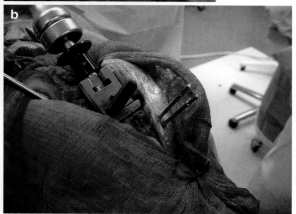

**Fig. 25.9** (**a**) Small tear at patellar tendon. (**b**) Protection of the extensor mechanism throughout the procedure with two pins

- In fixed valgus deformity, proceed in multiple horizontal incisions at posterior capsule, lateral collateral ligament, and iliotibial band.

## Implant Removal

- Evaluate the components for loosening, malposition, or impingement.
- Use special instruments:
  - Extraction devices (Fig. 25.10a, b)
  - Osteotomes (Fig. 25.11a, b)
  - Gigli saw (Fig. 25.12)

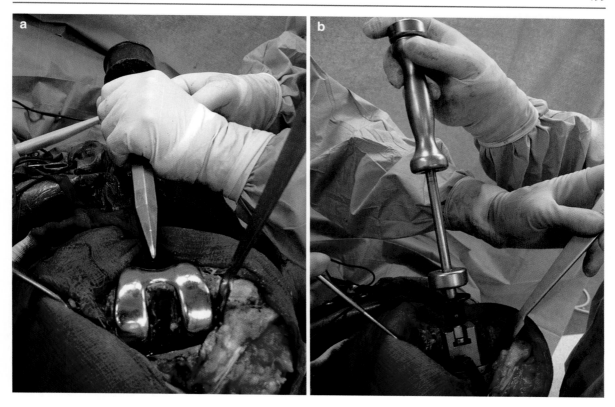

**Fig. 25.10** (**a**, **b**) Extraction devices

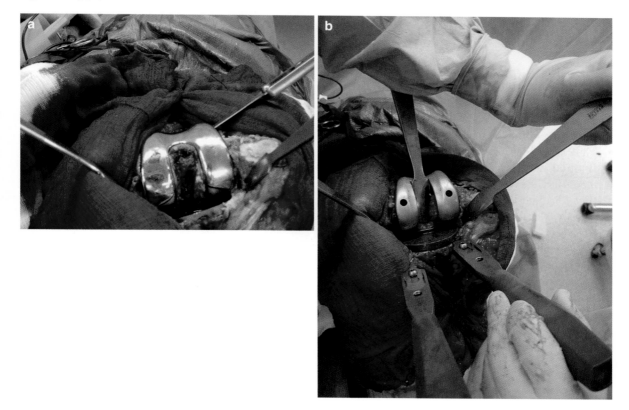

**Fig. 25.11** (**a**, **b**) Osteotomes

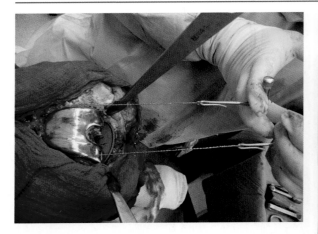

**Fig. 25.12** Gigli saw

- – Small oscillating saw
- – Diamond-tipped drill
- Remove femoral component first (leave cement on femur to facilitate tibial subluxation) (Fig. 25.13a) and then the tibial component (Fig. 25.13b).
- Meticulous debridement should follow components removal (Fig. 25.14a–d).
- Once the components have been successfully removed, begin the reconstruction with the tibia. Tibia plateau affects both the flexion and the extension gap equally.

## Tibia Reconstruction

- Use reverse hook and reamers to remove any remaining fibrous tissue from the tibial canal.
- Tibia is brought forward with a PCL retractor.
- If tibial deformity is not severe, use an intramedullary stem to place the tibial resection block (Fig. 25.15a, b). In case of an excessive tibial bowing, use extramedullary guides.
- Bone loss should be addressed. Consider the use of:
  - – Cement
  - – A modular augmentation wedge block
  - – An allograft (cancellous or structural cortical)
  - – Modular tibial cone
- Final tibial preparation to accommodate the implant.
- Assess trial tibial component.
- After tibial reconstruction, the joint line should be within the midrange of polyethylene inserts available.

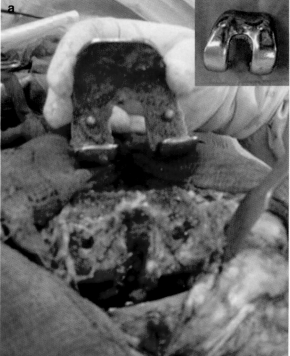

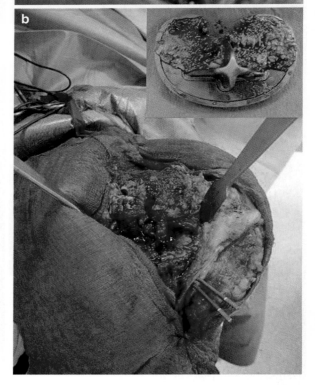

**Fig. 25.13** (**a**) Removed femoral component. (**b**) Removed tibial component

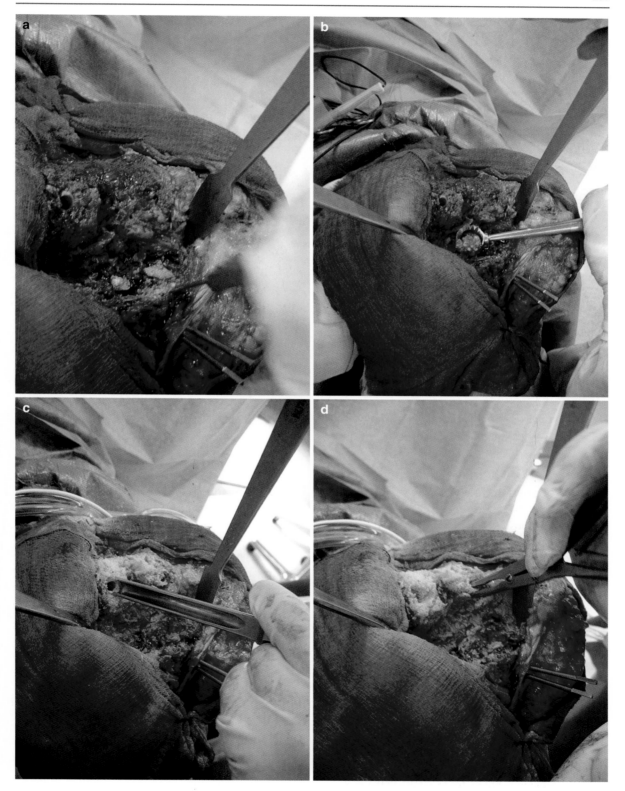

**Fig. 25.14** (**a**) Cement removal. (**b**) Debridement of tibial surface. (**c** and **d**). Cement removal from femoral peg holes

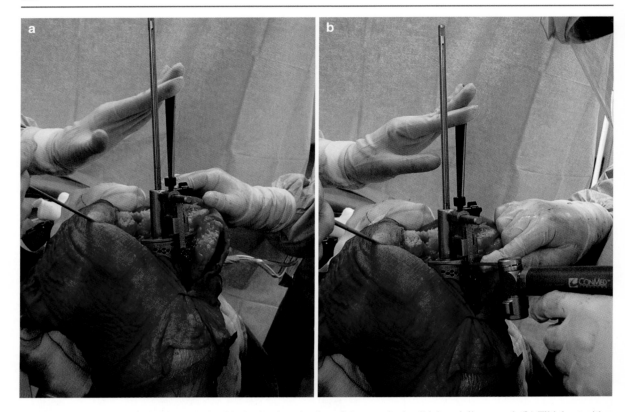

**Fig. 25.15** (**a**) Placement of tibial resection block after introduction of the stem in the tibial medullary canal. (**b**) Tibial cut with a saw blade

## Femur Reconstruction

- Start with a posterior capsular release.
- Distal, anterior, and posterior femoral bone cuts in succession (Fig. 25.16a–f).
- Address any osseous defects. Consider the use of:
  - Cement
  - A modular augmentation wedge block (Fig. 25.17)
  - An allograft (cancellous or structural cortical)
- In most cases, use a femoral stem extension (Fig. 25.18).
- Assess trial femoral and tibial components (Fig. 25.19).

## Patella Reconstruction

- Following component insertion, check patella tracking.
- If maltracking is noted, try to establish the problem and consider:
  - Lateral release
  - Alter femoral and tibial component position
  - Patellar ligament lengthening or tibial tubercle advancement
  - Patelloplasty
- Using a prosthetic patellar component depends on patellar position and bone stock. Contradictions are insufficient bone stock (<10 mm) or of very poor quality.

## Implant Selection

- Choose the correct size of components:
  - Preoperatively:
    Notes from previous procedure
    Template the opposite site/guide only
  - Intraoperatively:
    Size of removed components.
    For femur, you can use epicondylar width.
    Trial reduction to assess stability, flexion–extension gap, patella tracking, and range of movements (Fig. 25.19).

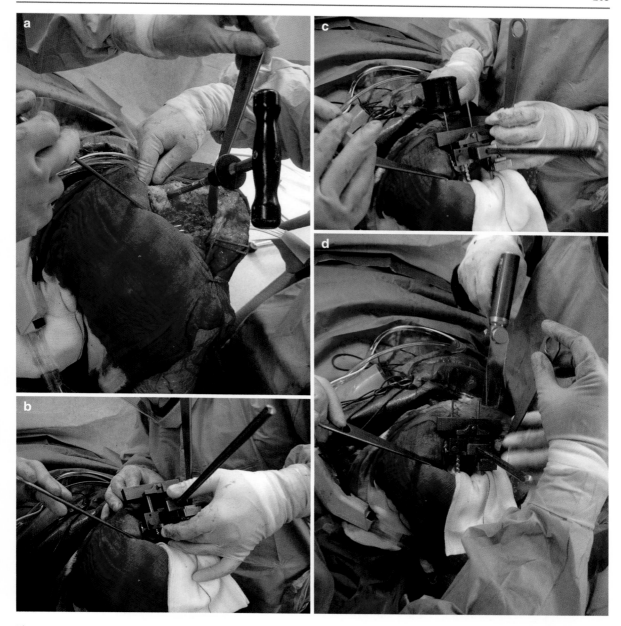

**Fig. 25.16** (**a**) Introduction of stem in femoral medullary canal. (**b**) Placement of femoral resection block for the distal cut. (**c**) Fixation of the femoral resection block with pins. (**d**) Distal femoral cut with a saw blade. (**e**) Placement of femoral resection block for the anterior and posterior cut. (**f**) Posterior femoral cut with a saw blade. (**g**) Resection of femoral intracondylar bone stock

- Stem extensions:
  - In revision arthroplasty, it is preferable to use stem extensions (Fig. 25.18).
  - Advantages:
    Transfer stress from the proximal part of the tibia more distally
    Provide additional surface area for fixation
    Assist with component orientation

## Cement Use (Authors' Preference)

- Use pulse-lavage irrigation to remove fat and debris from the cut surfaces and the medullary canals of the femur and tibia prior to cementation (Fig. 25.20).
- Dry surface must be obtained to provide an optimal surface for cement injection.
- The tibia is cemented first:

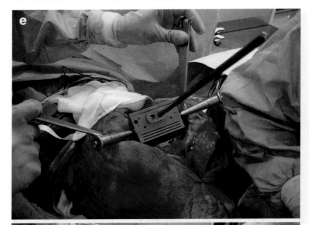

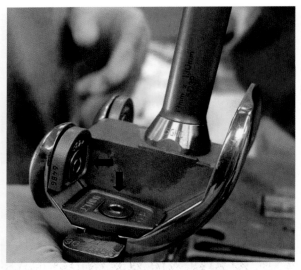

**Fig. 25.17** Modular augmentation wedge blocks at the femoral component (black arrows)

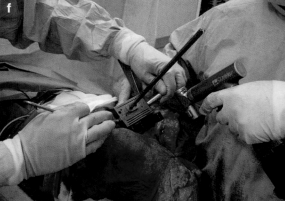

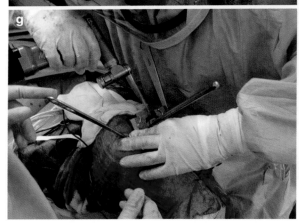

**Fig. 25.16** (continued)

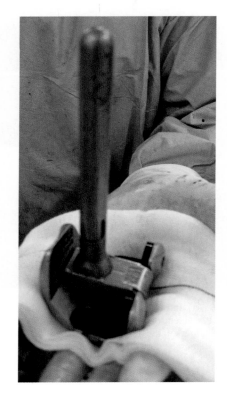

**Fig. 25.18** Femoral stem extension

- Insertion of cement restrictor (Fig. 25.21).
- Cement is applied intramedullary and at the tibial surface with a cement gun (Fig. 25.22a, b).
- Cement is also placed evenly to the tibial component,
  and it is then delivered on to the tibia (Fig. 25.23a).
- Excess of cement released from the interfaces
  removed (Fig. 25.23b).

- Assess final position of tibial component
  (Fig. 25.24).
- Femoral component cemented in a similar fashion
  (Fig. 25.25).

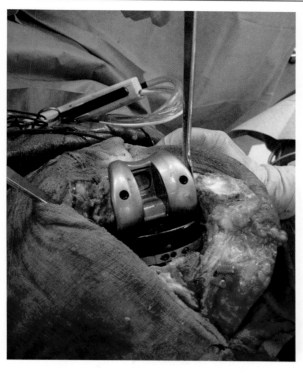

**Fig. 25.19** Trial femoral and tibial components with a trial polyethylene insert in place

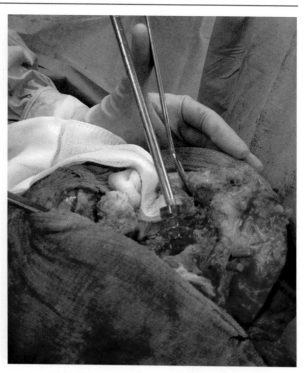

**Fig. 25.21** Insertion of cement restrictor into the tibial medullary canal

- The knee is extended (Fig. 25.26). One size bigger plastic trial may be used at this stage to maximize cement penetration. Excess of cement removed.
- Patella if replaced, cemented accordingly.
- Assess final components (Fig. 25.27a, b).

## Closure

- Irrigation.
- Infiltration with local anesthetic and epinephrine.
- Drain.
- Closure in layers: deep fascia with PDS 0 or 1, subcutaneous tissues with Vicryl 2/0, and skin with either staples or nonabsorbable sutures. It is advisable for interrupted sutures.
- Wound is covered with a bulky dressing – wool and crepe – that is reduced few days after surgery.
- Tourniquet is deflated, and drain is opened.

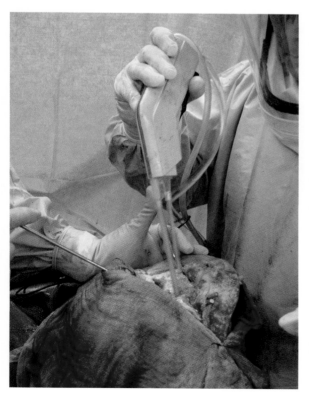

**Fig. 25.20** Pulse-lavage irrigation to remove fat and debris from the cut surfaces and the medullary canals prior to cementation

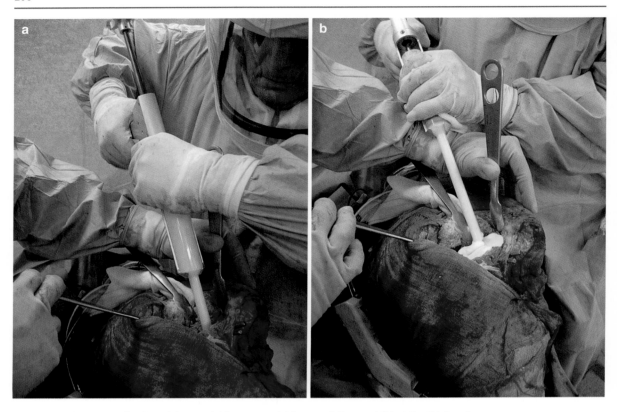

**Fig. 25.22** Cement application with a special instrument (**a**) intramedullary and (**b**) at the tibial surface

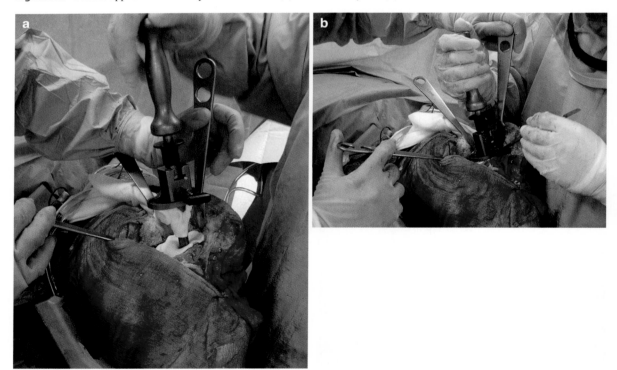

**Fig. 25.23** (**a**) Insertion of tibial component. (**b**) Removal of excess of cement from tibial component

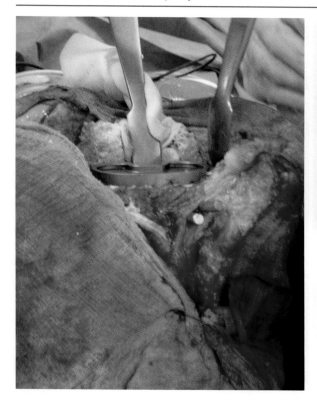

**Fig. 25.24** Final position of tibial component

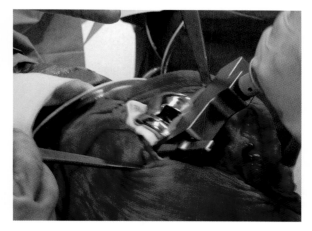

**Fig. 25.25** Insertion of femoral component after insertion of cement restrictor into the femoral medullary canal

## Tips and Tricks

- Reconstruct tibial surface first and then the femoral surface.
- Femoral component rotation is determined by identification of epicondylar axis. Usually, for correct

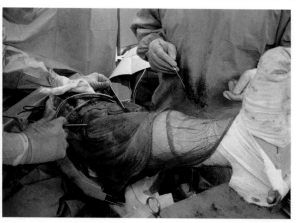

**Fig. 25.26** Knee extension during cement setting

femoral component rotation, augmentation of posterolateral condyle is essential.
- Recreate the joint line as close to the anatomic state as possible. Landmarks available:
  - The fibular head (1 cm above)
  - The inferior pole of the patella (1 cm below)
  - The lateral epicondyle (2.5 cm below)
  - The medial epicondyle (3 cm below)
- Create equal flexion and extension gaps. To address any imbalance, see Table 25.1.
- Bone loss management:
  - Depends on whether it is contained or not and to the size of the defect (small <5 mm, intermediate 5–10 mm, and large >10 mm)
    <5 mm + contained: cement or morselized bone graft
    >10 mm + contained: autogenous bone graft or allograft
    <5 mm + uncontained: cement
    5–10 mm + uncontained: modular wedges
    >10 mm + uncontained: modular augments or structural allografts

## Postoperative Care

- Observe blood loss and requirements for analgesia.
- Monitor vascular and neurological status of the leg.
- Check X-rays (Fig. 25.28a, b) and FBC.
- Start mechanical VTE prophylaxis at admission. Continue mechanical VTE prophylaxis until the patient no longer has significantly reduced mobility. Start pharmacological VTE prophylaxis after surgery.

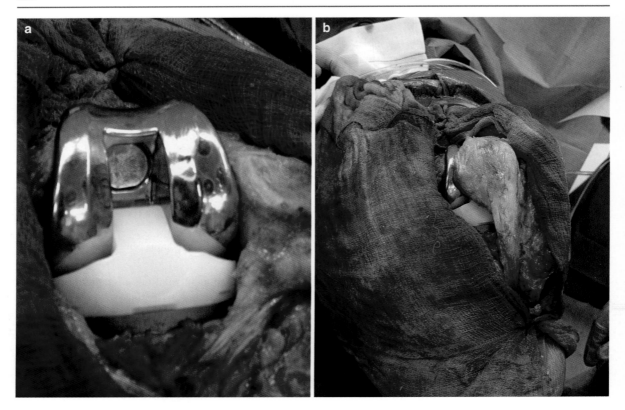

**Fig. 25.27** (**a**, **b**) Final components in place

**Table 25.1** Treatment algorithm of flexion–extension gap imbalance

| Flexion | Extension | Action |
|---------|-----------|--------|
| Tight | Tight | • Downsize tibial component thickness |
| Tight | Ok | • If femoral component is positioned posteriorly at the sagittal plane, use an offset femoral stem extension (care not to overstuff patellofemoral joint)<br>• Downsize femoral component |
| Tight | Loose | • If femoral component is positioned posteriorly at the sagittal plane, use an offset femoral stem extension (care not to overstuff patellofemoral joint) and use a thicker tibial component<br>• Downsize femoral component and use a thicker tibial component<br>• Augment distal femur and use a thinner tibial component |
| Ok | Tight | • Resect more distal femur or reduce distal femoral augmentation<br>• Release posterior capsule |
| Ok | Loose | • Augment distal femur |
| Loose | Tight | • If femoral component is positioned anteriorly at the sagittal plane, use an offset femoral stem extension<br>• Resect more distal femur or reduce distal femoral augmentation<br>• Upsize femoral component size<br>• Use a constrained prosthesis<br>• Collateral ligament reconstruction |
| Loose | Ok | • Advance femoral component proximally and use a thicker tibial component |
| Loose | Loose | • Use a thicker tibial component |

**Fig. 25.28** (**a**) AP and (**b**) lateral postoperative X-rays

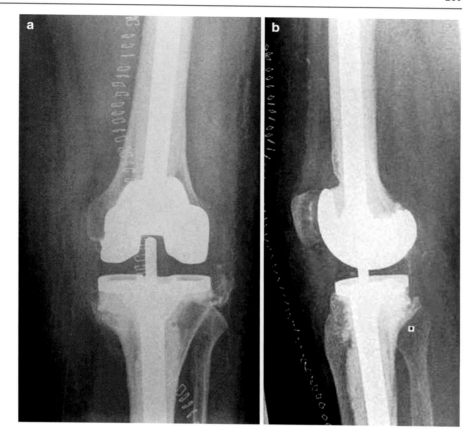

Continue pharmacological VTE prophylaxis for 10–14 days.

- Mobilize weight-bearing and start ROM exercises with physiotherapist as early as possible, usually 1 day after surgery. Zimmer frame is helpful at this stage.
- Alter postoperative mobilization protocol in case of questionable fixation of tibial tubercle osteotomy (limit motion and quadriceps exercise for 6–8 weeks).

## Complications

- Wound healing
- Infection
- Fractures
- Patella clunk syndrome
- Stiffness
- Thromboembolism
- Extensor mechanism rupture
- Instability and flexion–extension inequality
- Neurovascular injury

## Follow-up

- Patients are assessed clinically and radiographically at 3, and 12 months and every 5 years thereafter, unless at GP's request. Ideally, indefinite follow up is required.

## Further Reading

Jacofsky DJ, Della Valle CJ, Meneghini RM, Sporer SM, Cercek RM. Revision total knee arthroplasty: What the practicing orthopaedic surgeon needs to know". J Bone Joint Surg Am. 2010;92:1282–92.

Lewallen DG, Fehring TK, Dennis DA, Scuderi GR. Revision total knee arthroplasty: surgical techniques. J Bone Joint Surg Am. 2009;91 Suppl 5:69–71.

Lonner JH, Fehring TK, Hanssen AD, Pellegrini Jr VD, Padgett DE, Wright TM, et al. Revision total knee arthroplasty: the preoperative evaluation. J Bone Joint Surg Am. 2009;91 Suppl 5:64–8.

Mulhall KJ, Ghomrawi HM, Scully S, Callaghan JJ, Saleh KJ. Current etiologies and modes of failure in total knee arthroplasty revision. Clin Orthop Relat Res. 2006;446:45–50.

Nice clinical guideline 92 – Venous thromboembolism: reducing the risk. Reducing the risk of venous thromboembolism (deep vein thrombosis and pulmonary embolism) in patients admitted to hospital. (www.nice.org.uk/guidance/CG92) Accessed Jan 2010.

# Tibial Shaft Nonunion: Exchange Nailing

# 26

Peter V. Giannoudis and Theodoros I. Tosounidis

## Indications

- Tibial diaphyseal symptomatic aseptic nonunions.
- Tibial diaphyseal asymptomatic aseptic nonunions (after consultation with the patient).
- Tibial diaphyseal septic nonunions (temporary antibiotic-impregnated polymethylmethecrylate followed by permanent nail) (two-stage operation).
- Correctable alignment.

## Preoperative Planning

### Clinical Assessment

- Complete patient history. Age, occupation, past medical history, general health status (systematic diseases such as diabetes), nutritional status, medications, habits (such as smoking and drug abuse), previous fractures, and their "history until union."
- Complete injury history. Events surrounding the initial injury such as number of other fractures, open fracture, classification of the fracture, and trauma at other body areas (polytrauma). Treatment of the initial fracture: find the previous file of the patient and the surgical notes.

P.V. Giannoudis (✉)
Academic Department of Trauma and Orthopaedic Surgery,
School of Medicine, University of Leeds, Leeds, UK
e-mail: pgiannoudi@aol.com

T.I. Tosounidis
Department of Trauma and Orthopaedic Surgery,
Leeds Teaching Hospitals NHS Trust,
Leeds, UK

- Perform a complete physical examination of the patient (identify signs of systematic diseases that may inhibit fracture healing).
- Perform a thorough examination of the extremity (deformity and alignment of the limb, gross instability, skin condition, draining sinuses, signs of underlying infection, checking and documentation of the neurovascular status of the extremity, measurement and documentation of limb length, identification of previous wounds and incisions, and examination of the neighboring joints and the contralateral limb).

### Imaging Assessment

- Anteroposterior, lateral and oblique radiographs including knee and ankle joints to identify nonunion morphology (Fig. 26.1a, b).
- In the presence of deformity, perform a scanogram compare the limbs.
- Document bone loss and bone deformity.
- In elusive cases, perform a high-resolution CT of the nonunion site.
- Try to clearly define the plane of nonunion.
- In suspected infection, an MRI can determine the bone involvement.
- A bone scan and a radiolabel white cell scan can be helpful.

### Laboratory Tests

- Routine labs (FBC and biochemistry).
- In suspected infection, evaluate the ESR and CRP.

P.V. Giannoudis (ed.), *Practical Procedures in Elective Orthopaedic Surgery*,
DOI 10.1007/978-0-85729-814-0_26, © Springer-Verlag London Limited 2012

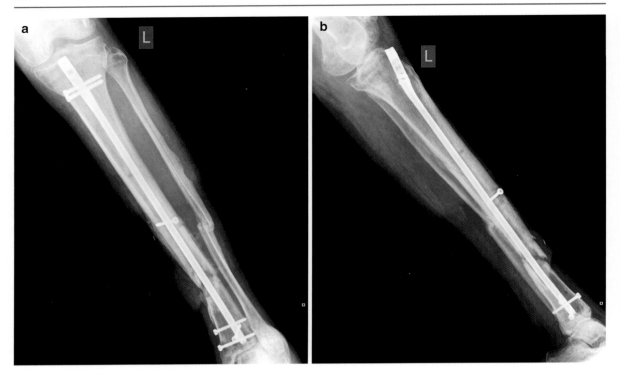

Fig. 26.1 (a) AP and (b) lateral x-rays of a tibial shaft nonunion

## Classifying the Nonunion and Planning for Action

- Infected vs noninfected nonunions.
- Hypertrophic vs oligotrophic vs atrophic.
- Determine the biologic potential of the nonunion, e.g., hypertrophic nonunions are characterized by their normal biologic potential, but are biomechanically unstable.
- Check from the patient's records the size of the nail that was used and estimate the size of the exchange nail. Usually, the exchange nail should be at least 1–2 mm larger in diameter.
- Plan for grafting procedures or fibula osteotomy.
- Familiarize yourself with the available equipment and inform the operating theater personnel about your plan of action.
- If necessary, consult a more experienced colleague.

## Operative Treatment

### Anesthesia

- Regional (spinal/epidural) and/or general anesthesia.
- Administration of prophylactic antibiotics is held before the acquisition of intraoperative cultures.

## Table and Equipment

- Nail removal set or screw removal set for locked screws.
- Locked nailing set. All implants and instruments should be available (Fig. 26.2a, b).
- Nailing on flat table (performing a nailing on flat table is technically more demanding).
- Check that additional material such as BMP or other grafts are available.
- Image intensifier and experienced radiographer.
- If a tourniquet is used, it is advisable to be inflated up to 350 mmHg.

### Advantages of Nailing Table

- Can be performed with relatively little need of a surgical assistant.
- The knee can be flexed to 90–110°.
- Tibial traction is constantly maintained.
- The reduction is maintained.

### Disadvantages of Nailing Table

- The debridement of the nonunion site is more difficult.

**Fig. 26.2** The tray with (**a**) the tibial nails and (**b**) instruments. It is appropriate to insert a nail bigger by 2 mm than the extracted

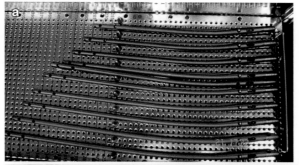

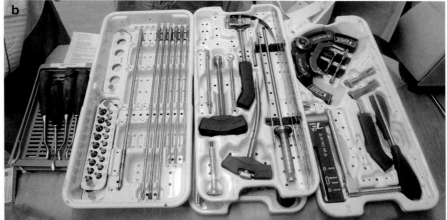

- Excessive traction may inadvertently be applied, and consequently, the incidence of compartment syndrome is increased.

## Table Setup

- Scrub nurse and instrumentation on the same side of non-united lower extremity.
- Image intensifier and radiographer across the operating side.
- Check that anteroposterior and lateral view can be readily performed and that there is ample space for the image intensifier to move freely.

## Draping

- If you use a flat table, place a radiolucent bolster or triangle under the distal thigh.
- The entire area from lower thigh to submalleolar region should be prepped with an antiseptic solution.
- If you are planning for a graft application procedure, prep and drape the area for bone harvesting accordingly (see bone harvesting procedures).

- Four large drapes around foot and lower thigh and over other leg are cautiously placed. Place a large drape at the opposite site to protect from the image intensifier when performing lateral x-rays.
- Place sterile cover over head of C-arm.
- Tourniquet not required. If used, deflate it while exposing the nonunion site for distinguishing the vital bone from the nonvital.

## Removing Previous Implants

- In the case of a fracture treated initially with a nail, remove the distal and proximal locking screws utilizing the previous stab incisions. Through the previous knee incision (either longitudinal or transverse), approach the proximal part of the nail. Remove the end cap. Mount the extraction handle onto the nail and use a hammer to gently tap backwards (Fig. 26.3).
- After nail removal, intramedullary irrigation with sterile saline solutions using either a syringe or a bag (Fig. 26.4a, b).
- Find the plane of nonunion. Use a rongeur or an osteotome or a curette to debride the nonunion (Fig. 26.5).
- Perform meticulous elevation of the periosteum.

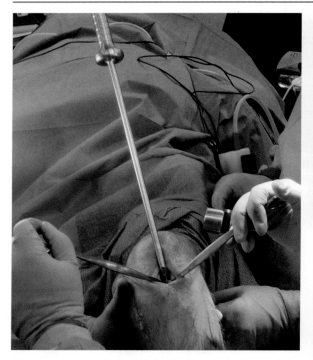

**Fig. 26.3** Removal of the nail using the nail extractor

- Send intraoperative tissue sample from the non-union site for microbiology and histology to detect indolent infection.
- Irrigate copiously the nonunion area with adequate amount of normal saline.
- AVOID devitalizing the nonunion site.

## Surgical Approach

- Longitudinal approach
  - 8–10-cm incision from tibial tuberosity to patella
  - Crosses Langer's lines
  - Risk of damage to lateral geniculate nerve
  - Easier exposure
- Transverse approach
  - 6–8-cm incision halfway between joint line and tibial tuberosity
  - Parallel to Langer's lines (heals better)
  - No nerve damage
  - Transverse incision recommended
- Subcutaneous dissection. 1.5–2-cm longitudinal incision just medial to patellar tendon, down to bone (some surgical techniques require the insertion of the nail through the patellar tendon).

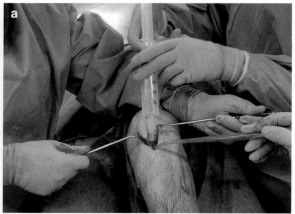

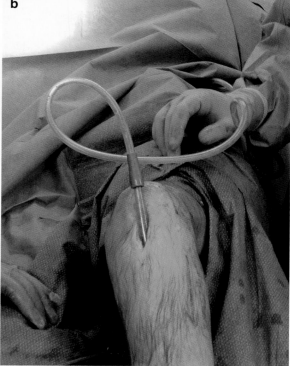

**Fig. 26.4** (**a**) Intramedullary irrigation with sterile saline solutions using a syringe. (**b**) Aspiration of washout solution

## Surgical Technique

### Initial Instrumentation

- Insert small pre-bent hand reamer into proximal intramedullary canal and breach the proximal tibial metaphysis.

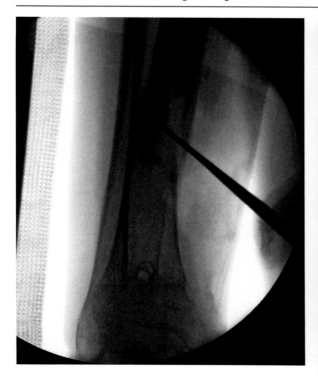

**Fig. 26.5** The nonunion site is prepared by removing the non-vital tissues with a curette

- Insert the ball-tipped guide wire down to the intramedullary canal.
- Check the trajectory of the guide wire in both AP and lateral views as this is passed through the proximal tibia canal. Check the position of the guide wire just before you advance it at nonunion site. Varus or valgus angulation and deformities can be reduced by a laterally or medially applied force, poller screws, or manipulation of the fracture parts with Schanz screws.
- Reinsert the guide wire if it is not central in the distal tibia. If it cannot be centralized, use a bent olive-tipped guide wire. Rotate under intensifier control to centralize guide wire.
- The guide wire should be central in AP and lateral planes.

## Reaming (Fig. 26.6a, b)

- Ream in 0.5-mm increments. Confirm with image intensifier that the tibia is reduced when the reamer passes the nonunion.

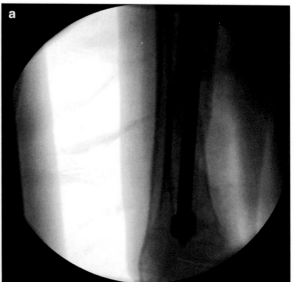
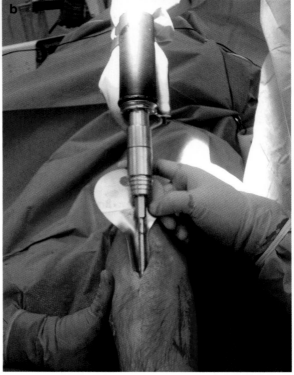

**Fig. 26.6 (a, b)** The tibial medullary canal is reamed; it is advisable to use the reaming products only if infection is excluded

- Ream at least 2 mm more than the size of the initial nail.
- The exchange nail should be at least 2 mm wider, larger than the initial nail.

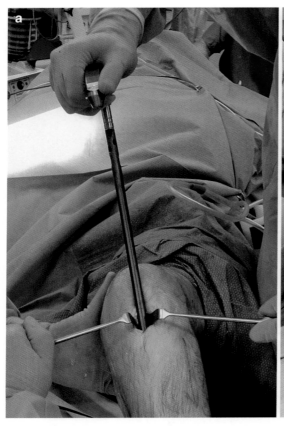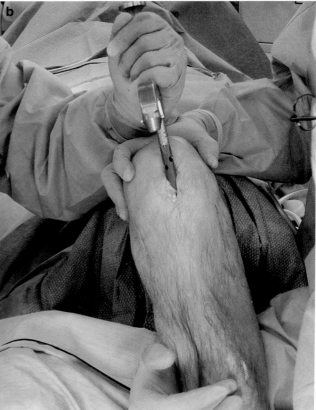

**Fig. 26.7** (**a, b**) The new nail is inserted

- Use sharp reamers. Do not forcefully advance the reamer. Ream slowly and gradually to avoid thermal necrosis and the reamer becoming stuck.
- Ream the full length of the nail.

## Nailing

- Change guide wire if so needed according to manufacturer's instructions. Use the exchange tube to insure correct reposition of the guide wire.
- Calculate length of nail. Usually, a measuring device is supplied, but the guide wire can be measured. Take into account the biomechanics of the nonunion and any previous overdistraction in order to apply compression at the nonunion, utilizing the appropriate nail length.
- Tightly mount the nail to the introducer.
- Insert the nail into the tibia. Avoid rotation of the nail as this often makes the correct insertion of the nail at the distal tibia more difficult (Fig. 26.7a, b).

- Check that the nonunion is reduced before the nail is passed.
- Do not overcountersink the nail and do not forcefully tap it.
- Check the nail length on image intensifier.
- Insert at least two proximal cross screws utilizing the appropriate jig (Fig. 26.8a, b).

## Distal Screw Insertion: Free-Hand Technique
(Fig. 26.9a, b, c)

- Align C-arm exactly at 90° to the leg.
- Rotate table and patient if required.
- Adjust image intensifier so the screw holes in nail appear as perfect circles.
- Insert cross screws from medial side to avoid fibula.
- Place sharp point on skin so that it is central in one of the screw holes.
- Make 1-cm skin incision.

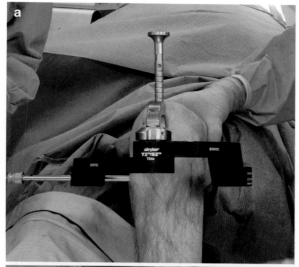

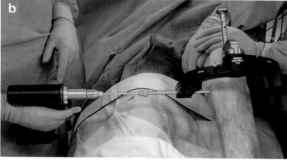

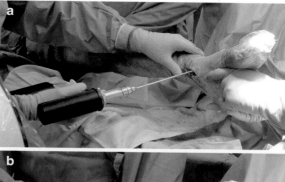

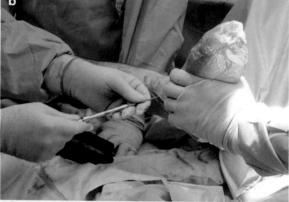

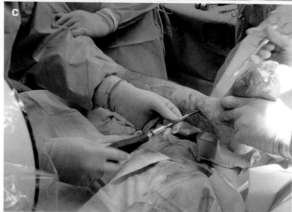

Fig. 26.8 (a, b) The proximal locking is performed with the specific targeting device. Make sure that the nail holder is locked firmly over the nail and the targeting devise is calibrated prior to the insertion of the nail

- Replace sharp point on bone to appear in center of screw hole.
- Make a divot or screw hole in bone in line with C-arm.
- Complete screw hole.
- Measure screw length.
- Insert screw(s).

Fig. 26.9 (a) Free-hand drilling of distal holes. (b) Screw length measurement and (c) screw insertion

## Bone Grafting (see Bone Graft Harvesting Procedures)

- Intramedullary grafting. Deliver bone graft into the canal at the site of nonunion.
- Posterolateral grafting. Use the posterolateral approach at the site of nonunion. Make a longitudinal incision of adequate length just posterior to the fibula. Identify and protect the cutaneus branch of the peroneal nerve.

The plane is between the peroneal muscles and the superficial posterior compartment. The soleus is detached from the fibula (beware of the peroneal artery). Detach tibialis posterior from the intraosseous membrane. Apply the bone graft to tibia.

- After debridement of the nonunion site (Fig. 26.10a, b), perform open bone grafting (place autologous bone graft or products of reaming at the site of the nonunion or growth factors) (Fig. 26.11a). Apply the graft material subperiosteally. Carefully contain the graft into a bone-periosteal envelope (Fig. 26.11b, c).

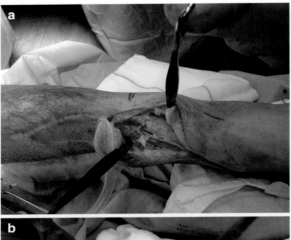

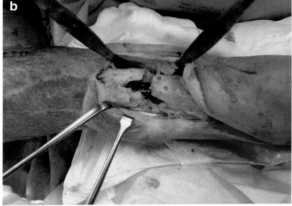

Fig. 26.10 (a) The nonunion site and (b) after the debridement

## Closure

- Continuous or interrupted suturing with Vicryl 0 or 1 for the patellar tendon.
- No subcutaneous sutures are needed although they are often used.
- Staples, nonabsorbable sutures, or subcuticular suturing are used (Fig. 26.12a, b).
- Replace compartment monitor after nailing operation is finished.

## Postoperative Treatment

- Anteroposterior and lateral x-rays (Fig. 26.13a, b).
- Monitor the neurovascular status for possible compartment syndrome.
- Remove compartment monitor when compartment pressure stabilizes.

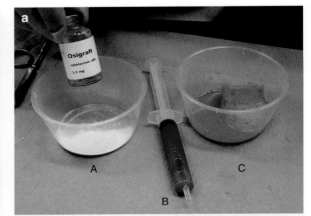

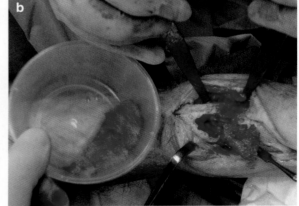

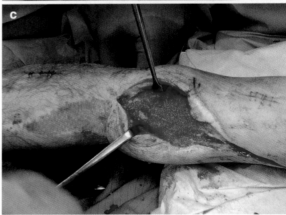

Fig. 26.11 (a) Bone grafts (A = BMP-7, B = concentrated bone marrow aspirate containing MSC, C = RIA graft). (b) Application of grafts. (c) Nonunion site after bone graft application

- Two further doses of prophylactic antibiotics. Chase the results of tissue samples taken intraoperatively and act accordingly.

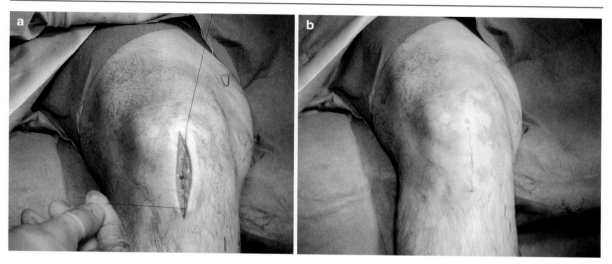

**Fig. 26.12** (**a, b**) Continuous suturing is an option for the skin closure

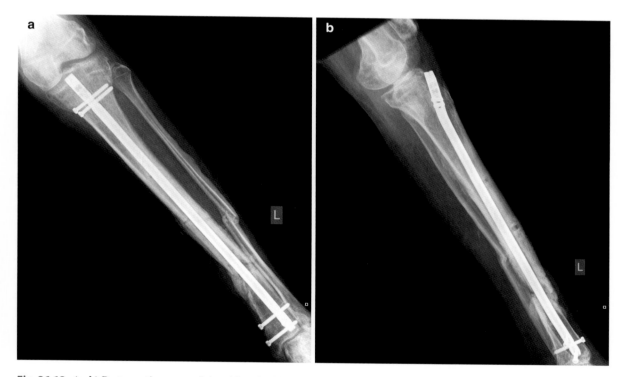

**Fig. 26.13** (**a, b**) Postoperative x-rays. It is evident the bigger thickness of the nail

- Start mechanical VTE prophylaxis at admission and continue until the patient no longer has significantly reduced mobility, based on an assessment of risks. Start pharmacological VTE prophylaxis after surgery and continue until the patient no longer has significantly reduced mobility.

**Postoperative Rehabilitation**

- Mobilize weight-bearing as pain allows.
- There is no need for cast as this only adds to stiffness.
- Physiotherapy may be required particularly in older patients.

## Outpatient Follow-up

- Follow up at 2 weeks with AP and lateral radiographs of tibia.
- Thereafter, follow up every 4 weeks.
- Union rates of 95–100% have been reported in association with reamed nailing for tibial nonunions.
- Discharge after union.

## Implant Removal

- Mainly removed because of knee pain.
- No other good reason to remove tibial nails.

## Further Reading

Court-Brown CM, Keating JF, Christie J, McQueen MM. Exchange intramedullary nailing. Its use in aseptic tibial nonunion. J Bone Joint Surg Br. 1995;77(3):407–11.

Zelle BA, Gruen GS, Klatt B, Haemmerle MJ, Rosenblum WJ, Prayson MJ. Exchange reamed nailing for aseptic nonunion of the tibia. J Trauma. 2004;57(5):1053–9.

Wiss DA, Stetson WB. Tibial nonunion: treatment alternatives. J Am Acad Orthop Surg. 1996;4(5):249–57.

Richmond J, Colleran K, Borens O, Kloen P, Helfet DL. Nonunions of the distal tibia treated by reamed intramedullary nailing. J Orthop Trauma. 2004;18(9):603–10.

# Tibial Shaft Nonunion: Plating

# 27

Peter V. Giannoudis, Theodoros I. Tosounidis, and George M. Kontakis

## Indications

- Tibial diaphyseal symptomatic aseptic nonunions.
- Tibial diaphyseal asymptomatic aseptic nonunions (after consultation with the patient).
- Tibial nonunion with closed intramedullary canal.
- Stiff tibial nonunions.
- Need for bone graft application, e.g., for atrophic nonunions or to address the biomechanics of a nonunion e.g., hypertrophic nonunions.

## Preoperative Planning

### Clinical Assessment

- Complete patient history. Age, occupation, past medical history, general health status (systematic diseases such as diabetes), nutritional status, medications, habits (such as smoking and drug abuse), previous fractures, and their "history until union."

P.V. Giannoudis (✉)
Academic Department of Trauma and Orthopaedic Surgery, School of Medicine, University of Leeds, Leeds, UK
e-mail: pgiannoudi@aol.com

T.I. Tosounidis
Department of Trauma and Orthopaedic Surgery, Leeds Teaching Hospitals NHS Trust, Leeds, UK

G.M. Kontakis
Academic Department of Trauma and Orthopaedic Surgery, School of Medicine, University of Crete, Crete, Greece

- Complete injury history. Events surrounding the initial injury, such as the number of other fractures, open fracture, classification of the fracture, trauma at other body areas (polytrauma). Treatment of the initial fracture: find the previous file of the patient and the surgical notes.
- Perform a complete physical examination of the patient (identify signs of systematic diseases that may inhibit fracture healing).
- Perform a thorough examination of the extremity (deformity and alignment of the limb, gross instability, skin condition, draining sinuses, signs of underlying infection, check and document the neurovascular status of the extremity, measurement and documentation of limb length, identification of previous wounds and incisions, and examination of the neighboring joints and the contralateral limb).

## Imaging Assessment

- Anteroposterior and lateral and oblique radiographs including knee and ankle joints to identify nounion morphology (Fig. 27.1).
- In the presence of deformity, perform a scanogram and compare the films.
- Establish the true plane of nonunion so that you can plan your incision-plate placement accordingly.
- Document bone loss and bone deformity.
- In elusive cases, perform a high-resolution CT of the nonunion site.
- In suspected infection, perform an MRI can determine the bone involvement. A bone scan and a radiolabeled white-cell scan can be helpful.

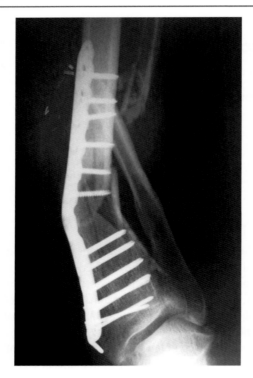

**Fig. 27.1** A preoperative X-ray of an atrophic nonunion with a broken plate

## Laboratory Tests

- Routine labs (FBC and biochemistry).
- In suspected infection, evaluate the ESR and CRP.

## Classify the Nonunion and Plan for Action

- Infected vs noninfected nonunions.
- Hypertrophic vs oligotrophic vs atrophic.
- Determine the biologic potential of the nonunion, e.g., hypertrophic nonunions are characterized by their normal biologic potential, but mechanical instability.
- Check from the patient's records the materials which were used in the primary operation (type and characteristics of nail or plate) and plan accordingly for removal if so needed.
- Plan for grafting procedures or fibula osteotomy.
- Familiarize yourself with the available equipment, and inform the operating theater personnel about your plan of action.
- If necessary, consult a more experienced colleague.

## Operative Treatment

### Anesthesia

- Regional (spinal/epidural) and/or general anesthesia.
- At induction, administer prophylactic broad spectrum antibiotic. Usually second or third generation cephalosporin.
- In cases of infected nonunions, do not administer antibiotics at the induction to anesthesia.

### Table and Equipment

- Use a flat table.
- Nail removal set or screw and plate removal set. Remember that locked plates need special instrumentation.
- Full range of plates including 4.5-mm DCP, 4.5-mm LC-DCP and LCP. Use locking plates if considering proximal or distal tibial with metaphyseal involvement.
- Complete instrumentation available.
- Check that additional material, such as BMP or other grafts are available.
- Image intensifier and experienced radiographer.

### Table Setup

- Scrub nurse and instrumentation on side of affected limb.
- Image intensifier and radiographer across the operating site.
- Check that anteroposterior and lateral view can be readily performed and that there is ample space for the image intensifier to move freely.

### Draping

- If you are planning for an autologous bone-harvesting procedure, prep and drape the harvesting donor site accordingly (see bone harvesting procedures).
- Place a tourniquet at the thigh and inflate it if needed.
- The entire area from toes to groin should be prepped with an antiseptic solution.

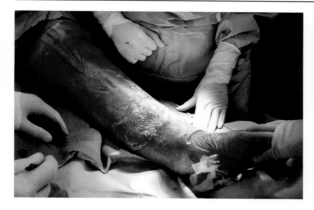

Fig. 27.2 Skin preparation and covering of the toes with a sterile drape

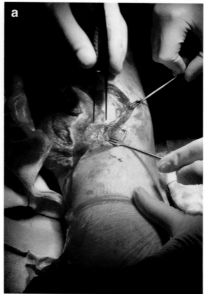

- Four large drapes around foot and lower thigh and over other leg should be placed cautiously (Fig. 27.2). Place a large drape at the opposite site to protect from the image intensifier when performing lateral x-rays.
- Sterile cover over head of C-arm.

**Remove Previous Implants**
- In the case of an initial plate osteosynthesis, utilize the previous incision(s) to remove the screws and the plate (Fig. 27.3a–c). Remember that the locking plates/screws need specialized instruments for removal.

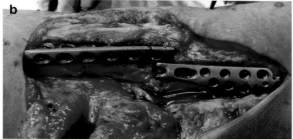

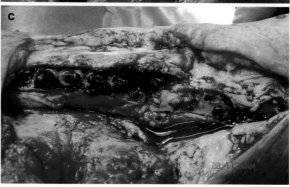

Fig. 27.3 (a) Skin incision over the previous one, removing also the scar of the first operation. (b) The broken plate is exposed completely, and (c) removed

**Surgical Technique**

**Approach and Exposure of Nonunion**

- The approach is preferably determined by the true plane of the nonunion.
- Most of the times the classical anterior tibial approach is used.
- Incision is placed 1–2 cm lateral to the crest of the tibia. Proximally, it curves laterally toward the head of the fibula, and, distally, it curves toward the medial malleolus.
- The length of the incision is determined from the nonunion morphology and the plate that will be used.
- Extend the incision so that you can have enough space to mobilize the nonunion.

- Sharp dissection down to fascia without raising skin flaps.
- Incise deep fascia.
- Use no-touch technique and sharp extraperiosteal dissection to mobilize the skin at the medial site if you need to apply the plate medially.

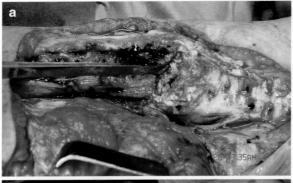

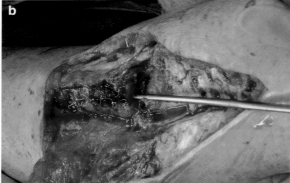

**Fig. 27.4** (**a**). The nonunion site is exposed and an osteotome is used to remove the non vital bone parts. (**b**) A hand reamer or a 2.5 mm drill is used to re-open the tibial medullar canal

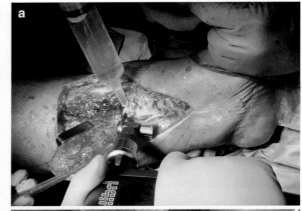

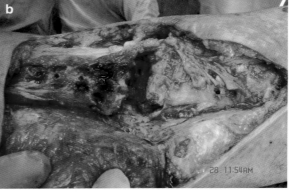

**Fig. 27.5** (**a**) An oscillating saw is often used for removing non vital bone. (**b**) The nonunion area is exposed completely and a vital bed is prepared for bone graft application + BMP

- Perform meticulous elevation of the periosteum if you are planning for bone grafting. Otherwise keep your dissection extraperiosteal.
- Find the plane of the nonunion.
- Debride the area around the nonunion. Remove preexisting fibrous tissue and dead bone. Use a rongeur or a currete or an osteotome appropriately (Fig. 27.4a, b).
- Sent intraoperative tissue sample for microbiology and histology to detect indolent infection.
- Irrigate copiously the nonunion area with adequate amount of normal saline (Fig. 27.5a, b).
- AVOID devitalizing the nonunion site.

## Stabilization of the Nonunion

- Follow standard osteosynthesis principles.
- Carefully realign the nonunion by the means of pointed reduction clamps or indirect techniques.
- The plate should ideally be placed at the tension site of nonunion (either laterally or medially). Most of the times, the lateral tibial surface is chosen due to its soft-tissue coverage.
- Insert a lag screw perpendicular to the plane of nonunion, if this is >30°.
- Apply a neutralization plate in a standard mode.
- If the plane of nonunion is <30º, apply a plate to compress the nonunion site.
- Prebend the LCD plate. The LC-DCP and the LCP plates do not need prebending.
- Insert the first screw at the center of the proximal hole at one site of nonunion. Eccentrically insert the second screw at the other site of nonunion.
- Insert the third screw eccentrically. Before tightening of this screw the adjacent screw at the same site needs to be loosened.
- Apply the rest of the screw centrically. You cannot achieve any additional compression.
- Usually six cortices at each fracture site suffice for adequate stability, (Fig. 27.6).

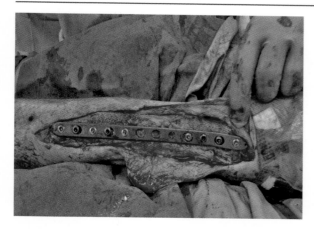

**Fig. 27.6** Tibial non-union stabilised with a locking plate

- If the fracture of nonunion is perpendicular to the tibial shaft, do not insert compression screw.
- If you use the LC-DCP or the LCP plating system, use the locking screws based on the quality of the bone. These plates are mostly advantageous in the treatment of metaphyseal nonunions.

## Bone Grafting (see Bone-Graft Harvesting Procedures)

- Posterolateral grafting. Use the posterolateral approach at the site of nonunion. Make a longitudinal incision of adequate length just posterior to the fibula. Identify and protect the cutaneus branch of the peroneal nerve. The plane is between the peroneal muscles and the superficial posterior compartment. The soleus is detached from the fibula (beware of the peroneal artery). Detach tibialis posterior from the intraosseous membrane. Apply the bone graft to tibia.
- Open bone grafting (place autologous bone graft or products of reaming or growth factors at the site of the nonunion). Apply the graft material subperiosteally. Carefully contain the graft into a bone–periosteal envelope.

## Closure

- No subcutaneous sutures are needed although they are often used.

- Staples, non-absorbable sutures, or subcuticular suturing used.
- Replace compartment monitor after nailing operation finished.

## Postoperative

- Neurovascular check for compartment syndrome.
- Start mechanical VTE prophylaxis at admission and continue until the patient has no longer significantly reduced mobility based on an assessment of risks. Start pharmacological VTE prophylaxis after surgery and continue until the patient no longer has significantly reduced mobility.
- Anteroposterior and lateral X-rays.
- Remove compartment monitor when compartment pressure stabilizes.
- Two further doses of prophylactic antibiotics. Chase the results of tissue samples taken intraoperatively and act accordingly.
- On the first postoperative day, the patient is treated with a hinged knee brace or a walking fracture boot, and continuous passive mobilization (CPM) is initiated. The rehabilitation protocol included gentle active and active assisted range of motion and touch-down weight-bearing under the close supervision of a physical therapist.
- There is no need for a cast, as this only adds to stiffness.

## Outpatient Follow-up

- Follow up at 2 weeks with AP and lateral radiographs of tibia, (Fig 27.7).
- Thereafter, follow up every 4 weeks.
- Union rates up to 100% have been reported in association with plating for tibial nonunions.
- Discharge after union.

## Implant Removal

- Implant removal is not justified in a routine basis.
- Implant can be removed if they irritate the surrounding soft tissues or according to patient's desire.

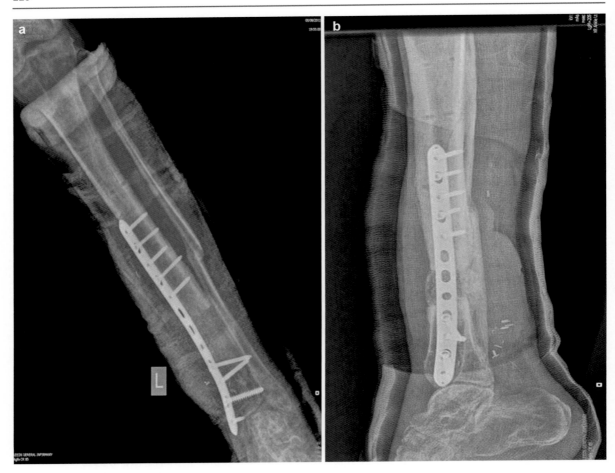

**Fig. 27.7** Post-operative radiographs, AP (**a**) and lateral (**b**) of the tibial non-union stabilised with plating (bone grafting seen in situ)

## Further Reading

Gardner MJ, Toro-Arbelaez JB, Hansen M, Boraiah S, Lorich DG, Helfet DL. Surgical treatment and outcomes of extraarticular proximal tibial nonunions. Arch Orthop Trauma Surg. 2008;128(8):833–9.

Wiss DA, Stetson WB. Tibial nonunion: treatment alternatives. J Am Acad Orthop Surg. 1996;4(5):249–57.

Wiss DA, Johnson DL, Miao M. Compression plating for nonunion after failed external fixation of open tibial fractures. J Bone Joint Surg Am. 1992;74(9):1279–85.

# Masquelet Technique for Distal Tibial Infected Non-union

### Peter V. Giannoudis

## Introduction

- The Masquelet technique implies the insertion of cement spacer loaded with or without antibiotics.
- Such an approach maintains the space of reconstruction.
- It facilitates the induction of a pseudo-synovial membrane.
- The membrane delivers growth factors.
- The membrane avoids the resorption of the bone graft and promotes the revascularization of the graft.

## Indications

- Non-unions aseptic or infected associated with bone defect more than 2 cm.

## Preoperative Planning

### Clinical Assessment

- Full history.
- Physical examination (assess leg length discrepancy, rotational deformity, mechanical axis).
- Assess state of soft tissue envelope and the need for reconstruction (Fig. 28.1a).
- Pus swab in case of active discharge – culture sensitivity.

- Evaluate the presence or absence of neuropathy.
- Presence of associated comorbidities.
- Request baseline blood investigations (FBC, U/Es, LFT, Clotting screen).
- CRP, ESR.

## Radiological Assessment

- Anteroposterior (AP) and lateral views of the tibial non-union (Fig. 28.2b, c) including the adjacent joints.
- Obtain long leg views to assess mechanical axis and the extent of the deformity.
- CT scan to evaluate the presence of sequestrum.
- MRI for soft tissue assessment and bone marrow state.

## Timing of Surgery

- Aseptic non-union of duration of more than 6–9 months.
- Active infection with discharge ± failure of metal work anytime following initial surgery, usually within 6–16 weeks or even longer.

## Operative Treatment

### Anesthesia

- Spinal or general anesthesia.
- Do not administer prophylactic antibiotic until tissue biopsies have been obtained.

P.V. Giannoudis
Academic Department of Trauma and Orthopaedic Surgery,
School of Medicine, University of Leeds, Leeds, UK
e-mail: pgiannoudi@aol.com

P.V. Giannoudis (ed.), *Practical Procedures in Elective Orthopaedic Surgery*,
DOI 10.1007/978-0-85729-814-0_28, © Springer-Verlag London Limited 2012

**Fig. 28.1** Soft tissue state on the non-union illustrating the deformity and the presence of erythema and active discharge due to underlying sepsis

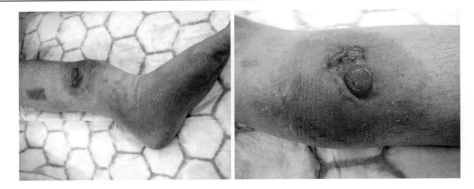

**Fig. 28.2** (**a**) AP X-ray of left distal tibial illustrating non-union with failure of the nail in situ. (**b**) Lateral X-ray of left distal tibial demonstrating the non-union and the broken nail

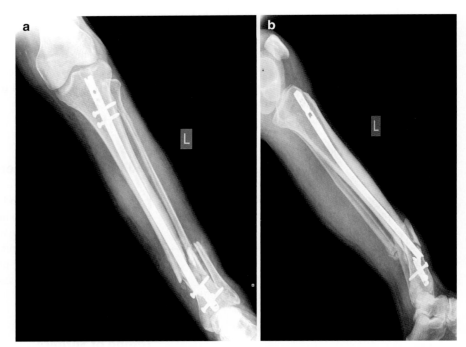

## Table and Equipment

- Appropriate extraction kit for removal of implant in situ.
- Any external fixator kit – Hoffman II Stryker.
- PMMA cement to be loaded with 2 g of vancomycin.
- Image intensifier and a competent radiographer.

## Table Setups

- The instrumentation is set up on the side of the operation and at the foot of the operating table.
- Image intensifier is from the contralateral side.
- Position the table diagonally across the operating room so that the operating area lies in the clean air field.

## Patient Positioning

- The patient is positioned supine on a radiolucent table.
- Place a pneumatic tourniquet and inflate if needed.

## Draping and Surgical Approach

### Part A: Removal of Implant, Debridement, Cement Spacer Implantation, and Induction of the Induced Membrane

- Prepare the skin over lower leg, ankle, and entire foot with usual antiseptic solutions (aqueous/alcoholic povidone–iodine). Prepare skin between toes thoroughly.
- Apply standard draping above knee.

**Fig. 28.3** (**a**) Using an S-shaped incision, necrotic skin edges and underlying necrotic subcutaneous tissue are removed. (**b**) Illustrating removal of dead bone from the infected non-union site

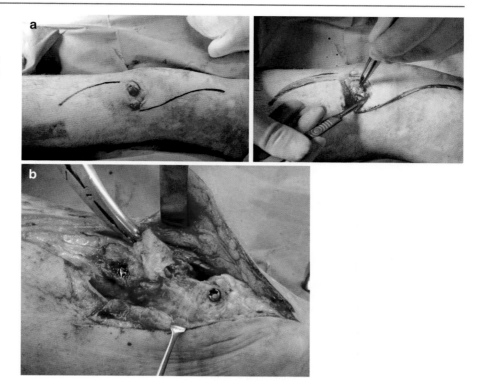

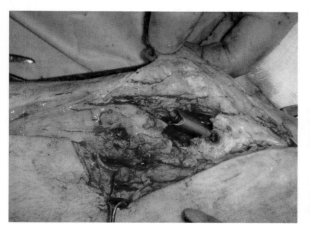

**Fig. 28.4** Distal broken part of the nail is retrieved from the canal

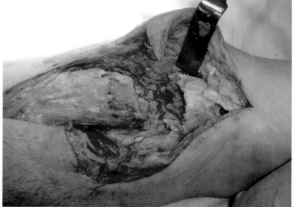

**Fig. 28.5** Following debridement, a healthy bed of the non-union site is shown

- Apply tape around toes to minimize the risk of infection.
- Use an S-shaped incision and remove necrotic skin edges and underlying necrotic subcutaneous tissue (Fig. 28.3a).
- Take tissue biopsies.
- Remove dead bone and exposed non-union site (Fig. 28.3b).
- Remove broken distal nail part with locking screws (Fig. 28.4).

- Irrigate area with 6 lit of warm Normal Saline solution (N/S).
- Bone edges of proximal and distal tibia should be healthy with a viable bleeding bed (Fig. 28.5).
- Incise previous midline incision at the level of the knee joint.
- Flex knee and identify entry point, remove end cap of nail.
- Screw extraction rod at the tip of the nail. Remove proximal locking screws and extract nail from intramedullary canal.

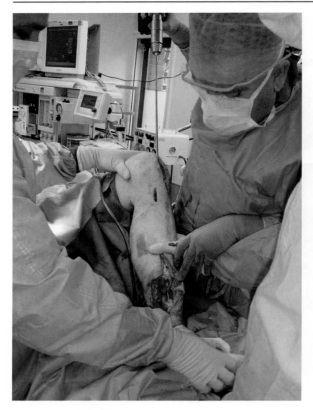

**Fig. 28.6** Reaming of the medullary canal for debridement is illustrated

- Ream tibial canal (for debridement) (Fig. 28.6) at least more that 2–3 mm of the previous reaming steps performed during the acute stabilization of the fracture with the nail.
- Irrigate intramedullary canal with 3–6 lit of N/S.
- Stabilize proximal and tibial non-union edges with external fixator, paying attention to restore the length and the rotation of the limb.
- Mix PMMA cement with the 2 g of vancomycin.
- Insert cement between the bone edges and make sure that part of the cement is inserted within the bone canal for better stability of the construct (Fig. 28.7a, b).
- Close wound with interrupted mattress 2/0 nylon sutures.

## Postoperative Care

- Elevate limb and watch neurovascular status.
- Chase microbiology results and start appropriate antibiotic treatment for a minimum of 6–8 weeks (max 12 weeks).

- Start mechanical VTE prophylaxis at admission and continue until the patient no longer has significantly reduced mobility, based on an assessment of risks. Start pharmacological VTE prophylaxis after surgery and continue until the patient no longer has significantly reduced mobility.
- Mobilize patient N/W bearing.
- Assess patient clinically and radiologically in the outpatient clinic at 2, 4, and 8 weeks.
- Readmit patient between 10 and 12 weeks for second-stage procedure.

## Part B: Removal of Cement Spacer, Grafting of the Defect, and Stabilization with Appropriate Implant

- Patient is positioned supine in a fracture table. The affected limb is placed on a leg support to keep it away from the operative field for harvesting of autologous RIA graft from the contralateral femur (Fig. 28.8) (autologous graft can be harvested also from the pelvis, but if a substantial volume is necessary, then consider the RIA option technique).
- Administer one dose of prophylactic antibiotics as per local hospital policy after acquisition of samples for culture has been obtained to exclude persistence of infection in previously infected cases.
- Following harvesting of the RIA graft, the affected limb is placed on the operating table.
- Using a brush, wash the pins sites with local antiseptic and remove external fixator prior to draping (Fig. 28.9).
- Patient positioning and draping is similar as previously described above.
- Incise previous incision and elevate the induced membrane (Fig. 28.10).
- Remove cement spacer while protecting the membrane (Fig. 28.11).
- Open the medullary canal proximally and distally with hand reamers.
- Irrigate and remove any nonvital tissue.
- Implant growth factor (BMP-7 on this occasion) inside the medullary canal and in the bed of the defect.
- Implant the RIA graft (Fig. 28.12).
- Close the induced membrane with 2/0 vicryl (Fig. 28.13) and apply locking plate under image

**Fig. 28.7** (**a**) Cement spacer between the bone edges is shown. (**b**) Postoperative radiographs AP and lateral showing stabilization of the non-union site with the external fixator and the cement spacer in situ.

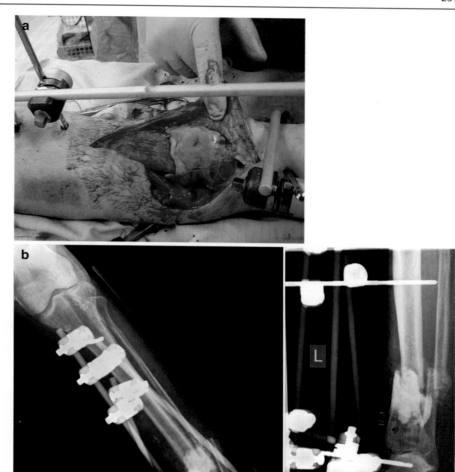

intensifier control (Fig. 28.14a, b). Pay attention to restore the length and the rotation of the limb.

- Closure of skin and subcutaneous tissue with 2/0 interrupted nylon sutures (Fig. 28.15).

## Postoperative Care

- Two more prophylactic doses of antibiotics are administered if intraoperative cultures are negative.
- Start mechanical VTE prophylaxis at admission and continue until the patient no longer has

significantly reduced mobility, based on an assessment of risks. Start pharmacological VTE prophylaxis after surgery and continue until the patient no longer has significantly reduced mobility.

- Apply a posterior splint with the foot in 90° dorsiflexion.
- Elevate the limb for a time period of 48 h.
- Carefully assess the neurovascular status of the extremity.
- Begin ankle motion only when the surgical wound has sealed and the soft tissue condition has improved.

**Fig. 28.8** The affected limb is placed on a leg support to keep it away from the operative field for harvesting of autologous RIA graft from the contralateral femur

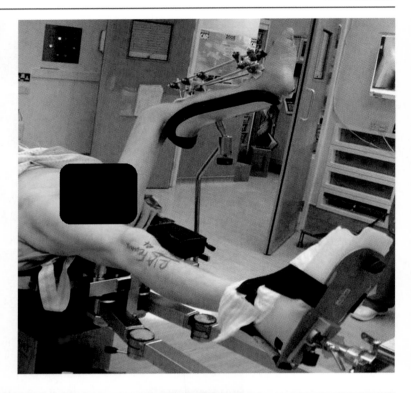

**Fig. 28.9** Using a brush, wash the pin sites with local antiseptic, and remove external fixator prior to draping

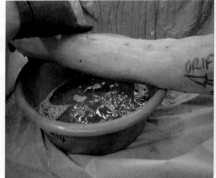
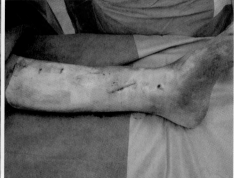

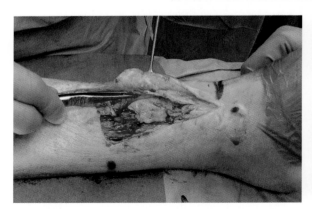

**Fig. 28.10** Elevation of the induced membrane is noted

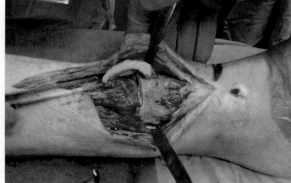

**Fig. 28.11** Cement spacer is removed while the induced membrane is protected

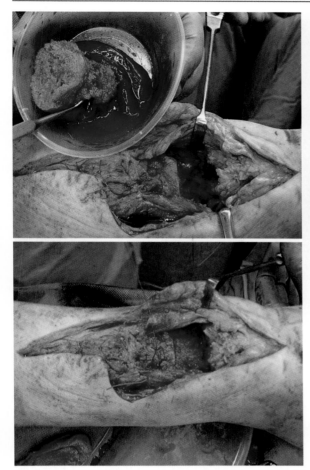

**Fig. 28.12**  Illustration of implantation of the RIA graft

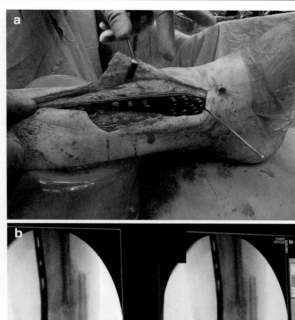

**Fig. 28.14**  (**a**) Intraoperative picture of stabilization of the non-union with locking plate. (**b**) Fluoroscopic images showing stabilization of the non-union with locking plate

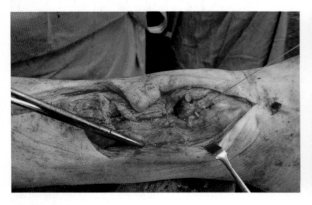

**Fig. 28.13**  Closure of the induced membrane is shown for containment of the graft

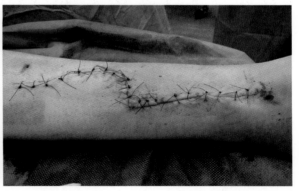

**Fig. 28.15**  Skin closure with interrupted 2/0 nylon sutures

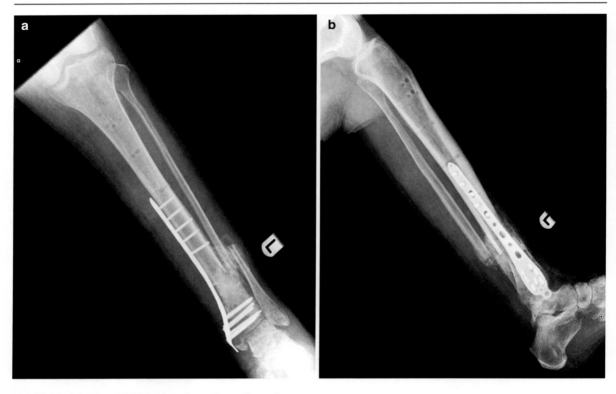

**Fig. 28.16** (**a**) AP and (**b**) lateral postoperative radiographs

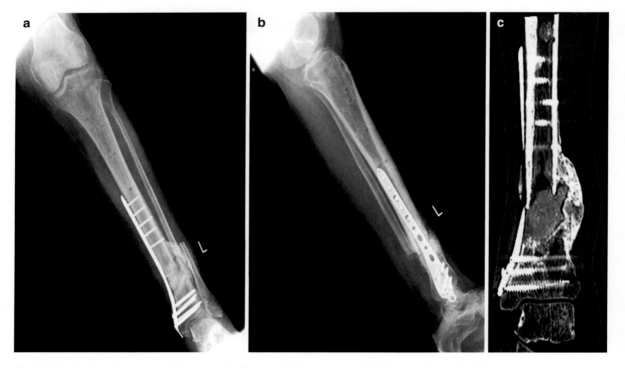

**Fig. 28.17** Radiological union is illustrated. (**a**) AP view. (**b**) Lateral view. (**c**) CT scan at 4 months follow up

## Outpatient Follow up

- Review in outpatient clinic after 2 weeks, with X-rays on arrival (Fig. 28.16a, b) and thereafter at 6 weeks, 3 months, 4 months, 6 months, 9 months and at 12 months.
- Allow ambulation with crutches only after swelling diminution and wound healing.
- After 2 weeks, begin active range of motion.
- Toe-touch weight bearing is instituted for 8 weeks.
- Full weight bearing is allowed between 3 and 4 months postoperatively and when radiological progression of union is evident (Fig. 28.17a–c).

## Further Reading

Pelissier P, Masquelet A, Bareille R, et al. Induced membranes secrete growth factors including vascular and osteoinductive factors, and could stimulate bone regeneration. J Orthop Res. 2004;22:73–9.

Masquelet A, Beque T. The concept of induced membrane for reconstruction of long bone defects. Orthop Clin North Am. 2010;41:27–37.

# Corrective Osteotomies About the Knee: Opening Wedge High Tibial Osteotomy

# 29

Stuart J. Calder, Fragkiskos N. Xypnitos, and Peter V. Giannoudis

## Indications

- Pain relief for osteoarthritis (OA) associated with malalignment.
- Mechanical axis correction.
  - Where there is varus (lateral) thrust with ACL and posterolateral laxity ± ligamentous reconstruction.
  - In association with cartilage or meniscal transplantation.

## Relative Contraindications in OA

- Non-specific knee pain.
- Patellofemoral symptoms.
- Arthrosis or meniscectomy in the compartment intended for weight bearing.
- Inflammatory disease.
- Age > 50 years. This is surgeon dependant.
- Fixed varus deformity > 15°.
- Range of motion less than 90°.
- Ligamentous instability.
- Tibio-femoral subluxation > 1 cm.
- Obesity.

S.J. Calder (✉) • F.N. Xypnitos
Department of Trauma and Orthopaedic Surgery,
Leeds Teaching Hospitals NHS Trust,
Leeds, UK
e-mail: stuart.calder@leedsth.nhs.uk

P.V. Giannoudis
Academic Department of Trauma and Orthopaedic Surgery,
School of Medicine, University of Leeds,
Leeds, UK
e-mail: pgiannoudi@aol.com

## Clinical Assessment

- Detailed clinical examination of the knee should be performed.
  - Check for previous skin incisions.
  - Deformity, contractures.
  - Ligamentous stability.
  - Knee range of motion.
- Examine ipsilateral hip function.
- Assess neurovascular status of the entire extremity.
- Consider the patient's weight.
- Discuss all treatment options with patient.

## Radiological Assessment

- Radiographs of the knee:
  - Standing anteroposterior view (Fig. 29.1).
  - Lateral view.
  - Intercondylar notch view.
  - Skyline patellar view.
- Full-length weight-bearing radiograph (hip-knee-ankle) to assess the mechanical axis and reveal femoral and/or tibial deformities, (Fig. 29.2).

## Background Biomechanics

- Normal knee: loads 2–4 times body weight on tibiofemoral joint.
  - 70% of load is on medial compartment when mechanical axis central.
  - 75% of load is on medial compartment when in single leg stance.
  - 6° valgus of mechanical axis: 40% medial load, 60% lateral load.

P.V. Giannoudis (ed.), *Practical Procedures in Elective Orthopaedic Surgery*,
DOI 10.1007/978-0-85729-814-0_29, © Springer-Verlag London Limited 2012

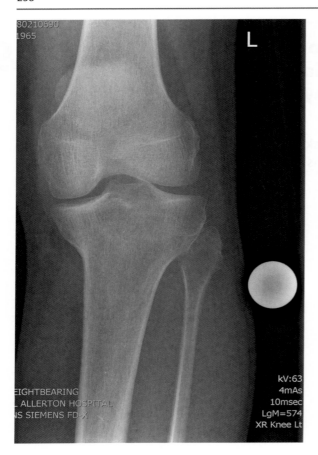

**Fig. 29.1** Pre-operatively standing AP x-ray

## Types of Osteotomies

Most commonly done to correct varus deformity – either due to reduced medial joint space or dynamic varus thrust (ligamentous).

- Proximal Tibial (High Tibial Osteotomy – HTO)
  - Medial opening wedge.
  - Lateral closing wedge.
  - Dome-shaped proximal.
  - Open wedge by callus distraction.
  - Oblique metaphyseal.
- Femoral – generally done for valgus deformity, much less common than HTO
  - Medial closing wedge supracondylar.
  - Lateral opening wedge supracondylar.
- Dual (distal femur and proximal tibia) for severe deformities.

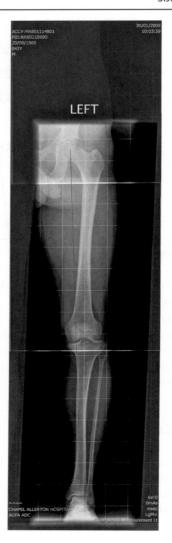

**Fig. 29.2** Long leg x-ray

## Opening Wedge High Tibial Osteotomy

### Indications

- Medial compartment OA.
  - Where arthroplasty not considered appropriate.
- Varus thrust associated with complex ligament laxity.
  - Postero-lateral and lateral instability with a varus thrust.
  - Lateral soft tissue surgery alone will stretch.
  - ACL reconstruction alone will fail.

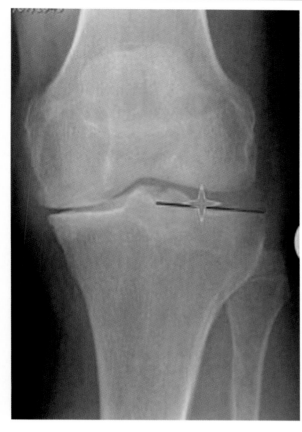

**Fig. 29.3** Fujisawa point

## Preoperative Assessment

- See above

## How Much Correction?

- Depends if done for pain or instability

## For Pain

- Normal femoro-tibial angle (FTA): 5–7° valgus.
- Aim post op FTA: 10–13° (overcorrect 3–5°).
- Fujisawa point – point of new mechanical axis (Fig. 29.3).
- Commonest error is under-correction.

## For Instability

- For dynamic varus thrust, it is acceptable to correct to neutral, or just beyond.

## Operative Treatment

### Anaesthesia

- Regional or General Anaesthesia ± nerve blocks (may want to avoid sciatic nerve block to allow assessment of common peroneal nerve post-operatively).
- Antibiotic prophylaxis according to the hospital protocol, prior to tourniquet inflation.

### Theatre Preparation

- Confirm the correct patient and side.
- Ideally operating theatre should use ultra clean air system.
- Implants and instruments specific to the operation must be available.
- Image intensifier – unless using computer navigation.

### Patient Positioning

- Should be done by the operating surgeon.
- Supine position.
- Lateral support and foot roll.
- Hip/knee ankle accessible to the image intensifier, AP views.
- Check correct proximal thigh position of tourniquet, diathermy plate, flowtron and pressure sore prevention gel pad to the contralateral leg.

### Draping

- Skin preparation with the use of antiseptic solutions (Fig. 29.4).
- Surgical site isolated with sterile drapes.
- Inflate tourniquet (300–350 mmHg).

**Fig. 29.4** Set up and skin preparation

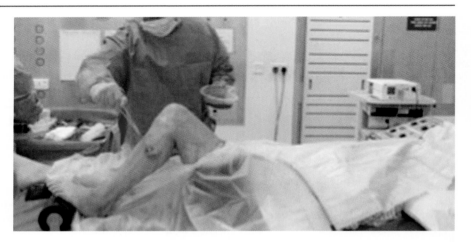

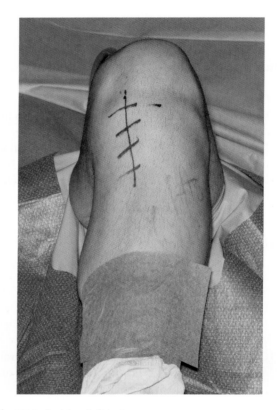

**Fig. 29.5** Incision (left leg)

## Surgical Approach

- Longitudinal incision of approximately 12 cm, starting just below the joint line, over the anteromedial aspect of the tibia; over the pes anserinus insertion, in-between the medial border of the patellar

ligament and the posterior margin of the tibia (Fig. 29.5).
- Care should be taken to provide adequate skin bridges to accommodate any future midline or parapatellar approach, e.g. for total knee replacement.
- Expose and incise the sartorial fascia, to allow surface placement of the plate.
- Careful placement of retractors anterior and posterior to protect the patellar tendon, the posterior neurovascular structures, MCL and hamstrings tendons.
- MCL – release by elevation or partially divide if very tight.

## Osteotomy

- Osteotomy site should be carried out above the tibial tuberosity as it is closer to the site of the deformity and the healing is better in metaphyseal bone.
- Under fluoroscopic control, initial guide wire positioning across the proximal tibia (Fig. 29.6a, b) from medial on the flare of the metaphysis, aimed proximally to lateral cortex about 1 cm below joint line, ensuring the wire passes on or above patellar tendon insertion on the AP view.
- The starting point on the medial cortex is usually about 4 cm below the joint line, mid-flare.
- The fibula and the tibiofibular joint do not need to be disturbed.
- The medial tibial cortex is cut with osteotomes or the osteotomy can be initiated with an oscillating saw (Fig. 29.7a, b).

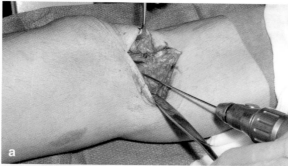

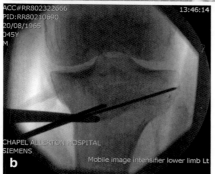

**Fig. 29.6** (**a, b**): Guide pin insertion

- The saw cut is made using the pin as a guide, and advanced within 1 cm of the lateral cortex of the tibia. The lateral tibial cortex should remain intact. Consideration is given to the plane of the osteotomy.
- Ensure completion of osteotomy posteriorly. Protect posterior structures by flexing to 90° and putting, e.g., a Bristow elevator behind (Fig. 29.8a, b).
- Gradual opening up of osteotomy site with wedges or a bony spreader to avoid fracture (Fig. 29.9a, b).
- Fluoroscopic control is used intra-operatively to assess the mechanical axis (Fig. 29.10).
- Fixation of osteotomy with a plate with the leg in extension, when the desired opening is achieved (Fig. 29.11a, b) – in this case a tomofix plate is used.
- The osteotomy site may be grafted with autologous bone graft, or bone substitute (Fig. 29.12).

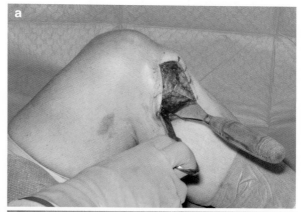

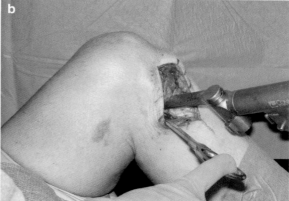

**Fig. 29.8** Osteotome (**a**) or saw (**b**) at 90°, with protective retractor posteriorly

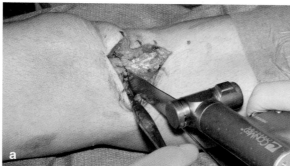

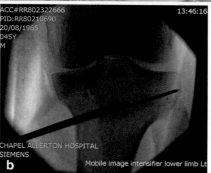

**Fig. 29.7** (**a, b**) The medial tibial cortex is cut with oscillating saw

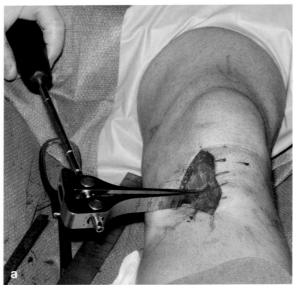

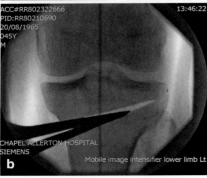

**Fig. 29.9** (**a**, **b**) Gradual opening up of osteotomy site with a bony spreader

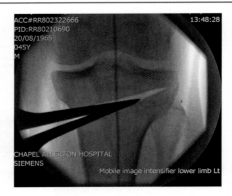

**Fig. 29.10** Intra-operative films to confirm new mechanical axis. Wire lying between hip and ankle, overlying knee

## Implant Positioning

- Often has to be placed slightly antero-medial.
- In ACL or PCL laxity, the slope of the HTO may be adjusted.
- Ensure not encroaching above joint line.
- Check screw positions with lateral screening.

## Opening Versus Closing Wedge

- For
  - Corrects bony deformity.
  - Restores MCL tension.
  - Less chance peroneal nerve injury.
  - Avoids fibular osteotomy.
  - More per-op adjustability.
- Against
  - Higher risk of union problems.
  - Slower weight bearing.
  - May over lengthen the extremity.
  - May reduce patella height, but rarely significant.

## Calculation of Wedge Size

- Measure anatomic axis' angle from standing radiographs. Calculate the amount of correction required to restore this angle to normal (5–7° of valgus), or to take the axis through fujisawa point if doing HTO for pain. Rule of thumb to estimate the height of tibial osteotomy's wedge (1 mm ≈ 1°). Accurate only when tibial flare's width is 56 mm.
- Use of mechanical axis is more accurate.
  - Trigonometric method
  - Weight bearing line method
- Final adjustment of alignment using imaging.
- Computer navigation may also be used.

## Closure

- Irrigation, infiltration with local anaesthetic ± epinephrine, ± drain.
- Tack down tibial anterior fascia over the plate if possible.
- Closure in layers, deep fascia, subcutaneous tissues and skin.

**Fig. 29.11** (**a, b**) Fixation of osteotomy with a plate with the leg in extension

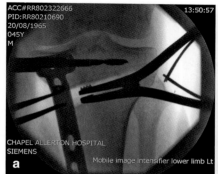

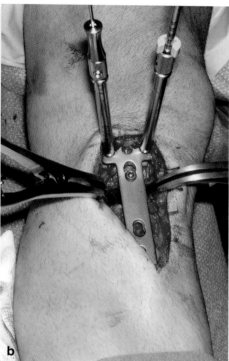

- Wound is covered with a bulky dressing/wool and crepe/that is reduced few days after surgery.
- Tourniquet is deflated and drain is opened (if used).

## Postoperative Care

- Routine antibiotic according to local protocols.
- Start mechanical VTE prophylaxis at admission. Continue mechanical VTE prophylaxis until the patient no longer has significantly reduced mobility. Start pharmacological VTE prophylaxis after surgery. Continue pharmacological VTE prophylaxis for 10–14 days.
- Monitor vascular and neurological status of the leg.
- Post-operative X-ray (Fig. 29.13a, b).
- Early ROM.
- Crutches non-weight-bearing for 6 weeks.
- Then x-ray.
- Protected weight bearing for 6 weeks.
- Period depends on size of osteotomy, fixation device, and patient habitus.

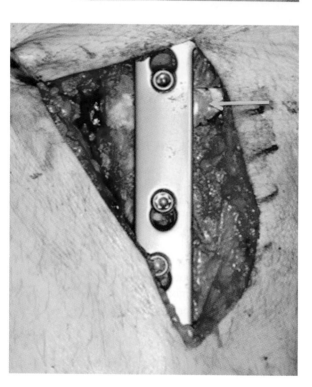

**Fig. 29.12** Fixation is complemented usually with a bone graft or a bone substitute (*yellow arrow*).

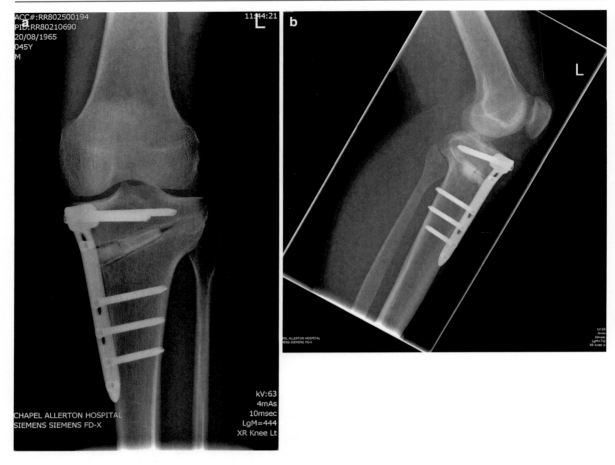

Fig. 29.13  (a, b) Post-operative AP-lateral – x-rays of HTO with tomofix plate

## Complications to Look for

- Plateau fracture.
- Screw in joint.
- Breaching the lateral cortex (unstable).
- Vascular compromise.
- Compartment syndrome.
- Wound infection.
- Nerve damage (foot drop).
- Delayed or non-union. Revision surgery is needed.
- Osteonecrosis of proximal fragment.
- Breakage of plate or screws.
- Patella tendon scarring, patella baja.
- In ex-fix technique:
    - Pin site infection – up to 50%.
    - Risk of infection after TKR years later.
    - Loss of correction, if fixator is removed < 3 months.

## Follow up

- At 2–3 weeks, 6 weeks (x-ray), 12 weeks (x-ray), 6 months.
- Discharge when clinical and radiological evidence of union and satisfactory ROM is present.

## Implant Removal

- If the implant is prominent or irritating.
- If arthroplasty planned.

## Further Reading

Amendola A, Bonasia DE. Results of high tibial osteotomy: review of the literature. Int Orthop. 2010;34(2):155–60.

Jenny JY. The current status of computer-assisted high tibial osteotomy, unicompartmental knee replacement, and revision total knee replacement. Instr Course Lect. 2008;57:721–6.

Brouwer RW, van TM Raaij, Bierma-Zeinstra SM, Verhagen AP, Jakma TS, Verhaar JA. Osteotomy for treating knee osteoarthritis. Cochrane Database Syst Rev. 2007;18(3):CD004019.

Jackson DW, Warkentine B. Technical aspects of computer-assisted opening wedge high tibial osteotomy. J Knee Surg. 2007;20(2):134–41.

Giffin JR, Shannon FJ. The role of the high tibial osteotomy in the unstable knee. Sports Med Arthrosc. 2007;15(1): 23–31.

# Part V

# Lower Extremity: Ankle – Foot

# Ankle Arthroscopy

# 30

Kurt Haendlmayer and Nick Harris

## Indications

- The commonest indications are impingement and osteochondral injuries. Impingement can be soft tissue or bony, anterior or posterior. We will concentrate on anterior ankle arthroscopy in this chapter.
- Other indications are removal of loose bodies, synovitis, meniscoid lesions, septic arthritis, and arthroscopic ankle fusion for degenerative arthritis.
- Contraindications include soft tissue infection superficial to the joint and arterial insufficiency.

## Preoperative Planning

### Clinical Assessment

- A detailed history will often guide the clinician to the diagnosis. Pain with reduced dorsiflexion and pain with extreme plantar flexion are typical of anterior and posterior impingement. Instability may contribute to anterolateral impingement. Persistent pain following an ankle sprain felt deep in the joint is typical of an osteochondral lesion.
- Examination looking in particular at hindfoot alignment, local tenderness and swelling, range of movement, and stability are important in focusing the clinician to the area of concern.

K. Haendlmayer • N. Harris (✉)
Department of Trauma and Orthopaedic Surgery,
Leeds Teaching Hospitals NHS Trust, Leeds, UK
e-mail: nick.harris@leedsth.nhs.uk

### Radiological Assessment

- Weight bearing X-rays will show the joint alignment and joint space.
- An MRI is the investigation of choice and is often used to confirm the initial diagnosis.

## Operative Treatment Procedure

### Anesthesia

- General anesthesia combined with intra-articular local anesthetic at the end of the procedure.
- An examination under anesthetic should be performed once the patient is anesthetized, looking at range of movement and stability.

### Table and Equipment

- Must have facility to lower foot end of table relative to the rest of the table to apply traction when needed.
- Leg support (sternal retractor), plus ankle distractor.
- 4.0-mm 30° arthroscope is the mainstay of treatment. Smaller arthroscopes are available with 30° and 70° options.
- Instrumentation includes shavers (4.5-mm soft tissue incisor, Fig. 30.1a, and 4-mm burr), intra-articular diathermy (side effect probe, Fig. 30.1b), punch (Fig. 30.1c) and graspers, and microfracture picks.

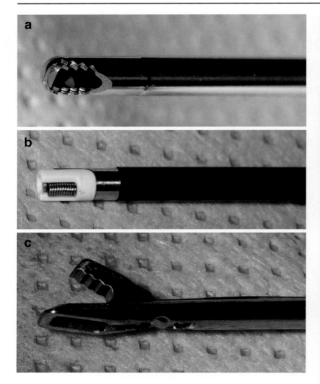

**Fig. 30.1** (**a**) A 4.5-mm soft tissue incisor. (**b**) A side effect diathermy probe. (**c**) A straight punch

## Patient Position and Setup

- A thigh tourniquet is applied.
- The patient is positioned supine with the operated leg over a thigh support.
- The ankle distractor is placed around the foot and secured to the table. No traction is applied to start with (Fig. 30.2a). This allows better visualization of the anterior joint space. When necessary, the foot end of the table can be lowered, applying traction to allow better visualization of the joint itself.
- The skin is prepared as far as the tourniquet, and the leg is draped (Fig. 30.2b).

## Portals and Landmarks

- Preoperatively landmarks are identified and clearly marked. The most important landmarks are the tendons of tibialis anterior (TA), and peroneus tertius (PT). Flexing the fourth toe should demonstrate the superficial peroneal nerve.

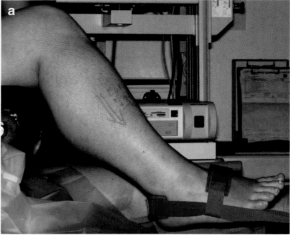

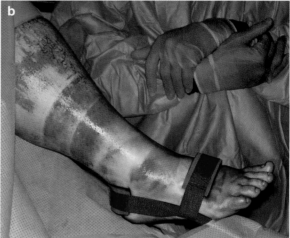

**Fig. 30.2** (**a**) Initial patient setup. (**b**) Ankle after prepping and draping

- The commonest anterior portals are the anteromedial portal, which is located just medial to the TA tendon in the notch of Harty, and the anterolateral portal, lateral to the PT. The less common anterocentral portal lies between the EDC tendons.
- Structures at risk with the most common portals are saphenous vein and nerve, TA tendon, and EHL for the anteromedial portal, and superficial peroneal nerve, EDC, and PT for anterolateral portal.

## Surgical Technique

- A vertical anteromedial skin incision of about 1 cm is made just medial to the tibialis anterior tendon. The soft tissues are then dissected down to the

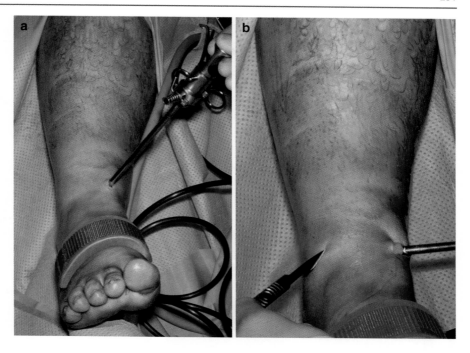

**Fig. 30.3** (**a**) Introduction of 4.0-mm arthroscope anteromedially. (**b**) Creation of anterolateral portal

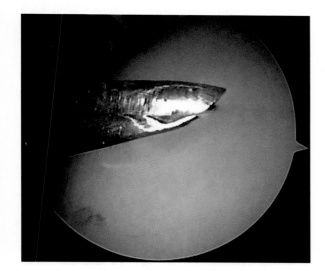

**Fig. 30.4** Scapel enter joint under direct vision

capsule. An incision is then made in the capsule, and the blunt trochar, inserted followed by the arthroscope (Fig. 30.3a).

- The light from the arthroscope can then be used to illuminate the skin laterally to help locate the anterolateral portal (Fig. 30.3b). A vertical incision is made anterolaterally in the skin, lateral to the peroneus tertius. The soft tissues are dissected and a

vertical incision is then made in the capsule. It should be possible to visualize the blade as it enters the joint (Fig. 30.4).

- Through the anteromedial portal the anterolateral part of the joint is inspected. Traction can then be applied to allow better visualization of the central and posterior aspects of the joint. It is often necessary to perform an anterior synovectomy to gain a good field of vision (Fig. 30.5a). This is usually performed with a soft tissue shaver. A side effect intra-articular diathermy probe (Fig. 30.5b) and straight punch may also be helpful in removing prominent anterior soft tissue which may be either obscuring the field of view or causing impingement.
- Once the lateral aspect of the joint has been dealt with, the arthroscope is then introduced through the anterolateral portal to allow visualization of the anteromedial aspect of the joint (Fig. 30.6a, b). The foot can be passively dorsiflexed to give a clearer picture of any soft tissue or bony impingement.
- Bony prominences are resected using a 4-mm acromionizer.
- The joint is thoroughly washed out.
- Postoperatively, intra-articular Marcaine is injected into the joint to help with pain relief.

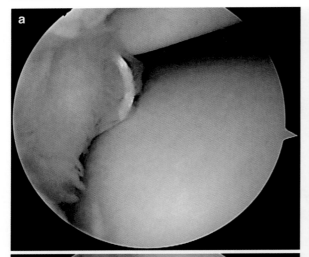

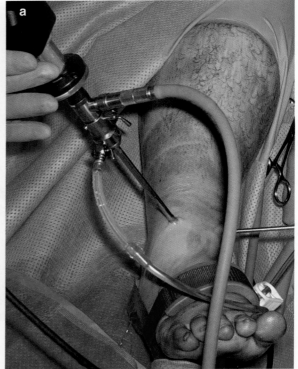

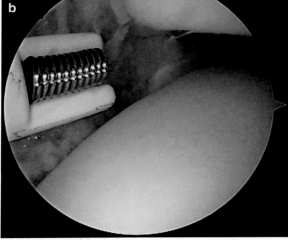

**Fig. 30.5** (**a**) Soft tissue shaver resecting prominent anterolateral soft tissues. (**b**) Side effect diathermy probe used to reduce prominent soft tissues

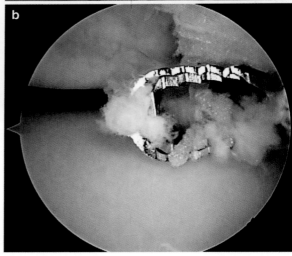

**Fig. 30.6** (**a**) Introduction of arthroscope anterolaterally. (**b**) Resection of prominent soft tissue anteromedially with a shaver

## Closure

- The portals are closed either with a suture or Steri-Strip and a sterile adhesive dressing applied.
- A compression bandage is then applied.

## Postoperative Course

- The ankle is initially immobilized in a walker boot.
- Once the portals are dry, physiotherapy is commenced.
- Surgery is performed as a day case.

- Start mechanical VTE prophylaxis at admission and continue until the patient no longer has significantly reduced mobility, based on an assessment of risks. Start pharmacological VTE prophylaxis after surgery and continue until the patient no longer has significantly reduced mobility.

## Outpatient Follow-Up

- The outpatient follow-up depends entirely on intra-operative findings and the procedure performed. Therefore this has to be individualized, and no global recommendation can be given.

## Complications

- Neurologic injury (nearly half of all complications, mainly injury to the superficial peroneal nerve)
- Vascular injury
- Tendon injury
- Septic arthritis and soft tissue infection around portals
- Thromboembolic events mainly in immobilized, non-weight-bearing patients
- Iatrogenic injury to articular structures

## Further Reading

Glazebrook MA, Ganapathy V, Bridge MA, et al. Evidence-based indications for ankle arthroscopy. Arthroscopy. 2009; 25(12):1478–90.

Allegra F, Maffulli N, Cerza F, et al. Postero-medial approach procedure in the supine position for one-step anterior and posterior ankle arthroscopy. Sports Med Arthrosc. 2009;17(3): 185–9.

Van Dijk CN, Van Bergen CJ. Advancements in ankle arthroscopy. J Am Acad Orthop Surg. 2008;16(11):635–46.

Lui TH. Arthroscopy and endoscopy of the foot and ankle: indications for new techniques. Arthroscopy. 2007;23(8):889–902.

# Ankle Joint Fusion

**31**

Peter V. Giannoudis

## Indications

- Chronic arthritis
- Posttraumatic arthritis
- Postinfection arthritis
- Neuromuscular disorders
- Postpoliomyelitis

## Clinical Symptoms

- Pain localized at ankle joint on active movement.
- Painful walking and decreased walking capacity.
- Reduced range of ankle joint motion.
- Residual foot swelling may be present.

## Preoperative Planning

### Clinical Assessment

- Assess any structural deformity.
- Evaluate range of motion of both ankle and subtalar joint.
- Assess the presence of equinus (Achilles tendon shortening) which may necessitate Achilles tendon lengthening.
- Assess state of surrounding soft tissues.
- Palpate dorsalis pedis and tibialis posterior pulses.
- Any underlying toe inflammation must be excluded.

P.V. Giannoudis
Academic Department of Trauma and Orthopaedic Surgery,
School of Medicine, University of Leeds, Leeds, UK
e-mail: pgiannoudi@aol.com

- Patients with a positive diabetes family history should be screened.

### Radiological Assessment

- Arthritic joint changes are evident in plain X-rays (exception of those cases with neuromuscular disorders and polio).
- Obtain AP and lateral views of the joint (Fig. 31.1a, b). If there is metal work in situ, this needs to be removed either prior to surgery or during the same surgical setting (ankle fusion). On the case shown here, the medial malleolar screws were removed 6 months prior to ankle fusion.

## Operative Treatment

### Anesthesia

- General, spinal, or epidural anesthesia can be discussed with the patient.
- If possible, avoid giving regional blocks as they could prevent prompt assessment of clinical features consistent with compartment syndrome.
- Antibiotic prophylaxis according to the hospital protocol.
- Antibiotic administration prior to tourniquet inflation.

### Table/Equipment

- Radiolucent table.
- Imaging intensifier.
- Small fragment set and cannulated screw system (6.5 mm).

P.V. Giannoudis (ed.), *Practical Procedures in Elective Orthopaedic Surgery*,
DOI 10.1007/978-0-85729-814-0_31, © Springer-Verlag London Limited 2012

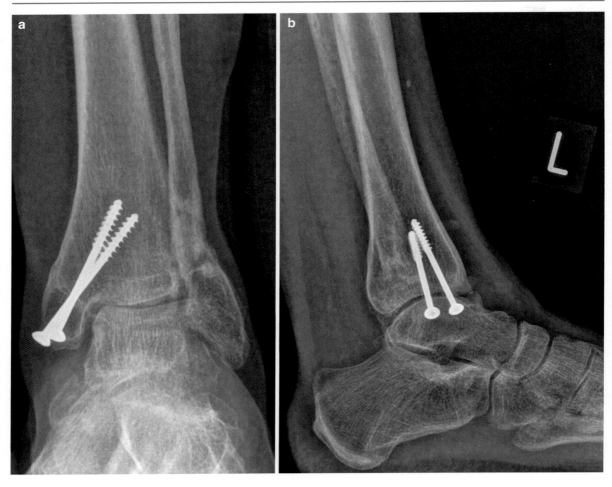

**Fig. 31.1** (**a**) AP and (**b**) lateral X-rays of a patient with posttraumatic arthritis of the ankle joint

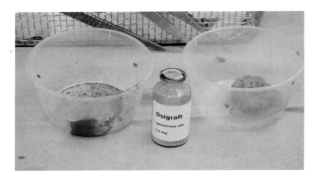

**Fig. 31.2** Grafts that can be used in ankle fusion

- Inflate thigh tourniquet to 300 mmHg.
- Bone substitutes should be available to facilitate fusion (consider autologous iliac crest graft, BMP-7 or RIA graft) (Fig. 31.2).

## Patient Positioning (Fig. 31.3)

- Supine positioning.
- Above knee tourniquet applications – be aware that in obese people the tourniquet could slip and not be effective.

## Marking and Draping

- Palpate vessels and mark the incision (Fig. 31.4).
- Extensive below-knee skin preparation with the use of antiseptic solutions (alcoholic povidone/iodine). Extra care in the web spaces of the toes (Fig. 31.5a).
- Sterile drape or glove could be used to cover the toes as an extra precaution (Fig. 31.5b).

**Fig. 31.3** Supine position and application of the tourniquet

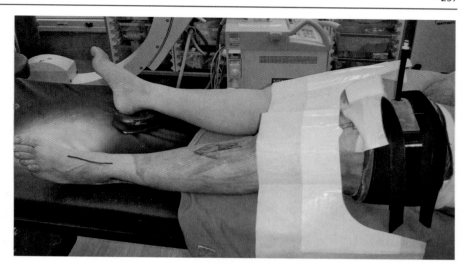

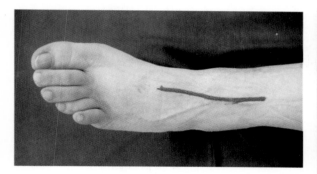

**Fig. 31.4** Skin marking with a permanent marker

## Surgical Exposure

- Straight incision is performed over the dorsum of the ankle joint, expanded proximally by 10 cm (Fig. 31.6a).
- The superficial peroneal nerve is indentified and retracted laterally. The extensor retinaculum is incised longitudinally.
- Develop interval between extensor hallucis longus (EHL) laterally and tibialis anterior (TA) medially (Fig. 31.6b).
- Take caution to protect the neurovascular bundle medially. As the NV adheres to the deep tissues, mobilization is advisable. (Deep peroneal nerve and anterior tibial artery).
- Proceed with subperiosteal elevation to expose the distal tibia.

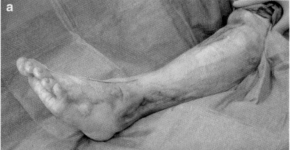

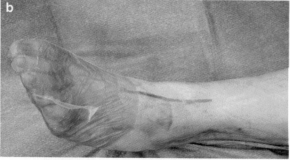

**Fig. 31.5** (**a**) Below-knee skin preparation with antiseptic solution, paying extra attention at the web spaces. (**b**) A sterile drape isolating the toes

- Incise and excise joint capsule to expose the ankle joint.
- Using small osteotomes, proceed with decortication of the tibial and talar joint surfaces including the inner medial and lateral malleolus areas (Fig. 31.7a).

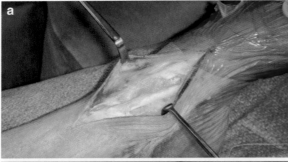

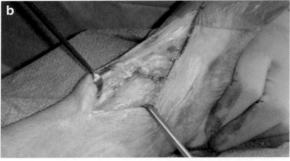

**Fig. 31.6** (**a**) A straight skin incision is performed, and the extensor retinaculum is incised longitudinally accordingly. (**b**) The extensor hallucis longus (EHL) is retracted laterally and tibialis anterior (TA) medially. Take caution to protect the NV bundle medially

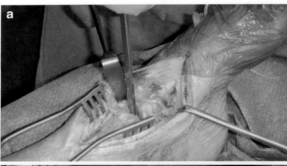

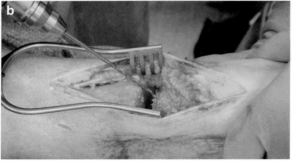

**Fig. 31.7** (**a**) Decortication performed with an osteotome. (**b**) Bony drilling holes with 2.5-mm drill to enhance the biological activity

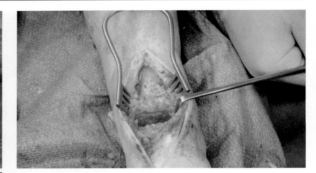

**Fig. 31.8** Evaluation of the bony edges to be clear from cartilage and parallel

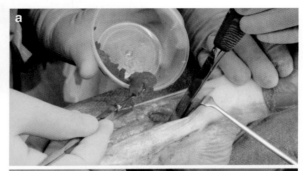

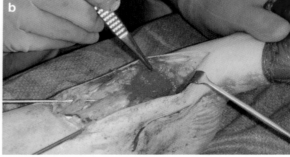

**Fig. 31.9** (**a**) Graft positioning. (**b**) Graft packed at the fusion site

- Complete cartilage removal is desirable down to bleeding bone.
- The two surfaces must be parallel (Fig. 31.8), while the joint is inspected with the image intensifier.
- Use of lamina spreader for facilitation of decortication of the posterior malleolus.
- Prepare the bed of the fusion (joint surfaces) by making multiple bony drilling holes with 2.5-mm drill to enhance the biological activity of the bed (Fig. 31.7b).
- Graft is positioned between the well-prepared and cleaned bony edges (Fig. 31.9a, b).

**Fig. 31.10** (**a**) Intra-operative fluoroscopic images demonstrating the insertion of K-wires (**b**) followed by cannulated screw insertion and (**c**) Fluoroscopic images after screw insertion

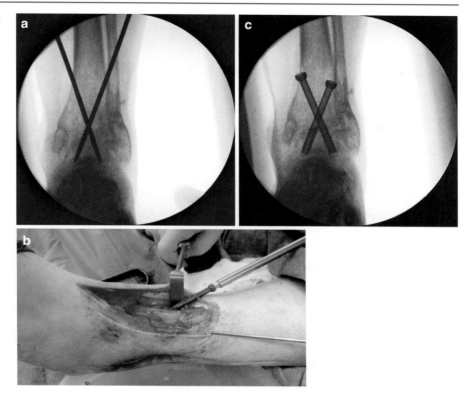

## Implant Positioning

- Before insertion of K-wires, position the ankle joint passively at 90°.
- Placement of K-wires under direct vision and image intensifier control (Fig. 31.10a). Position of K-wires should be aimed towards medial anterior and lateral posterior direction.
- Be aware that talus in narrower that distal tibia, and the temporary fixation must be controlled with X-rays.
- Using the depth gage, measure the desirable of the screws.
- Use the cannulated drill to prepare the tunnel for easy insertion of the two partially threaded 6.5-mm cannulated screws (Fig. 31.10b).
- Compress the bony edges of the joint surfaces to optimize bone contact.
- Be aware that the screws must not protrude into the subtalar joint.
- X-ray certification/documentation for the final screw positioning is advised prior of closure (Fig. 31.10c).

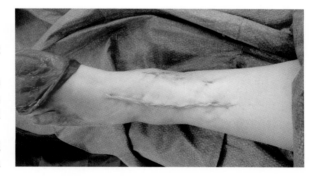

**Fig. 31.11** Skin closure with absorbable sutures

## Closure

- Release tourniquet and check for any sources of bleeding.
- Irrigate wound with caution.
- Use 2/0 Vicryl interrupted sutures for closure of the subcutaneous layer.
- 3/0 Monocryl absorbable suture is used for skin closure (Fig. 31.11).

- Wound dressing and wool application prior to stabilization of the fused ankle joint with a back slab for support (Fig. 31.12).
- Be cautious not to apply the back slab tightly.

## Postoperative Care Rehabilitation

- Elevation of the foot.
- Watch neurological status.
- Start mechanical VTE prophylaxis at admission and continue until the patient no longer has significantly reduced mobility, based on an assessment of risks. Start pharmacological VTE prophylaxis after

surgery and continue until the patient no longer has significantly reduced mobility.
- Wound inspection within 48 h.
- Application of below-knee cast.
- Obtain radiographs AP/lateral of ankle joint.
- Mobilize non-weight bearing for 4 weeks with the aid of crutches.
- Proceed to partial weight bearing between 4 and 8 weeks.
- After 8 weeks, full weight bearing can be allowed.

## Complications

- Wound infection
- Compartment syndrome
- Deep vein thrombosis
- Nonunion/high incidence in smokers

## Follow-Up

- On discharge, prescribe chemical thromboprophylaxis as per local hospital policy for a period of 6 weeks.
- Outpatient follow-ups at 4, 8, and 12 weeks for clinical and radiological assessment (AP/lateral X-rays).

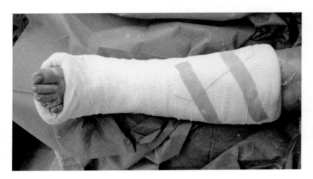

**Fig. 31.12** Final dressing with back slab in place

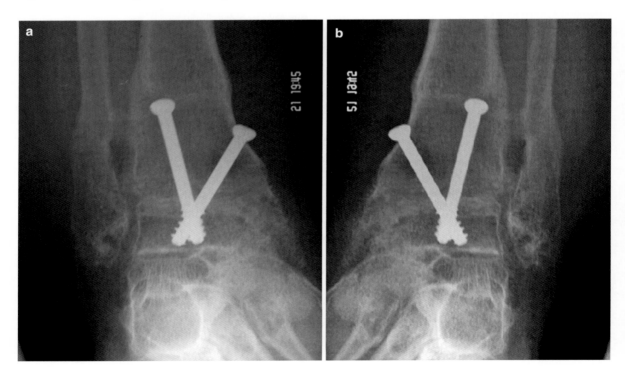

**Fig. 31.13** (**a, b**) X-rays (AP and lateral) confirming the ankle joint fusion

- Patient can be discharged when union has been confirmed both clinically and radiologically (Fig. 31.13a, b).

## Implant Removal

- It is not routinely performed.
- If there is soft tissue irritation, screws can be removed after establishment of a joint fusion.

## Further Reading

Marsh JL, Rattay RE, Dulaney T. Results of ankle arthrodesis for treatment of supramalleolar nonunion and ankle arthrosis. Foot Ankle Int. 1997;18(3):138–43.

Muir DC, Amendola A, Saltzman CL. Long-term outcome of ankle arthrodesis. Foot Ankle Clin. 2002;7(4):703–8.

Nihal A, Gellman RE, Embil JM, Trepman E. Ankle arthrodesis. Foot Ankle Surg. 2008;14(1):1–10.

Zwipp H, Rammelt S, Endres T, Heineck J. High union rates and function scores at midterm follow up with ankle arthrodesis using a four screw technique. Clin Orthop Relat Res. 2009;468(4):958–68.

# Subtalar Joint Fusion

# 32

## Peter V. Giannoudis and Nikolaos K. Kanakaris

## Indications

- Posttraumatic osteoarthritis
- Multi-fragmented intra-articular calcaneal fractures not amenable to reconstruction
- Lesions limited to the subtalar joint, including talocalcaneal bars

## Preoperative Planning

### Clinical Assessment

- Assess swelling and state of soft tissues.
- Evaluate deformity, gait pattern, and neurovascular status.
- In the acute setting, be aware of associated fractures in the adjacent foot and ankle.

### Radiological Assessment

- Plain radiographs (lateral view of the hindfoot, axial view of the calcaneus) and CT (Fig. 32.1)

P.V. Giannoudis (✉)
Academic Department of Trauma and Orthopaedic Surgery,
School of Medicine, University of Leeds,
Leeds, UK
e-mail: pgiannoudi@aol.com

N.K. Kanakaris
Department of Trauma and Orthopaedic Surgery,
Leeds Teaching Hospitals NHS Trust,
Leeds, UK

## Operative Treatment

### Anesthesia

- Regional (spinal/epidural/popliteus) or general anesthesia
- Prophylactic antibiotic as per local hospital protocol

### Table and Equipment

- Small fragment set
- 3.5-mm cortical/cancellous screws
- 6.5-mm cannulated screw set
- Osteotomes
- Curettes
- Bone graft (see relevant chapter)
- A radiolucent table
- An image intensifier and a competent radiographer

### Table Setup

- The instrumentation set is at the foot end of the table.
- Image intensifier is from the contralateral side.

### Patient Positioning

- The patient is placed in the lateral decubitus position, with the affected side up.
- Use of tourniquet.

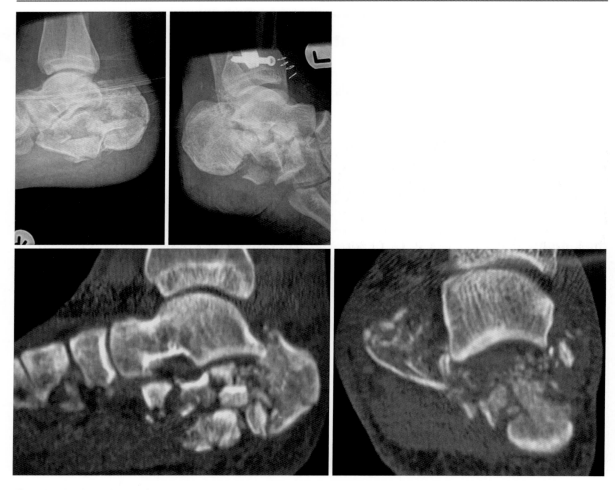

**Fig. 32.1** Radiographs and CT scan of a multi-fragmented calcaneal fracture following a fall from a height

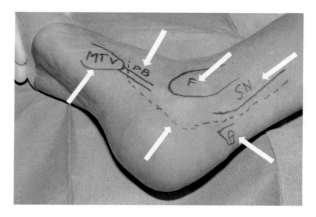

**Fig. 32.2** Extensile lateral approach. *Arrows* indicate: *MTV* fifth metatarsal base, *PB* peroneus brevis tendon, *F* fibula, *SN* sural nerve, *A* Achilles tendon. *Interrupted line*: incision

## Draping

- Prepare the skin over lower leg, ankle, and entire foot with usual antiseptic solutions (aqueous/alcoholic povidone-iodine). Prepare skin between toes thoroughly.
- Apply standard draping around lower leg in the middle between knee and ankle.
- Apply tape around toes.

## Approach

- Extensile lateral approach (Fig. 32.2).
- Make a curved incision with vertical and horizontal limbs.

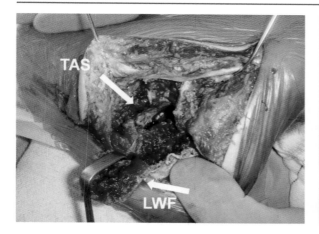

**Fig. 32.3** Acute fracture case. Lateral wall fragment of the calcaneum reflected following dissection. Visualization of the talar articular surface is shown. *LWF* lateral wall fragment, *TAS* talar articular surface

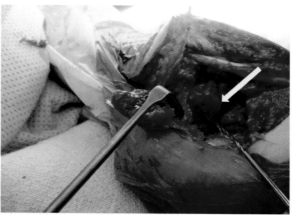

**Fig. 32.5** Drill holes made to the talar articular surface following removal of the cartilage

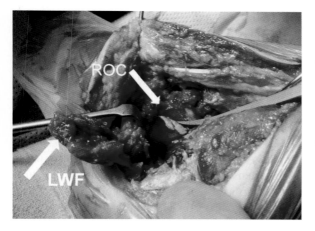

**Fig. 32.4** Using an osteotome, cartilage is removed from the talar articular surface. *ROC* removal of cartilage, *LWF* lateral wall fragment

- The vertical limb is oriented halfway between the posterior aspect of the peroneal tendons and the anterior aspect of the Achilles tendon.
- Be aware that at the superior margin of this incision, the sural nerve passes in the subcutaneous tissue.
- The horizontal limb of the incision parallels the plantar surface of the foot and is inclined slightly at the anterior margin.
- The sural nerve crosses at the junction of the middle and distal third of the horizontal limb of the incision. The sural nerve is very closely associated with the subcutaneous tissue above the peroneal tendons.

- Bring the incision sharply to bone on its vertical limb and on the curved portion of the incision and then carry more superficially and distally to the area of the peroneal tendons.
- Careful dissection should be performed near peroneal tendons and in the area of the sural nerve. The skin is dissected and raised as a full-thickness flap from the periosteum of the calcaneus and should include the calcaneofibular ligament.
- The subtalar joint can be seen as the flap is raised. Four 1.6-mm Kirschner wires (navicular, cuboid, talar neck, fibula) are placed to maintain retraction of the flap without excessive. Advance Kirschner wires into the bone approximately 1.5 cm, and then bent them to provide soft tissue retraction.
- In cases of an acute fracture subjected to primary fusion, elevate the lateral wall fragment of the calcaneum and expose the subtalar joint (Fig. 32.3).
- Remove the hematoma using suction and retrieve small fracture fragments using a pituitary rongeur.
- Using an osteotome or a curette, remove the cartilage from the talar surface down to bleeding bone (Fig. 32.4).
- Remove also the cartilage from the depressed segments of the posterior facet joint surfaces as well as the anterior facet.
- Make drill holes to talar articular surface following removal of the cartilage (Fig. 32.5).
- Using reduction instruments (pusher, 5-mm Schanz screw, K-wires, etc.), mobilize and reduce fragments (posterior facet) so that the shape of the foot is normal without any residual deformity (ankle in

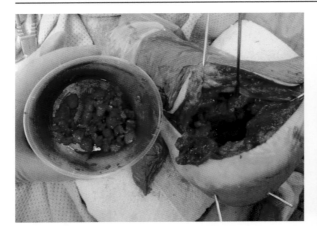

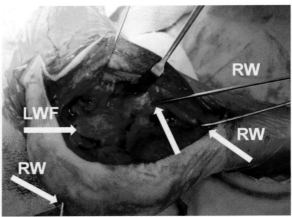

**Fig. 32.6** Using bone graft (autologous or synthetic), fill in the subtalar joint space

**Fig. 32.7** Flip the lateral wall fragment in place now, and using K-wires, secure the alignment of both calcaneum and the talus for fusion (LWF=lateral wall fragment; RW=reduction wire)

neutral dorsiflexion/plantar flexion; hindfoot in neutral or maximum in 5° of valgus; more valgus or any varus should be avoided).

- Using bone graft (autologous or synthetic), fill in the subtalar joint space (Fig. 32.6).
- Flip the lateral wall fragment in place now, and using K-wires, secure the alignment of both calcaneus and talus for fusion (Fig. 32.7).
- Different plates and/or cannulated screws can be used for the fusion.
- The preferred plate should have a low profile, particularly in the area of the peroneal tendons. The plate should be rigid enough to correct varus alignment.
- The plate includes fixation of both the talus and the calcaneum. Another 1/3 semitubal plate can be used to provide better stability between the talar and calcaneal bodies posteriorly (Fig. 32.8). On this occasion, 6.5-mm cannulated screws were not used due to the fragmentation of the body and the posterior facet of the calcaneum.
- In addition to the primary subtalar fusion for calcaneal fractures, this procedure can be performed in cases of chronic subtalar arthritis, after ineffective and prolonged conservative treatment:
- Halfway between the base of fifth metatarsal and the tip of lateral malleolus, an oblique incision is made, which parallels subtalar joint line over sinus tarsi. Alternatively, an incision from the tip of the fibula to the base of the fourth metatarsal can be performed. The sural nerve lies 1–2 cm beneath the distal tip of the fibula and must be avoided. The peroneal tendon

sheath is opened, and the extensor digitorum brevis tendon (EDB) is exposed. The extensor tendon sheath is partially opened, and the EDB is freed from its insertion & reflected distally (creation of a distally based EDB flap). Dissection is continued to cuboid and distal calcaneus, and the fibro-fatty content of the sinus tarsi is removed. The calcaneocuboid joint is identified just distal to the anterior beak of the calcaneus, as well as the neck of the talus. A bone lever is inserted over the neck or under the extensor tendons, which helps retract the neurovascular bundle. A curved elevator is inserted deep to the peroneal tendon and around calcaneus at the level of the subtalar joint, and the lateral talar process can be removed to better expose the posterior facet. The joint capsule of the talocalcaneal joint is incised, and a laminar spreader is inserted into sinus tarsi to expose the entire subtalar articular surface. The articular cartilage and subchondral bone of the subtalar joint are excised. Care should be taken to insure that the articular cartilage from anterior, middle, and posterior facet has been excised. All of the nonarticular surfaces are decorticated, but excessive bone resection should be avoided, as this may decrease the height of the subtalar joint. In cases of a fixed valgus or varus deformity, additional bone is removed from the medial or lateral sides of the joint, respectively. Bone graft is inserted and fixation is performed using one or two threaded lag screws (long or short). Screw insertion can be performed either from anterior to posterior or from posterior to

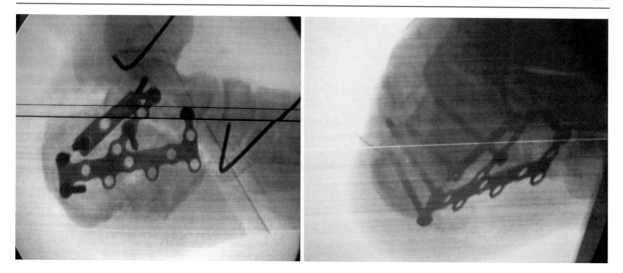

**Fig. 32.8** Image intensifier films showing the application of two plates to secure the talar and the calcaneus bodies for facilitation of fusion

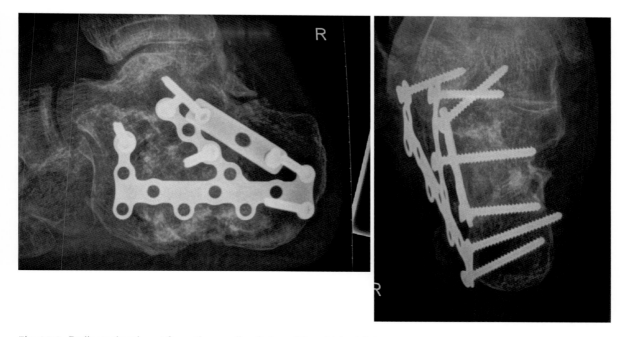

**Fig. 32.9** Radiographs taken at 3 months revealing fusion of the subtalar joint

anterior. For the latter, usually a short threaded lag screw is used and heel pad symptoms can be voided if the incision and screw are kept just above the heel pad. A guide pin is initially placed across the subtalar joint and usually a washer is used. For the anterior to posterior screw insertion, a pin is inserted medial to anterior tibial tendon from talar neck into calcaneus, while the surgeon's finger through the lateral incision palpates the drill to ensure that it is centered over the talar neck. A long threaded lag screw is inserted, located close to anterior margin of tibia.

## Closure

- Irrigate the wound thoroughly and achieve hemostasis.
- Close subcutaneous fascia (2.0 PDS/Vicryl) over a drain.
- Skin closure – monofilament nonabsorbable sutures.
- The sutures should start at the two ends of the incision and should be placed in a manner to allow absolute tension-free closure at the corner of the incision.
- Apply lower leg back slab.

## Postoperative Rehabilitation

- Remove drains and cast in 48 h. Prescribe chemical thromboprophylaxis for 6 weeks as per local hospital protocol.
- Apply jigsaw cast for regular inspection of wound and mobilize patient non-weight bearing for 4 weeks.
- Then, progress to partial weight bearing for another 4 weeks. Afterward, the patient can start full weight bearing.

## Outpatient Follow-Up

- Review at 6 and 12 weeks with radiographs • (Fig. 32.9) and longer as indicated until fusion has been achieved.
- Discharge from the follow-up after clinical and radiological evidence of fusion.
- Review again at request of the general practitioner.

## Further Reading

Scanlan RL, Burns PR, Crim BE. Technique tip: subtalar joint fusion using a parallel guide and double screw fixation. J Foot Ankle Surg. 2010;49(3):305–9.

Radnay CS, Clare MP, Sanders RW. Subtalar fusion after displaced intra-articular calcaneal fractures: does initial operative treatment matter? surgical technique. J Bone Joint Surg Am. 2010;92(Suppl 1 Pt 1):32–43.

Potenza V, Caterini R, Farsetti P, Bisicchia S, Ippolito E. Primary subtalar arthrodesis for the treatment of comminuted intra-articular calcaneal fractures. Injury. 2010;41(7):796–800.

Thomas PJ. Placement of screws in subtalar arthrodesis: a simplified technique. Foot Ankle Int. 1998;19(6):416–7.

Tuijthof GJ, Beimers L, Kerkhoffs GM, Dankelman J, Dijk CN. Overview of subtalar arthrodesis techniques: options, pitfalls and solutions. Foot Ankle Surg. 2010;16(3):107–16.

# Total Ankle Arthroplasty

**33**

## Nick Harris

## Indications

- Total ankle arthroplasty is indicated for painful arthritis of the ankle most commonly posttraumatic, primary, or rheumatoid. Other causes include psoriatic arthritis of the ankle, hemophilic arthropathy, and hemochromatosis.

## Preoperative Planning

### Clinical Assessment

- Assess hindfoot alignment with the patient standing. Severe malalignment is a contraindication to total ankle replacement surgery.
- Assess the soft tissues around the ankle. Previous scars associated with posttraumatic arthritis may compromise the incision used for the total ankle replacement. The soft tissues in the rheumatoid patient can be very fragile and great care must be taken.
- Assess the range of movement in the ankle. A very stiff ankle is a relative contraindication to a total ankle replacement.
- Assess the arterial and venous circulation in the limb. Arterial and venous insufficiency will affect wound healing.

N. Harris
Department of Trauma and Orthopaedic Surgery,
Leeds Teaching Hospitals NHS Trust, Leeds, UK
e-mail: nick.harris@leedsth.nhs.uk

## Radiological Assessment

- An AP and true lateral weight bearing X-rays of the ankle are mandatory (Fig. 33.1a, b).

## Operative Treatment

### Anesthesia

- Regional or general anesthesia with nerve blocks
- Thigh tourniquet
- Antibiotic prophylaxis at induction

### Table and Equipment

- Full set of total ankle replacement instruments
- Radiolucent table
- Image intensifier

### Table Set

- Instrumentation is set up on contralateral side.
- Image intensifier is set up on ipsilateral side.

### Patient Positioning

- Supine with supports on contralateral side.
- The table is tilted in the direction of the unoperated leg, which has the effect of rotating the leg into a neutral position.

**Fig. 33.1** (**a**) An AP weight bearing X-ray of the ankle. (**b**) A true lateral weight bearing X-ray of the ankle

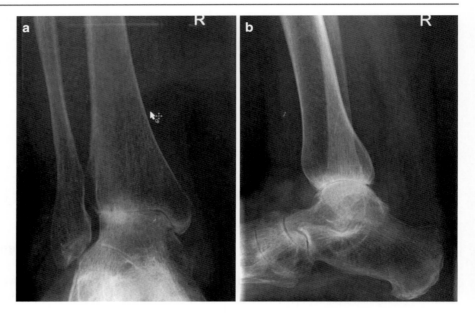

## Draping and Surgical Approach

- The skin is prepared over the foot and ankle with an appropriate antiseptic extending proximally above the knee.
- An anterior incision is used in the interval between tibialis anterior and extensor hallucis longus (Fig. 33.2).
- The neurovascular bundle is mobilized and retracted laterally.
- The medial and lateral malleoli are visualized.

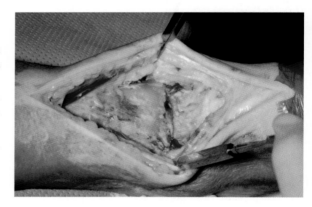

**Fig. 33.2** Anterior skin incision

## Operative Technique

- The tibial jig is applied under X-ray control and held with 2 or 3 pins.
- The distal end of the tibia is resected perpendicular to the long axis of the leg (Fig. 33.3).
- The tibia is sized and a tibial window is created (Fig. 33.4a).
- The tibial trial is then inserted with a spacer.
- Different-sized spacers are available depending on the size of the gap between tibia and talus.
- The talar cutting guide is then applied using two pins (Fig. 33.4b).
- Different amounts of talus can be resected using different talar cutting blocks.

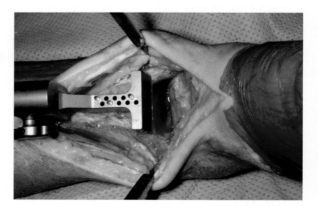

**Fig. 33.3** Tibial resection

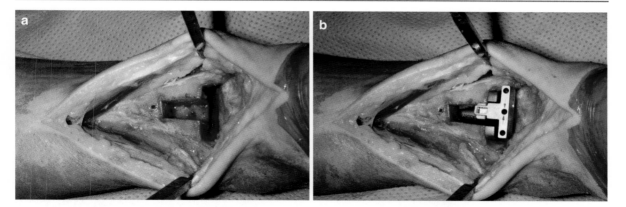

**Fig. 33.4** (**a**) Tibial window. (**b**) Talar cutting guide and spacer

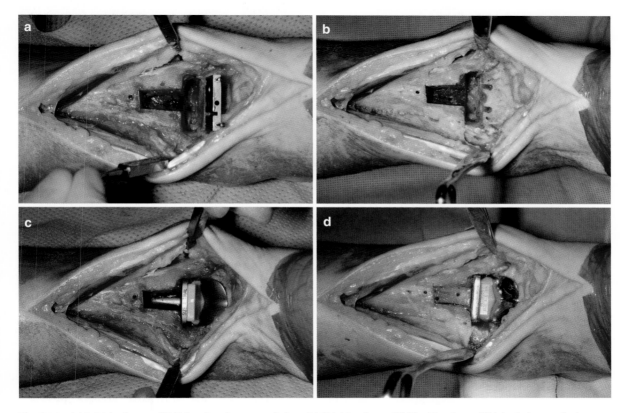

**Fig. 33.5** (**a**) Initial talar cut. (**b**) Talar chamfer cuts and slots. (**c**) Trial implants. (**d**) Final implants. Tibial window grafted

- A flat cut is then made on the superior surface talus parallel to the tibial cut (Fig. 33.5a).
- Anterior and posterior chamfer cuts are then made using jigs together with 2 slots for the talar implant (Fig. 33.5b).
- Trial implants are then inserted with a mobile polyethylene spacer (Fig. 33.5c).

- The joint and bony surfaces are then washed with pulsed lavage.
- The final implants are inserted uncemented and the tibial window grafted (Fig. 33.5d).
- The wound is closed in layers and a postoperative X-ray taken (Fig. 33.6a, b).

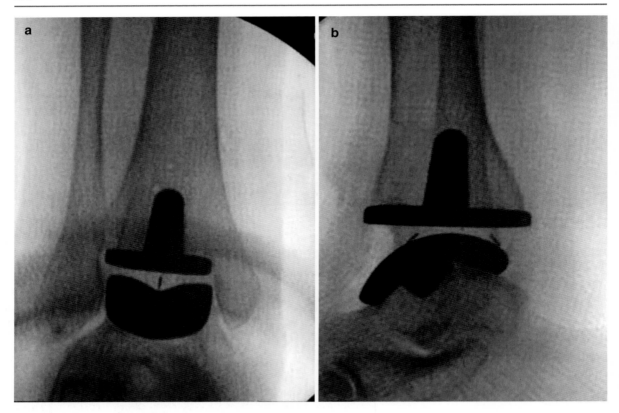

**Fig. 33.6** Postoperative (**a**) AP and (**b**) lateral X-ray of the ankle

## Postoperative Instructions

- The patient is immobilized in a below-knee plaster for 2 weeks while the wounds heal.
- Start mechanical VTE prophylaxis at admission and continue until the patient no longer has significantly reduced mobility, based on an assessment of risks. Start pharmacological VTE prophylaxis after surgery and continue until the patient no longer has significantly reduced mobility.
- Sutures are removed at 2 weeks.
- At 2 weeks, the patient is placed in a removable walker boot and allowed to weight-bear as symptoms permit.

## Follow-Up

- The regular appointments are a month postoperative and the following 3, 6, and12 months with X-rays on arrival.

- Usually, the patients were advised to have full weight bearing from the first post-op days while they are using a Zimmer frame.

## Further Reading

Kim BS, Choi WJ, Kim YS, et al. Total ankle replacement in moderate to severe varus deformity of the ankle. J Bone Joint Surg Br. 2009;91(9):1183–90.

Gougoulias N, Khanna A, Maffulli N. How successful are current ankle replacements?: a systematic review of the literature. Clin Orthop Relat Res. 2010;468(1):199–208.

Steck JK, Anderson JB. Total ankle arthroplasty: indications and avoiding complications. Clin Podiatr Med Surg. 2009;26(2):303–24.

Wood PL, Clough TM, Smith R. The present state of ankle arthroplasty. Foot Ankle Surg. 2008;14(3):115–9.

# Osteochondral Autograft Transfer for an Osteochondral Lesion of the Talus

# 34

Nick Harris

## Indications

- Osteochondral autograft transfer (OAT) for osteochondral lesions of the talus is a second line treatment for symptomatic lesions usually with a cystic element (Type V).

## Preoperative Planning

### Clinical Assessment

- Assess hind foot alignment – severe malalignment should be addressed prior to any OAT procedure.
- Assess range of movement and stability – marked stiffness is a relative contraindication to an OAT type procedure. Instability should be addressed prior to an OAT procedure.
- Assess arterial and venous circulation.

### Radiological Assessment

- An AP and true lateral weight-bearing radiograph of the affected ankle is mandatory.
- An MRI scan is also mandatory to localize and estimate the size of the osteochondral lesion (Fig. 34.1).

N. Harris
Department of Trauma and Orthopaedic Surgery,
Leeds Teaching Hospitals NHS Trust, Leeds, UK
e-mail: nick.harris@leedsth.nhs.uk

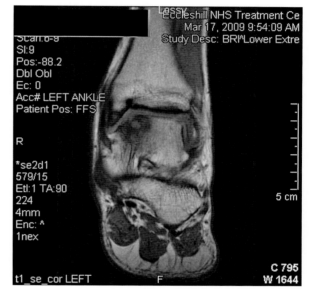

**Fig. 34.1** MRI showing a cystic osteochondral lesion affecting the medial dome of the talus

## Operative Treatment

### Anesthesia

- Regional or general anesthesia with nerve blocks
- High thigh tourniquet
- Antibiotic prophylaxis at induction

### Table and Equipment

- Radiolucent table
- Image intensifier

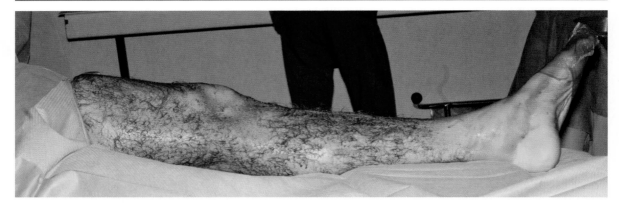

**Fig. 34.2** Preparation and draping of the leg in a supine position as far as thigh tourniquet

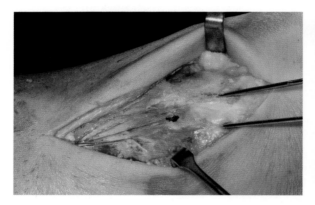

**Fig. 34.3** Skin incision over medial malleolus and insertion of two guide wires

- Sterile single use OATS set (Arthrex, Sheffield, UK) including sizes 6 mm, 8 mm, and 10 mm
- 4.5-mm knee arthroscope

## Table Setup

- Instrumentation is set up on ipsilateral side.
- Image intensifier is set up on contralateral side.

## Patient Positioning

- Supine with lateral support for ipsilateral thigh

## Draping and Surgical Approach

- The skin over the foot and ankle and knee is prepared with an appropriate antiseptic as far as the proximal thigh tourniquet (Fig. 34.2).

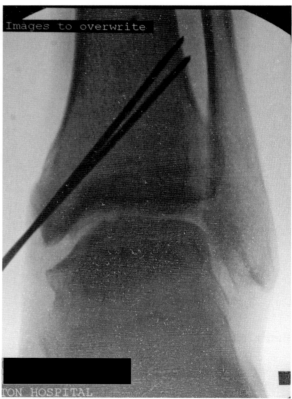

**Fig. 34.4** Two guide wires inserted into medial malleolus under image intensifier control

- A sterile drape is applied as far as the proximal thigh tourniquet.
- A medial incision is made over the medial malleolus (Fig. 34.3).
- The soft tissues are reflected medially and laterally.
- Under image intensifier control, two guide wires are passed up the medial malleolus (Fig. 34.4).

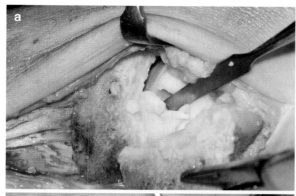

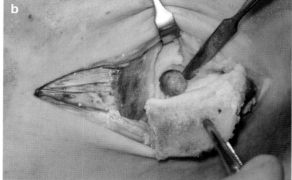

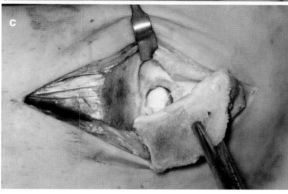

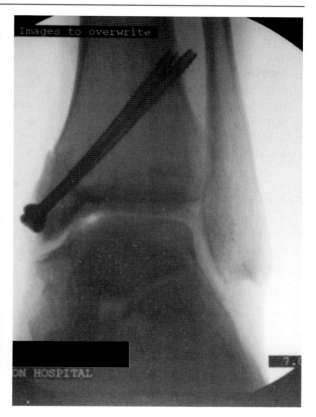

Fig. 34.6 Screws inserted after reduction of osteotomy

Fig. 34.5 (a) Osteotomy of medial malleolus exiting ankle joint at level of osteochondral lesion. (b) Talus following debridement of osteochondral lesion. (c) Talus after press fit of donor graft from intercondylar notch of knee

- The wires are then over drilled and tapped for two screws.
- The wires are then removed.
- An osteotomy is then made under image intensifier control of the medial malleolus exiting the ankle joint at the level of the osteochondral lesion of the talus (Fig. 34.5a).
- Care is taken to protect the tibialis posterior muscle/tendon.

- The osteochondral lesion of the talus is then debrided, sized, and drilled to healthy bone (Fig. 34.5b).
- A donor graft is then harvested arthroscopically from the lateral intercondylar notch of the ipsilateral knee.
- The donor graft should match the recipient defect both in diameter and depth.
- The donor graft is then press fit into the recipient defect in the talus (Fig. 34.5c).
- The joint surfaces are washed.
- The medial malleolus is replaced and fixed with the two screws which have already been pre-drilled and tapped (Fig. 34.6).
- The wound is closed in layers.

## Postoperative Instructions

- The operated leg is immobilized in plaster for 2 weeks followed by a walker boot for a further 4 weeks.

- The patient is kept non-weight-bearing for 6 weeks.
- Start mechanical VTE prophylaxis at admission and continue until the patient no longer has significantly reduced mobility, based on an assessment of risks. Start pharmacological VTE prophylaxis after surgery and continue until the patient no longer has significantly reduced mobility.
- Gentle range of movement exercises are commenced after 2 weeks.

## Follow-Up

- It is advisable to follow up the patients for in • 2 weeks, 4 weeks, 6 weeks, 3, 6, 12 months and thereafter as indicated.

## Further Reading

Scranton PE, Frey CC, Feder KS. Outcome of osteochondral autograft transplantation for type-V cystic osteochondral lesions of the talus. J Bone Joint Surg Br. 2006;88(5):614–9.

Choi WJ, Park KK, Kim BS, et al. Osteochondral lesion of the talus: is there a critical defect size for poor outcome? Am J Sports Med. 2009;37(10):1974–80.

Giannini S, Battaglia M, Buda R, et al. Surgical treatment of osteochondral lesions of the talus by open-field autologous chondrocyte implantation: a 10-year follow-up clinical and magnetic resonance imaging T2-mapping evaluation. Am J Sports Med. 2009;37 Suppl 1:112S–8.

# Achilles Tendon Lengthening

# 35

Peter V. Giannoudis and Efthimios J. Karadimas

## Indications

- Neuromuscular diseases
- Congenital equines foot
- Post-traumatic cases related usually with ankle fractures (Fig. 35.1)

## Clinical Symptoms

- Significantly reduced forefoot dorsiflexion
- Decreased walking ability

## Preoperative Planning

## Clinical Assessment

- The surgeon must assess the mobility of the joints and the strength of the Achilles tendon.

## Radiological Assessment

- A dynamic lateral X-ray could verify correction's range and ankle joint stiffness.

## Operative Treatment

### Anesthesia

- Regional or general anesthesia with nerve blocks
- Antibiotic prophylaxis according to the hospital protocol
- Antibiotic administration prior to tourniquet inflation

### Table/Equipment

- Surgical table
- General surgeons set
  - Thigh tourniquet

### Patient Positioning

- Prone position (Fig. 35.2a)
- Inflate thigh tourniquet to 300 mmHg

### Marking and Draping

- Extensive below knee skin preparation with the use of antiseptic solutions (alcoholic povidone/iodine) (Fig. 35.2b)
- Extra care in the web spaces between the toes

P.V. Giannoudis (✉)
Academic Department of Trauma and Orthopaedic Surgery,
School of Medicine, University of Leeds,
Leeds, UK
e-mail: pgiannoudi@aol.com

E.J. Karadimas
Department of Trauma and Orthopaedic Surgery,
Leeds Teaching Hospitals NHS Trust,
Leeds, UK

P.V. Giannoudis (ed.), *Practical Procedures in Elective Orthopaedic Surgery*,
DOI 10.1007/978-0-85729-814-0_35, © Springer-Verlag London Limited 2012

**Fig. 35.1** AP and lateral X-rays of a patient with post-traumatic arthritis of the ankle joint

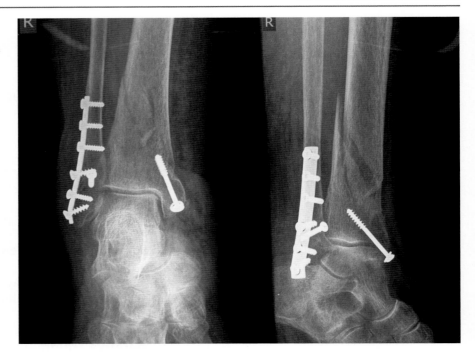

## Surgical Exposure

- There are several approaches through which Achilles tendon lengthening can be achieved.
- Percutaneous approach:
  - Create three small vertical stab cuts at both tendon sites.
  - Try to avoid being over the 50% of tendon thickness.
  - Dorsiflex the forefoot in order to achieve passive tendon stretching/lengthening.
- Z-plasty lengthening:
  - Involves an open approach at the posterior aspect of the ankle (Fig. 35.3a) which exposes the tendon (Fig. 35.3b).
  - Measure the length of the desirable tendon's elongation (Fig. 35.4).
  - Make a Z-cut in the tendon sheath.
  - Stretch the tendon apart to achieve the desirable length (Fig. 35.5).
  - Use nonabsorbable sutures to secure the lengthening (Fig. 35.6).
  - It is advisable that the assistant should hold the forefoot in dorsiflexion (over-correction) while the suturing is performed.

- Gastrocnemius recession:
  - Identify the gastrocnemius muscle and release its fibers.
  - Leave the soleus muscle untouched.
  - This method can be used for less severe contractures.

## Closure

- Release tourniquet and check for bleeding.
- Use 2/0 Vicryl interrupted sutures for closure of the subcutaneous layer.
- Use 3/0 Ethilon nonabsorbable interrupted suture for skin closure.
- A back slap or a full cast is applied, holding the leg in overcorrection.

## Postoperative Care/Rehabilitation

- Antibiotics (as per hospital protocol).
- Start mechanical VTE prophylaxis at admission and continue until the patient no longer has significantly reduced mobility, based on an assessment of

**Fig. 35.2** (**a**) Prone position. (**b**) Skin preparation

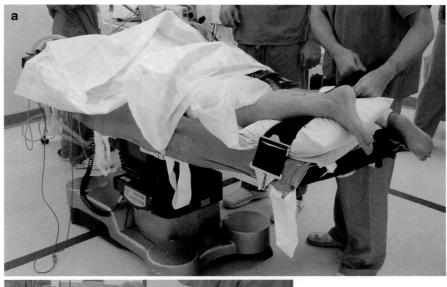

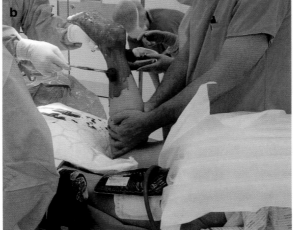

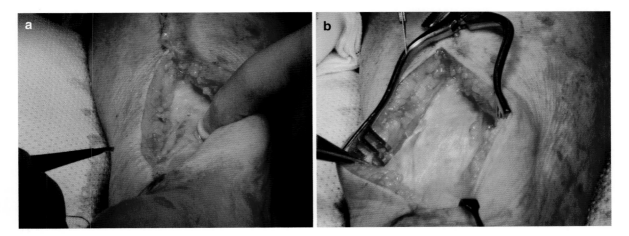

**Fig. 35.3** (**a**) A straight incision is performed (usually from the medial side). (**b**) The tendon is exposed

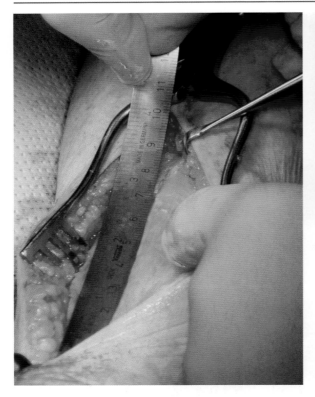

**Fig. 35.4** The lengthening required is measured

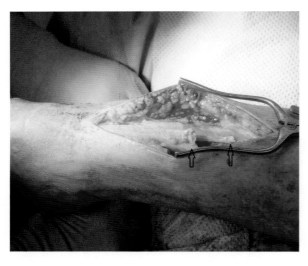

**Fig. 35.5** The desirable elongation is performed and controlled. It is evident in the distance between the *arrows*

risks. Start pharmacological VTE prophylaxis after surgery and continue until the patient no longer has significantly reduced mobility.
- Wound inspection within 48 h.

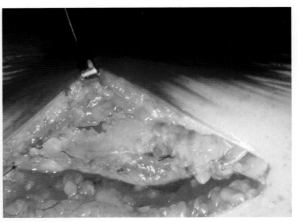

**Fig. 35.6** The lengthening is secured with sutures

- Full cast is applied for 6 weeks, non-weight-bearing for 6 weeks.
- Following that the cast is removed and physiotherapy can start.

## Complications

- Tendon mechanical failure/rupture
- Persistent pain and scar formation
- Joint stiffness
- Infection

## Follow-Up

- Outpatients follow up at 6, 12 weeks for clinical assessment.
- It is important to know that early mobilization and weight bearing may cause tendon rupture, and on the other hand, late mobilization can result in scar formation and stiffness.

## Further Reading

Chen L, Greisberg J. Achilles lengthening procedures. Foot Ankle Clin. 2009;14(4):627–37.

Schweinberger MH, Roukis TS. Surgical correction of soft-tissue ankle equinus contracture. Clin Podiatr Med Surg. 2008;25(4):571–85.

Meszaros A, Caudell G. The surgical management of equinus in the adult acquired flatfoot. Clin Podiatr Med Surg. 2007;24(4):667–85.

# Posterior Tibialis Tendon Transfer

# 36

## Peter V. Giannoudis and Efthimios J. Karadimas

## Indications

- Neuromuscular diseases
- Post-traumatic drop foot
- Congenital clubfoot

## Clinical Symptoms

- Incompetence to dorsiflex the forefoot
- Reduced ability of walking
- Drop foot in elderly increases the incident of falls

## Preoperative Planning

### Clinical Assessment

- The surgeon must assess the mobility of the joints and the strength of tibialis posterior muscle.
- With transposition, some muscular loss of functionality and strength is expected.

P.V. Giannoudis (✉)
Academic Department of Trauma and Orthopaedic Surgery,
School of Medicine, University of Leeds,
Leeds, UK
e-mail: pgiannoudi@aol.com

E.J. Karadimas
Department of Trauma and Orthopaedic Surgery,
Leeds Teaching Hospitals NHS Trust,
Leeds, UK

## Radiological Assessment

- A dynamic lateral X-ray could verify correction's range and joint's stiffness.

## Operative Treatment

### Anesthesia

- Regional or general anesthesia with nerve blocks
- Antibiotic prophylaxis according to the hospital protocol
- Antibiotic administration prior to tourniquet inflation

### Table/Equipment

- Surgical table
- Small fragment set/ wide drill set/ anchors or other system to hold the tendon in the new insertion point (Fig. 36.1)
- Thigh tourniquet

### Patient Positioning

- Supine position
- Inflate thigh tourniquet to 300 mmHg

P.V. Giannoudis (ed.), *Practical Procedures in Elective Orthopaedic Surgery*,
DOI 10.1007/978-0-85729-814-0_36, © Springer-Verlag London Limited 2012

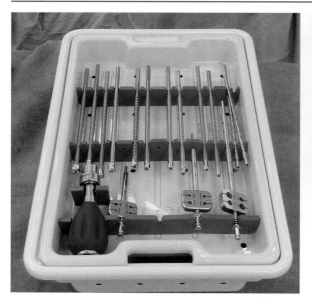

Fig. 36.1 Tray of instruments used for tendon fixation

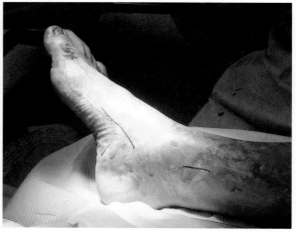

Fig. 36.3 Marking the incisions

## Marking and Draping

- Extensive below-knee skin preparation with the use of antiseptic solutions (alcoholic povidone/iodine) (Fig. 36.2)
- Extra care in the web spaces between the toes.
- Mark two incisions medially (the first over the navicular and the second one 5–6 cm proximal to the medial malleolus), a third incision laterally (5–6 cm proximal to the lateral malleolus), and a fourth incision over the 2nd or 3 rd cuneiform (Fig. 36.3)

## Surgical Exposure

- Posterior tibialis tendon is exposed initially at its insertion into the navicular and 1st–2nd MTT (Fig. 36.4a).
- The tendon is detached from its insertion (Fig. 36.4b). Suture placement at tendon edges will help with the transposition.
- Through the second incision, the tendon is retracted proximally up to one-third of the tibia (Fig. 36.5).
- Through the third incision, indentify the space between the anterior tibialis (deep fascia opened) and tibial crest, from where the tendon will be passed. The tendon is then transpositioned laterally (Fig. 36.6).
- The fourth incision is carried out; a tunnel connecting the 3rd and 4th incision is performed under the retinaculum of the extensor tendons (Fig. 36.7a). The tendon is retracted through the last incision (Fig. 36.7b).

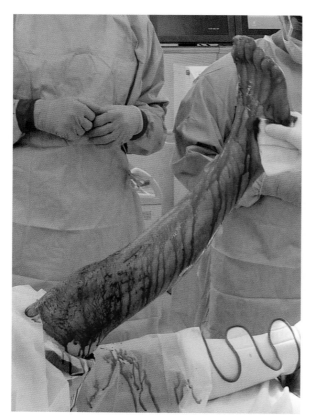

Fig. 36.2 Below-knee skin preparation

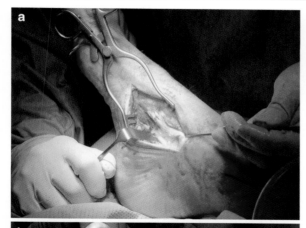

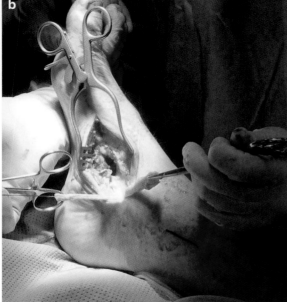

**Fig. 36.4** (**a**) First incision over navicular at the medial side. (**b**) Posterior tibialis tendon detachment

- With a drill, the new insertion point over the cuneiform is created (Fig. 36.8).
- The tendon of the posterior tibialis is delivered to its new insertion with the foot in dorsiflexed position.
- The fixation is secured either with the use of suture anchors (Fig. 36.9) or with a button on the plantar side of the foot.

## Closure

- Release tourniquet and check for bleeding.
- Use 2/0 vicryl interrupted sutures for closure of the subcutaneous layer.

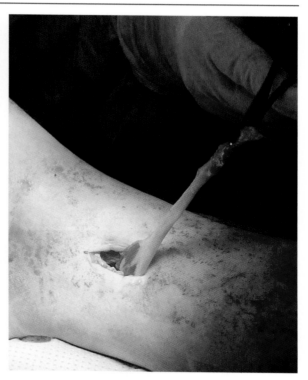

**Fig. 36.5** Posterior tibialis tendon is retracted through the second incision (proximally)

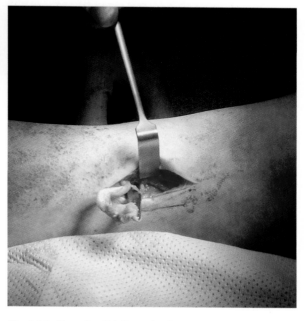

**Fig. 36.6** Posterior tibialis tendon is retracted through the third incision (laterally)

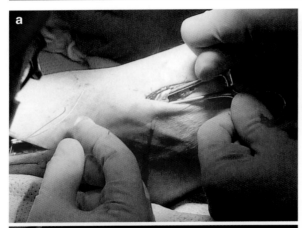

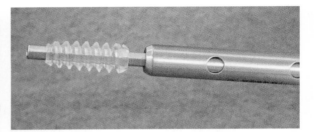

**Fig. 36.9** The anchoring system for tendon fixation

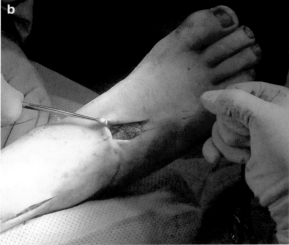

**Fig. 36.7** (**a**) Tunnel is performed connecting 3rd and 4th incisions. (**b**) Posterior tibialis tendon is retracted through the fourth incision

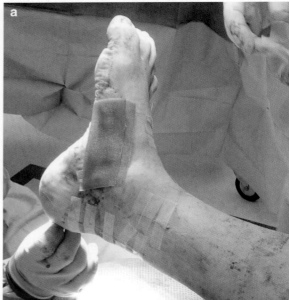

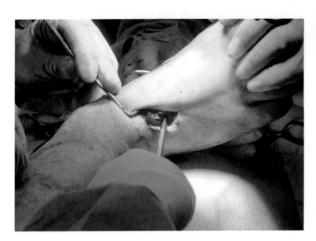

**Fig. 36.8** Creation of the new insertion point over the cuneiform with a drill

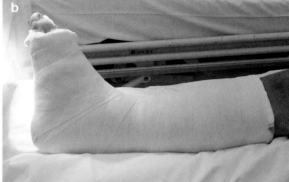

**Fig. 36.10** (**a**) Wound dressing. (**b**) Application of full non-weight-bearing cast

- Use 3/0 ethilon nonabsorbable suture or absorbable monocryl sutures for skin closure.
- Wound dressing and wool application (Fig. 36.10a).
- It is advisable to use swabs in the toes' web spaces.
- A back slap or a full cast is applied, holding the leg in overcorrection (Fig. 36.10b).

## Postoperative Care/Rehabilitation

- Antibiotics (as per hospital protocol).
- Start mechanical VTE prophylaxis at admission and continue until the patient no longer has significantly reduced mobility, based on an assessment of risks. Start pharmacological VTE prophylaxis after surgery and continue until the patient no longer has significantly reduced mobility.
- Wound inspection within 48 h.
- Full cast is applied for 6 weeks, non-weight-bearing for 6 weeks.
- Following that, the cast is removed and physiotherapy is started.

## Complications

- Tendon mechanical failure
- Joint stiffness

## Follow-Up

- Outpatients follow-up at 6, 12 weeks for clinical assessment.
- It is important to know that early mobilization and weight bearing may cause tendon rupture, and on the other hand, late mobilization can result in scar formation and stiffness.

## Further Reading

Yeap JS, Birch R, Singh D. Long-term results of tibialis posterior tendon transfer for drop-foot. Int Orthop. 2001;25(2):114–8.

Hove LM, Nilsen PT. Posterior tibial tendon transfer for drop-foot. Acta Orthop Scand. 1998;69(6):608–10.

Goh JC, Lee PY, Lee EH, et al. Biomechanical study on tibialis posterior tendon transfers. Clin Orthop Relat Res. 1995;319: 297–302.

# Triple Arthrodesis of the Foot

# 37

Panayiotis N. Soucacos and Rozalia I. Dimitriou

## Introduction

- The triple foot arthrodesis consists of fusion of the talonavicular, calcaneocuboid, and subtalar joints, aiming to achieve a stable, painless, and plantigrade foot.
- It is a technically demanding procedure with a prolonged recovery period.

## Indications

- Arthritis that involves the subtalar joint and either the talonavicular or the calcaneocuboid joint, or both, including post-traumatic degenerative and rheumatoid arthritis
- Unstable or/and deformed hindfoot secondary to congenital and acquired neuromuscular disorders such as poliomyelitis, Charcot-Marie-Tooth, posterior tendon dysfunction; nerve injury, and cerebral palsy
- End-stage posterior tibialis tendon rupture with fixed bone deformity
- Foot malalignment secondary to arthrofibrosis as a result of compartment syndrome, crush injury, or severe trauma

P.N. Soucacos (✉)
Professor of Orthopaedic Surgery,
University of Athens, School of Medicine, Director,
Orthopaedic Research & Education Center (OREC),,
Athens, Greece
e-mail: psoukakos@ath.forthnet.gr

R.I. Dimitriou
Department of Trauma and Orthopaedic Surgery,
Leeds Teaching Hospitals NHS Trust, Leeds, UK

- Symptomatic, previously resected or not, calcaneo-navicular coalition
- Severely symptomatic pes planus/cavus deformities

## Preoperative Planning

### Clinical Assessment

- Examine the affected foot for pain, motion, or any fixed deformity and assess the relationship between the forefoot and the hindfoot in pronation and supination deformities.
- Assess the circulation status. If pedal pulses are not palpable, preoperative arterial Doppler evaluation should be performed.
- Document sensation prior to surgery and if peripheral neuropathy is present.
- Assess secondary contracture of the gastrocnemius-soleus complex, or contraction of the plantar fascia.
- Examine the normal foot and note its alignment.

### Radiological Assessment

- Full weight-bearing anteroposterior, lateral (Fig. 37.1), and oblique plain radiographs of the foot and anteroposterior, lateral, and mortise views of the ankle.
- Valgus angulation of the talus in the ankle mortise is suggestive of deltoid ligament insufficiency, which may promote degenerative arthritic changes in the ankle joint postoperatively.

P.V. Giannoudis (ed.), *Practical Procedures in Elective Orthopaedic Surgery*,
DOI 10.1007/978-0-85729-814-0_37, © Springer-Verlag London Limited 2012

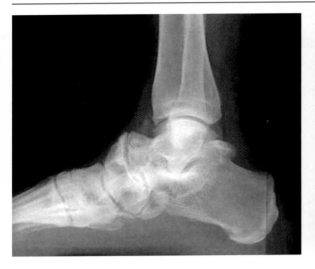

**Fig. 37.1** Preoperative lateral radiograph of the foot showing the arthritis of the subtalar and talonavicular joints

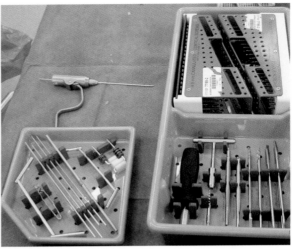

**Fig. 37.2** Tray of cannulated screws

- In cases of severe deformity, computer tomography with sagittal reconstruction may be helpful.

## Timing of Surgery

- It should be reserved as a salvage procedure for an end-stage painful, unstable foot or for a fixed and disabling deformed foot with degenerative changes of the hindfoot. Whenever possible, other procedures that preserve hindfoot motion and mechanics must be considered.

## Operative Treatment

### Anaesthesia

- Regional (spinal/epidural) and/or general anaesthesia
- Prophylactic antibiotics as per hospital protocol

### Table and Equipment

- Thigh tourniquet
- 4–4.5 mm and 7–7.3 mm cannulated screws, power staples, and a standard osteosynthesis set (Fig. 37.2)
- A radiolucent table
- An image intensifier

## Table Setup

- The instrumentation is at the foot end of the table.
- Image intensifier is at the contralateral site.

## Patient Positioning

- The patient is placed in a supine position with a support under the ipsilateral hip to improve visualization of the lateral aspect of the hindfoot. The respective leg is already marked.
- Tourniquet is applied.

## Draping

- Skin preparation over lower leg, ankle, and entire foot thoroughly, with usual antiseptic solutions.
- Standard draping around lower leg in calf region.
- Apply tape around toes to minimize the risk of infection.

## Surgical Approach and Technique

- A two-incision approach: one lateral and one medial.
- The first incision is the lateral (Fig. 37.3a, b), from the tip of the fibula down to the base of the fourth

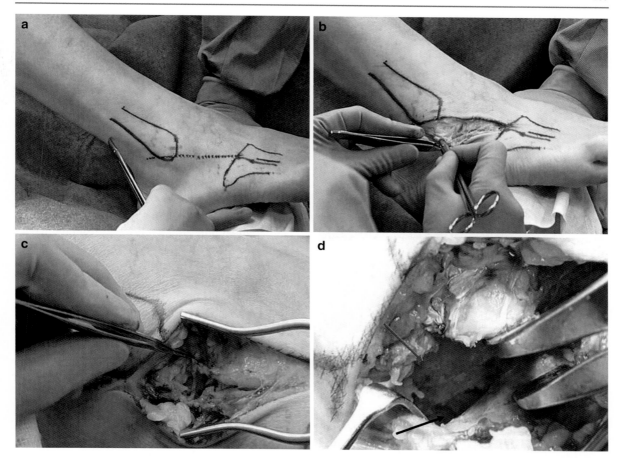

**Fig. 37.3** (**a, b**) The first incision is the lateral from the tip of the fibula down to the base of the fourth metatarsal. (**c**) The short extensor muscles are reflected dorsomedially and extensor digitorum brevis medially; the interosseous ligament is removed, and the subtalar joint is visualized. (**d**). Articular cartilage and subchondral bone to the level of the exposed cancellous surfaces are removed from the subtalar joint to allow fusion (*red arrow* shows the talus and *black arrow* the posterior facet of the os calcis)

metatarsal. Caution when deepening the incision at its distal part to avoid injury of an anterior branch of the sural nerve. The short extensor muscles are reflected dorsomedially and extensor digitorum brevis medially; the interosseous ligament is removed, and the subtalar joint is visualized (Fig. 37.3c). Articular cartilage and subchondral bone to the level of the exposed cancellous surfaces are removed (Fig. 37.3d) from the subtalar and calcaneocuboid joints, as well as from the lateral aspect of the talonavicular joint with the use of laminar spreader, a small osteotome and a curette. Attention must be paid not to injure flexor hallucis longus as it passes under the sustentaculum tali and to preserve the normal shape of the articular surfaces.

- The second incision is a dorsomedial incision (Fig. 37.4a) from the tip of the medial malleolus to the level of the navicular-cuneiform joint. The incision is deepened in the interval between the anterior and the posterior tibialis tendon, and care must be taken to avoid the saphenous nerve and vein. The talonavicular joint is identified by moving the forefoot in abduction and adduction. Dissection around the talar neck should be minimal to preserve the arterial branches of dorsalis pedis. Cartilage and subchondral bone are removed using a curette or an osteotome. Once more, the normal shape of the articular surfaces must be preserved.

- The hindfoot is manipulated first by bringing the subtalar joint into 3–5° of residual heel valgus, than the transverse tarsal joint into 0–5° of abduction, and the forefoot into less than 10° of varus. The foot cannot be manipulated if the joints have not been completely mobilized.

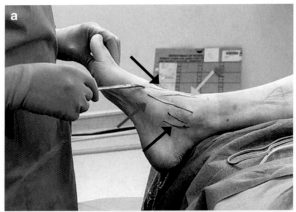

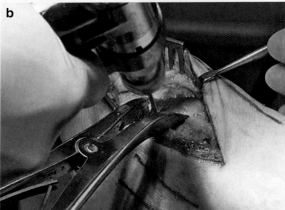

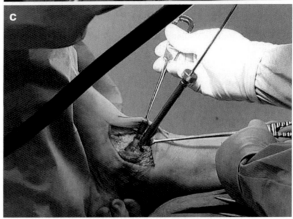

**Fig. 37.4** (**a**) The second incision is a dorsomedial incision from the tip of the medial malleolus to the level of the navicular-cuneiform joint (*red arrow*). The incision is deepened in the interval between the anterior and the posterior tibialis tendon (*black arrows*) and care must be taken to avoid the saphenous nerve and vein (*yellow arrow*). (**b**, **c**) After dissection, cartilage and subchondral bone are removed using a curette or an osteotome; the hindfoot is manipulated to achieve the appropriate position of arthrodesis, and a guide pin is introduced from the talar neck and directed inferiorly to the calcaneus. Fixation is performed with a cannulated screw (*dashed black arrow* in Fig. 37.5a)

- It is important to achieve proper reduction of the joints and good compression with rigid fixation. The position of arthrodesis is critical, because it provides a fixed position of the foot that cannot accommodate to the ground.
- It is easier to stabilize the subtalar joint first. A guide pin can be introduced either from the talar neck and directed inferiorly (Fig. 37.4b, c) or from the calcaneus and directed superiorly. Its position is verified by fluoroscopy. Fixation is performed with a cannulated screw (7.0–7.3 mm) with or without a washer, or with staples, driven from the neck of the talus through the posterior body of the calcaneus. Initial guide pins are then inserted from the naviculo-cuneiform joint and driven obliquely into the neck of the talus and from the calcaneus into the cuboid; and fixation of the talonavicular (Fig. 37.5a–c) and calcaneocuboid joints (Fig. 37.6a, b) respectively are then performed using a 4.5-mm or larger cannulated screw or staples.
- Bone grafting (usually autologous bone graft) may be required to bridge a large bone defect.
- The lateral talocalcaneal angle should be restored to prevent anterior tibiotalar impingement postoperatively.
- When Achilles tendon lengthening is required, a percutaneous technique of lengthening is preferred with three short transverse skin and tendon incisions.
- In more severe and fixed cavovarus deformities of the foot, a variation of triple arthrodesis, the Siffert beak-type triple arthrodesis, can be performed. After a lateral closing wedge osteotomy in the subtalar joint, the navicular is mortised beneath the head of the talus to reduce the longitudinal arch height. The residual forefoot adduction is corrected, and the shortening of the medial column is adjusted by removing a lateral wedge from the calcaneocuboid joint.
- Finally, partial resection of the talar head in the early intraoperative stages has been described to facilitate reduction of the deformity.

## Closure

- Over the lateral side, extensor digitorum brevis is sutured, followed by closure of the subcutaneous tissue and skin.
- On the medial side, capsular tissue over the talonavicular joint is preferably closed prior to subcutaneous tissue and skin closure.

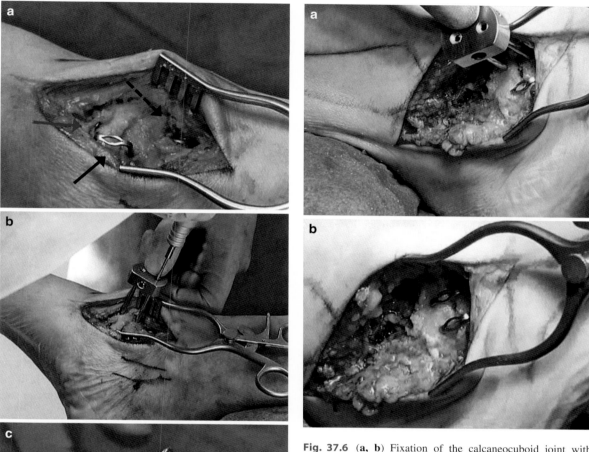

Fig. 37.6 (**a, b**) Fixation of the calcaneocuboid joint with staples

Fig. 37.5 (**a–c**) Fixation of the talonavicular joint with staples (*black arrow*) and a screw (*red arrow*) (*dashed black* shows the cannulated screw used for the subtalar joint)

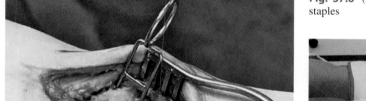

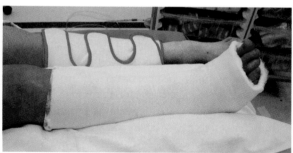

Fig. 37.7 Postoperatively, a below-knee plaster splint is applied

- Local anaesthetic (e.g., bupivacaine) can be instilled into the surgical wounds, or popliteal block can be performed, for initial postoperative analgesia.
- A compression dressing with a below-knee plaster splint is applied (Fig. 37.7).

## Postoperative Care and Rehabilitation

- Start mechanical VTE prophylaxis at admission and continue until the patient no longer has significantly reduced mobility based on an assessment of

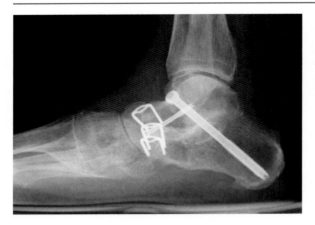

**Fig. 37.8** Postoperative lateral X-ray confirming fusion after triple foot fusion with staples and screws

risks. Start pharmacological VTE prophylaxis after surgery and continue until the patient no longer has significantly reduced mobility.

- Removal of sutures and change of initial plaster splint at 10–14 days after surgery.
- A short-leg removable cast is applied, and an elastic bandage is used to control oedema.
- Non-weight-bearing for 6 weeks.

## Outpatients Follow-Up

- X-rays at 6 weeks to assess the progression of fusion. If satisfactory, weight-bearing as tolerated is permitted with the removable cast.
- X-rays at 12 weeks, and if fusion is achieved (Fig. 37.8), the patient is allowed to bear weight as tolerated with an elastic stocking. If fusion is tenuous, the use of the cast must be prolonged.
- After solid union, a strengthening program for the muscles of the leg is recommended.

## Complications

- Nonunion of one of the fusion sites, and most often of the talonavicular joint. If asymptomatic, no treatment is indicated. If painful, but with satisfactory alignment of the foot, bone graft with or without reinforcement of the internal fixation is usually sufficient to achieve fusion. But if nonunion is symptomatic and the alignment is unsatisfactory, revision of the arthrodesis is required.
- Foot malalignment, under- or over-correction. Most frequent is residual varus of the calcaneus with a forefoot fixed in varus and adduction. Residual valgus may lead to lateral subfibular impingement and lateral pain, and if minor, it can be treated conservatively with a shoe insole. Residual varus may lead to lateral ankle instability and secondary ankle arthritis. Excessive hindfoot valgus or varus will result in abnormal gait pattern and may require either a medial or lateral displacement calcaneal osteotomy, respectively, or a revision of the triple arthrodesis.
- Secondary degenerative arthritis of the ankle and tarsometatarsal joints, and especially in patients with residual malalignment.
- Avascular necrosis of the talus. Initially, it can be treated with bracing, but if bracing is unsuccessful, ankle fusion should be considered.
- Recurrence of the deformity, especially in skeletally immature patients.
- Dysesthesias on the lateral side of the foot as a result of entrapment or injury of the sural nerve or its anterior branch, that may require neurolysis or nerve resection and burying of the stump under soft tissues or into bone.
- Achilles tendon over-lengthening.

## Implant Removal

- No implant removal is necessary, unless there is evidence of infection or soft tissue irritation.

## Further Reading

Coughlin MJ, Mann RA, Saltzman CL. Surgery of the Foot and Ankle, 8th edition (vol. II) Elsevier Mosby, Philadelphia, PA, 2007.

Figgie MP, O'Malley MJ, Ranawat C, Inglis AE, Sculco TP. Triple arthrodesis in rheumatoid arthritis. Clin Orthop Relat Res. 1993;292:250–4.

Scranton Jr PE. Results of arthrodesis of the tarsus: talocalcaneal, midtarsal, and subtalar joints. Foot Ankle. 1991;12(3):156–64.

Sullivan RJ, Aronow MS. Different faces of the triple arthrodesis. Foot Ankle Clin. 2002;7(1):95–106.

Thompson NS, Henderson SA. Talar head resection in difficult triple arthrodesis. Foot Ankle Surg. 2002;8(3):213–9.

Wapner KL. Triple arthrodesis in adults. J Am Acad Orthop Surg. 1998;6(3):188–96.

# Hallux Valgus Correction

**38**

Peter V. Giannoudis and Fragkiskos N. Xypnitos

## Introduction

- Hallux valgus (HV) is a medial deviation of the first metatarsal and lateral deviation and/or rotation of the hallux, with or without medial soft tissue enlargement of the first metatarsal head.
- This condition can lead to painful motion of the joint or difficulty with footwear.
- More than 100 procedures and variations have been developed for the correction of hallux valgus.
- It is more frequent in mid-aged women and there is also a familiar predisposing factor as well in patients with rheumatoid or gouty arthritis.
- Patients suffering from hallux valgus with concomitant deformities have a beneficial outcome following surgery, provided that simultaneous correction of the coexisting deformities will be performed at the same session.

## Indications

- Painful joint ROM.
- Deformity.
- Pain or difficulty with footwear.

P.V. Giannoudis (✉)
Academic Department of Trauma and Orthopaedic Surgery,
School of Medicine, University of Leeds,
Leeds, UK
e-mail: pgiannoudi@aol.com

F.N. Xypnitos
Department of Trauma and Orthopaedics Surgery,
Leeds Teaching Hospitals NHS Trust,
Leeds, UK

- Inhibition of activity or lifestyle.
- Overlapping/underlapping second digit.
- Bunion formation over the first metatarsal head (Fig. 38.1a).
- Ulceration.
- Inflammatory conditions of first metatarsal head.

## Contraindication

- Severe peripheral vascular disease.
- Active infection, septic arthritis.
- Lack of pain or deformity.

## Clinical Symptoms

- Pain localized over the first metatarsal head.
- Painful walking.
- Decreased walking capacity.
- Callosities formation (Fig. 38.1b).

## Preoperative Planning

### Clinical Assessment

- Assessment of resultant pathology.
- Assess any structural deformity and the ROM of the forefoot joints.
- Assess state of surrounding soft tissues.
- Any underlying toe inflammation must be excluded.
- Patients with a positive diabetes family history should be screened.

P.V. Giannoudis (ed.), *Practical Procedures in Elective Orthopaedic Surgery*,
DOI 10.1007/978-0-85729-814-0_38, © Springer-Verlag London Limited 2012

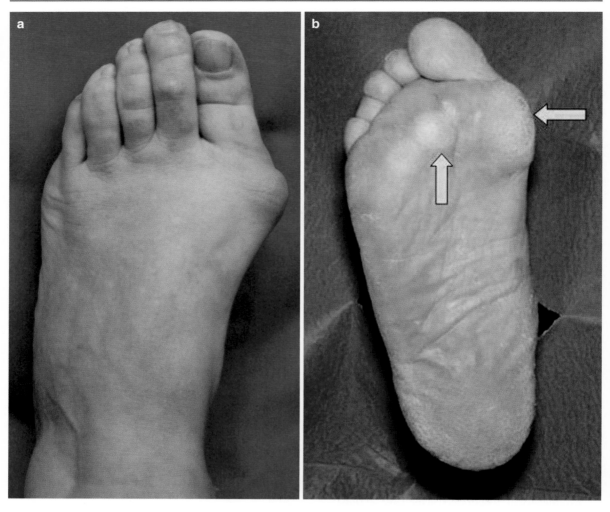

**Fig. 38.1** (**a**) Bunion formation over the first metatarsal head. (**b**) Callosity formation (*arrows*)

## Radiological Assessment

- Arthritic joint changes are evident in plain X-rays.
- Obtain AP (weight-bearing) and lateral views of the feet (Fig. 38.2a, b).
- Measure the HV angle and the intermetatarsal angle to estimate the correction needed.

## Pelmatography

- It is often needed to evaluate the necessity of any additional operation for concomitant deformities.

**Fig. 38.2** X-ray evaluation with (**a**) AP and (**b**) lateral images

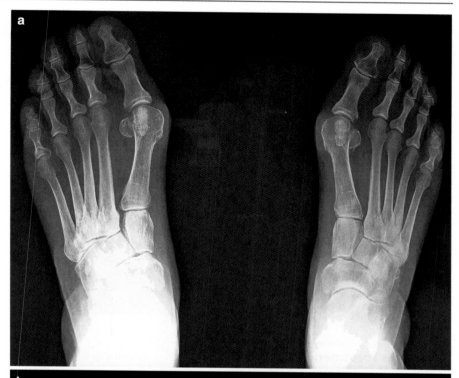

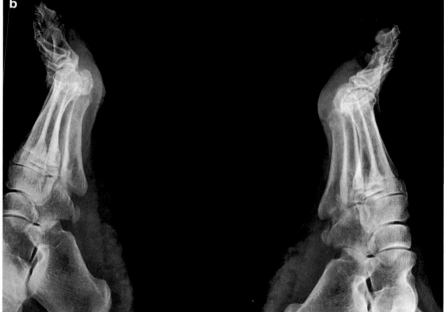

**Fig. 38.3** Marking the incision. In our case, the hallux valgus correction was combined with metatarsal head osteotomy

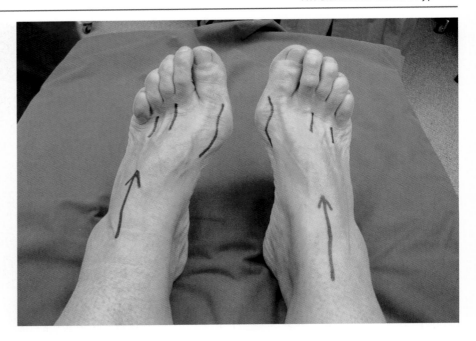

## Operative Treatment

### Anesthesia

- General anesthesia, spinal, or epidural can be discussed with the patient.
- Antibiotic prophylaxis according to the hospital protocol.
- Antibiotic administration prior to tourniquet inflation.

### Table/Equipment

- Radiolucent table.
- Imaging intensifier.
- Small fragment set/power saw with narrow blades.
- Thigh tourniquet.

### Patient Positioning

- Supine positioning.
- Inflate thigh tourniquet to 300 mmHg; be aware that in obese people, the tourniquet could slip and not be effective.

### Marking and Draping

- Mark the incision at the first metatarsal over the bunion (dorsomedial) (Fig. 38.3).
- Extensive below-knee skin preparation with the use of antiseptic solutions (alcoholic povidone/iodine); extra care in the web spaces between the toes.

## Surgical Exposure

### Mitchell Osteotomy

- Skin incision from the midshaft of the proximal phalanx up to the distal one-third of the first metatarsal (Fig. 38.4a) (be aware of the terminal branches of the medial division of the superficial peroneal nerve).
- Y-shape capsular incision over the bunion (Fig. 38.4b, c).
- The bunion is exposed (Fig. 38.4d), and with a power saw, the bony eminence is removed (Fig. 38.5a, b).
- Drill two holes vertical to the shaft from the dorsal to the plantar direction. The first one about 1.5 cm from the metatarsal head and more medially (Fig. 38.6a) and the second one 1 cm proximal to the first one and more lateral. Pass a no. 1 absorbable suture (Fig. 38.6b).

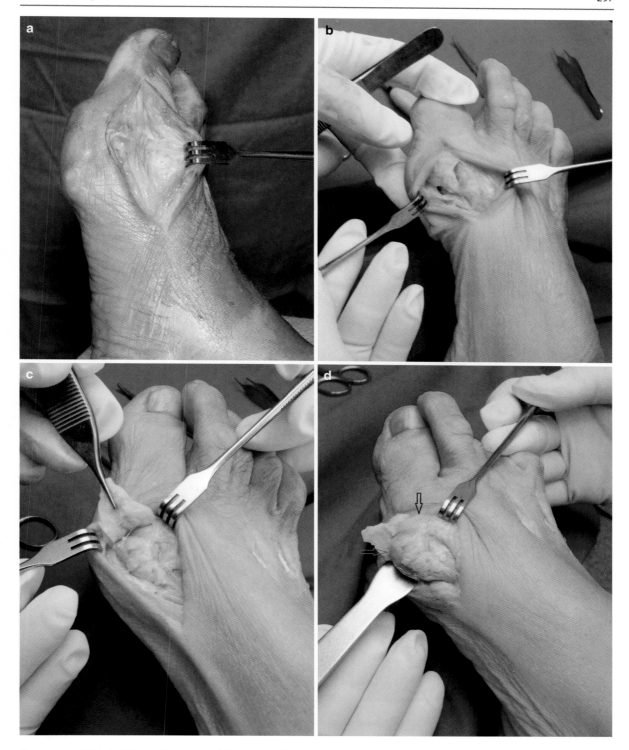

**Fig. 38.4** (**a**) Skin incision and exposure of the capsule. (**b**) Capsule was incised in Y shape and (**c**) retracted, and (**d**) the exposed bunion (the *black arrow* outlines the join surface and the *red* the bunion)

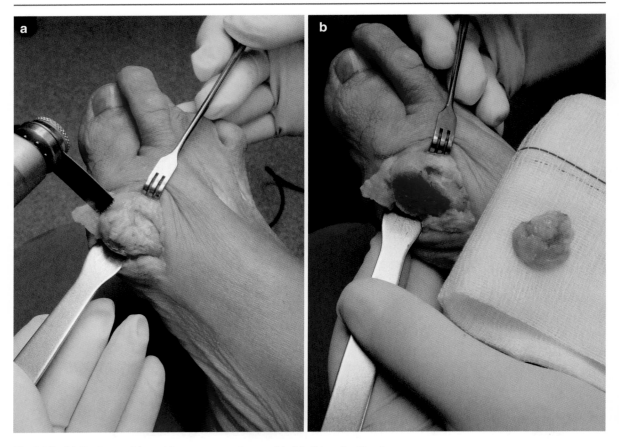

**Fig. 38.5** (**a**) Bunion excision with a power saw (narrow blade), (**b**) excised bunion

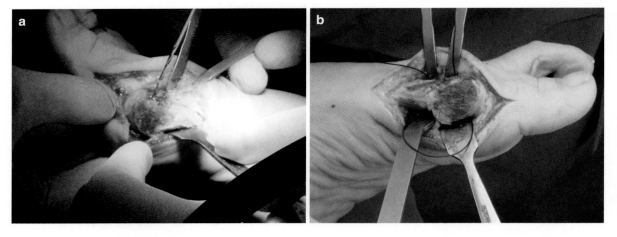

**Fig. 38.6** (**a**) Drilling of one of the two holes vertical to the shaft from the dorsal to the plantar direction. (**b**) Suture in place

- With a power saw, a double osteotomy is performed, the first incomplete, preserving a spike (step) in the lateral cortex (spike's size depends on the intermetatarsal angle: 10–12° angle = 3–4 mm spike), and the second complete, proximal to the first (Fig. 38.7a, b).

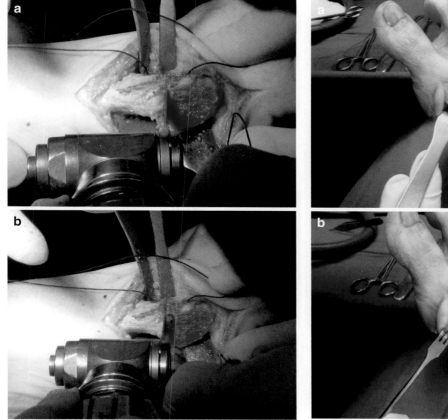

Fig. 38.7 Double osteotomy, (a) distal and (b) proximal

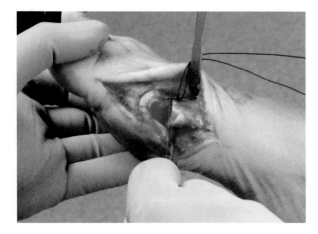

Fig. 38.8 Tying of suture

- Manually shift the distal fragment laterally until the spike rests opposite to the lateral cortex of the proximal fragment.

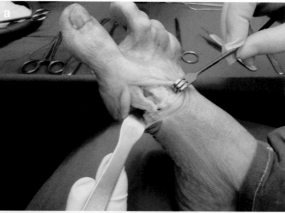

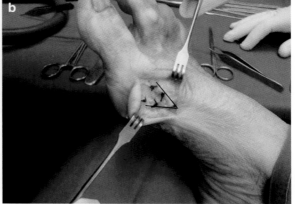

Fig. 38.9 Capsuloplasty: (a) the originally Y shape is sutured in (b) V shape

- Tie the suture with 10° of plantar flexion of the distal fragment (Fig. 38.8).
- The capsule is closed and the originally Y shape is sutured in V shape (capsuloplasty) (Fig. 38.9a, b).

## Wilson Osteotomy

- Skin incision from the midshaft of the proximal phalanx up to the distal one-third of the first metatarsal (Fig. 38.3).
- Y-shape capsular incision over the bunion (Fig. 38.4b, c).
- The bunion is exposed (Fig. 38.4d), and with a power saw, the bony eminence is removed (Fig. 38.5a, b).
- A 45° osteotomy is performed to the longitudinal axes with a narrow saw, preserving the lateral cortex (Fig. 38.10a).

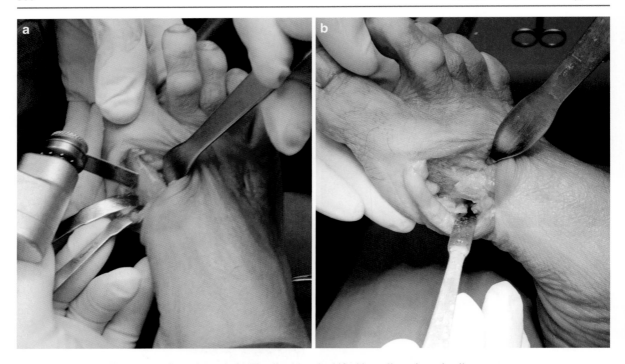

**Fig. 38.10** (**a**) A 45° osteotomy is performed. (**b**) The distal part is shifted laterally and proximally

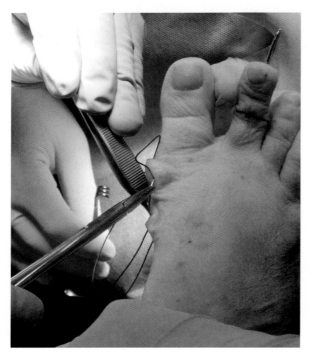

**Fig. 38.11** Varus position of hallux valgus during capsuloplasty

- A thin osteotome completes the osteotomy and as a fulcrum allows the transposition of the metatarsal head proximal and laterally (Fig. 38.10b).
- The osteotomy is held in place by holding hallux in varus position during capsuloplasty (Fig. 38.11).

## Closure

- Release tourniquet and check for any sources of bleeding.
- Use 2/0 Vicryl interrupted sutures for closure of the subcutaneous layer.
- Use 3/0 Ethilon nonabsorbable suture for skin closure (Fig. 38.12).
- Wound dressing and wool application are applied in a way to hold the first toe in varus (Fig. 38.13a, b).
- Depending on surgeon's preference, a custom made brace/shoe is applied.

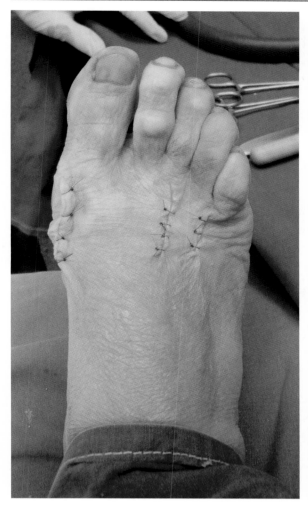

**Fig. 38.12** Skin closure with nonabsorbable sutures Ethilon 3/0

## Postoperative Care/Rehabilitation

- Antibiotics (as per hospital protocol).
- Start mechanical VTE prophylaxis at admission and continue until the patient no longer has significantly reduced mobility, based on an assessment of risks. Start pharmacological VTE prophylaxis after surgery and continue until the patient no longer has significantly reduced mobility.
- Wound inspection within 48 h.
- Obtain radiographs AP/lateral of forefoot.
- Pain management is obligatory.
- Weight bearing from the second week depending on pain and fixation type.

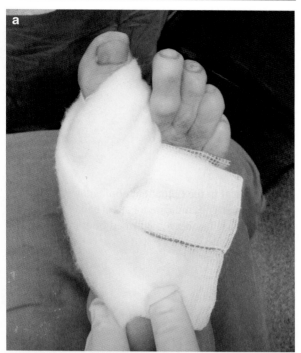

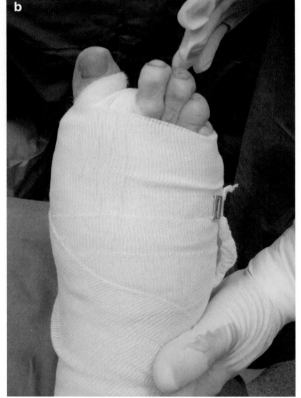

**Fig. 38.13** (**a**, **b**) Dressing is applied in such a fashion that holds the hallux row in varus position

## Complications

- Recurrence
- Development of hallux varus
- Wound infection
- Malunion, nonunion
- Metatarsalgia

## Follow-Up

- See patient in the outpatient clinic at 4, 8, 12 weeks and thereafter as indicated. Patient can be discharged when union has been confirmed both clinically and radiologically.

## Further Reading

Easley ME, Trnka HJ. Current concepts review: hallux valgus part II: operative treatment. Foot Ankle Int. 2007;28(6):748–58.

Madjarevic M, Kolundzic R, Matek D, et al. Mitchell and Wilson metatarsal osteotomies for the treatment of hallux valgus: comparison of outcomes two decades after the surgery. Foot Ankle Int. 2006;27(11):877–82.

Yildirim Y, Saygi B, Aydin N, et al. Components of the Wilson osteotomy that are effective on hallux valgus repair. J Foot Ankle Surg. 2007;46(1):21–6.

# Fusion of the 1st Metatarsophalangeal Joint

**39**

Peter V. Giannoudis and Efthimios J. Karadimas

## Indications

- Severe hallux deformity (an intermetatarsal angle of more than 20–22°, a hallux valgus angle of more than 45°, and severe pronation of the hallux)
- Degenerative arthritis with hallux valgus
- Recurrent hallux valgus (HV)
- Hallux valgus caused by muscle imbalance in patients with neuromuscular disorders, such as cerebral palsy, in order to prevent recurrence

## Clinical Symptoms

- Pain localized over the 1st metatarsal head
- Painful walking
- Decreased walking capacity

## Preoperative Planning

### Clinical Assessment

- Assessment of resultant pathology.
- Assess any structural deformity and the ROM of the forefoot joints.

P.V. Giannoudis (✉)
Academic Department of Trauma and Orthopaedic Surgery, School of Medicine, University of Leeds,Leeds, UK
e-mail: pgiannoudi@aol.com

E.J. Karadimas
Department of Trauma and Orthopaedic Surgery, Leeds Teaching Hospitals NHS Trust, Leeds, UK

- Assess state of surrounding soft tissues.
- Any underlying toe inflammation must be excluded.
- Patients with a positive diabetes family history should be screened.

### Radiological Assessment

- Arthritic joint changes are evident in plain X-rays with subluxation of the 1st metatarsophalangeal (MTP) joint (Fig. 39.1).
- Obtain AP (weight-bearing) and lateral views of the feet.
- Measure the HV angle and the intermetatarsal angle to estimate the correction needed.

### Pelmatography

- It is often needed to evaluate the necessity of any additional operation for concomitant deformities.

## Operative Treatment

### Anesthesia

- Regional or general anesthesia with nerve blocks
- Antibiotic prophylaxis according to the hospital protocol
- Antibiotic administration prior to tourniquet inflation

### Table/Equipment

- Radiolucent table
- Imaging intensifier

P.V. Giannoudis (ed.), *Practical Procedures in Elective Orthopaedic Surgery*,
DOI 10.1007/978-0-85729-814-0_39, © Springer-Verlag London Limited 2012

**Fig. 39.1** AP X-ray of the feet presenting bilateral arthritic joint changes with subluxation of the 1st MTP

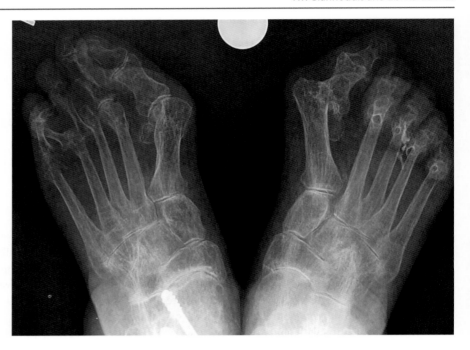

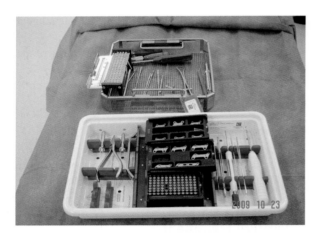

**Fig. 39.2** Specific plating system for the forefoot with 2.7-mm screws

- Small fragment set and 1.6-mm K-wires and plating system (Fig. 39.2)
- Thigh tourniquet

## Patient Positioning

- Supine positioning.
- Inflate thigh tourniquet to 300 mmHg.

## Marking and Draping

- Mark the incision at the 1st metatarsal over the bunion (dorsomedial).
- Extensive below-knee skin preparation with the use of antiseptic solutions (alcoholic povidone/iodine). Extra care in the web spaces between the toes (Fig. 39.3).

## Surgical Exposure

- Make a longitudinal incision dorsomedially over the 1st metatarsophalangeal joint. Similar cut over the capsule and exposure of the 1st MTP joint (Fig. 39.4).
- Together with exostosis removal, resect the articular cartilage from the metatarsal head and from the base of the proximal phalanx (Fig. 39.5), either with an osteotome or with a dental rongeur. The edge of the adjacent bones can have conical or parallel shape.
- Insert a K-wire through the 1st MTP joint, with direction from proximal medial to distal lateral, targeting the center of the distal phalanx. Make sure that the K-wire is sharp on both ends. In the same manner, drill a hole to insert a screw (cortical) to fix the fusion site (Fig. 39.6a).

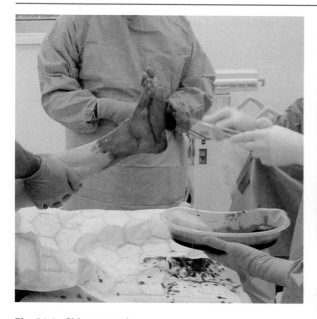

**Fig. 39.3** Skin preparation

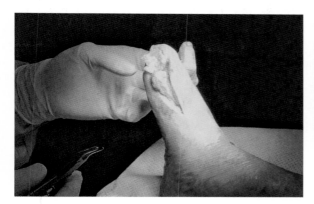

**Fig. 39.4** Exposure of the 1st MTP joint

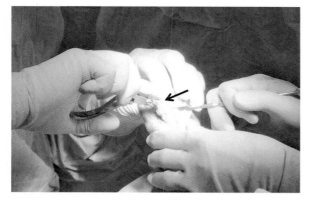

**Fig. 39.5** Trimming the exostosis and resection of the articular cartilage from the metatarsal head and the base of the proximal phalanx with a nibbler (*black arrow*)

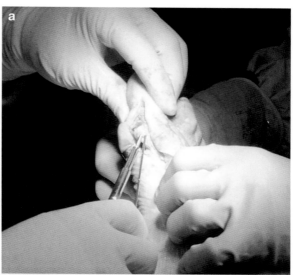

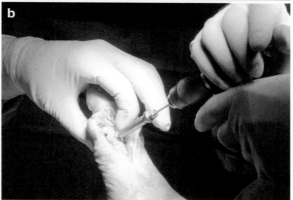

**Fig. 39.6** (**a**) Insertion of the cortical screw to fix the fusion site. (**b**) Application of the dorsal plate

- Following that, remove the K-wire and apply dorsally the specific plate and insert all the screws (Fig. 39.6b).
- X-ray certification/documentation for the final plate position is advised prior to closure (Fig. 39.7a, b).

## Closure

- Release tourniquet and check for any sources of bleeding.
- Use 2/0 Vicryl interrupted sutures for closure of the subcutaneous layer.
- Use 3/0 Ethilon nonabsorbable suture for skin closure.
- Wound dressing and wool application.

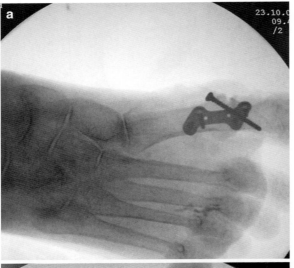

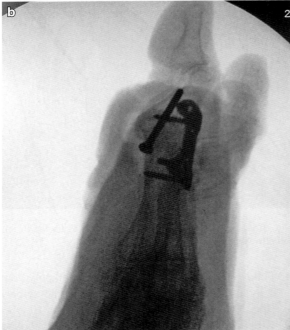

**Fig. 39.7** (**a**, **b**) Intraoperative X-ray evaluation of final plate position

- It is advisable to use swabs in between the toe web spaces.
- Depending on surgeon's preference, a custom made brace/shoe may be applied.

## Postoperative Care/Rehabilitation

- Antibiotics (as per hospital protocol).
- Start mechanical VTE prophylaxis at admission and continue until the patient no longer has significantly reduced mobility, based on an assessment of risks. Start pharmacological VTE prophylaxis after surgery and continue until the patient no longer has significantly reduced mobility.
- Wound inspection within 48 h.
- Obtain radiographs AP/Lateral of the forefoot.
- Pain management is obligatory.
- Weight bearing from the second week depending on pain and fixation type.

## Complications

- Wound infection
- Nonunion
- Malunion
- Degenerative arthritis of the interphalangeal joint of the hallux

## Follow-Up

- On discharge, DVT prophylaxis as per local hospital protocol.
- Outpatient follow-up at 4, 8, and 12 weeks for clinical and radiological assessment (AP/lateral X-rays).
- Patient can be discharged when union has been confirmed both clinically and radiologically.

## Further Reading

Bolland BJ, Sauvé PS, Taylor GR. Rheumatoid forefoot reconstruction: first metatarsophalangeal joint fusion combined with Weil's metatarsal osteotomies of the lesser rays. J Foot Ankle Surg. 2008;47(2):80–8.

Kadambande S, Debnath U, Khurana A, et al. Rheumatoid forefoot reconstruction: 1st metatarsophalangeal fusion and excision arthroplasty of lesser metatarsal heads. Acta Orthop Belg. 2007;73(1):88–95.

Trnka HJ. Arthrodesis procedures for salvage of the hallux metatarsophalangeal joint. Foot Ankle Clin. 2000;5(3):673–86.

# Claw/Hammer Toe Repair

40

Peter V. Giannoudis and Efthimios J. Karadimas

## Introduction

- Claw Toe (Fig. 40.1):
  - Abnormal flexion posture of the PIP joint that is often present in all toes.
  - Frequently caused by neuromuscular diseases.
  - The MTP joint is always in extension.
  - Often a flexion deformity at the DIP joint is present.
- Hammer toe:
  - Abnormal flexion posture of the PIP joint of one of the lesser four toes.
  - The flexion deformity may be fixed or flexible.
- Clinical Symptoms:
  - Pain localized at the dorsum of the PIP joint, plantar to the nail end (on DIP joint flexion) and beneath the metatarsal head (on proximal phalanx dorsal subluxation)
  - Hard corns of the toe/plantar callosities (Fig. 40.2)
  - Ulceration and deep infection (especially in patients with other co-morbidities such as diabetes mellitus or myelomeningocele)
  - Painful walking
  - Decreased walking ability

P.V. Giannoudis (✉)
Academic Department of Trauma and Orthopaedic Surgery,
School of Medicine, University of Leeds,Leeds, UK
e-mail: pgiannoudi@aol.com

E.J. Karadimas
Department of Trauma and Orthopaedic Surgery,
Leeds Teaching Hospitals NHS Trust,
Leeds, UK

- Conservative treatment usually is disappointing and unrewarding.
- The most commonly used procedures for the correction of the aforementioned pathologies are:
  - Soft tissue procedures (lengthening or tenotomy of EDL, EDB, MTP capsulotomy, collateral ligament sectioning)
  - Bone and joint procedures (e.g., partial or total resection of the proximal phalanx, arthrodesis, or resection of the PIP joint)
  - Combination of these

## Indications

- Pain
- Painful walking
- Decreased walking ability

## Preoperative Planning

### Clinical Assessment

- Assess any structural deformity and the ROM of the forefoot joints.
- Assess state of surrounding soft tissues.
- Any underlying toe inflammation must be excluded.

### Radiological Assessment

- AP (weight-bearing), lateral, and oblique X-rays of the foot

P.V. Giannoudis (ed.), *Practical Procedures in Elective Orthopaedic Surgery*,
DOI 10.1007/978-0-85729-814-0_40, © Springer-Verlag London Limited 2012

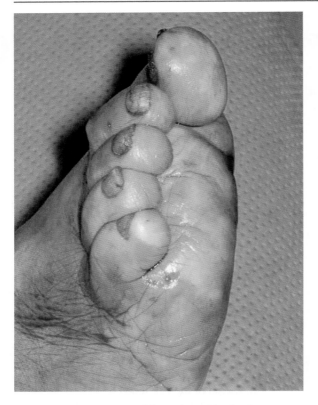

**Fig. 40.1** Claw toes in an oblique view of the forefoot

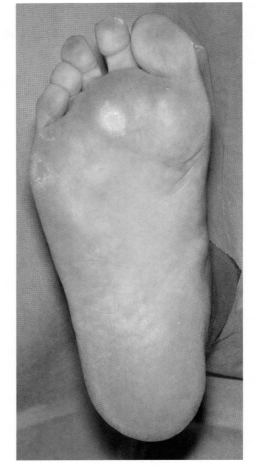

**Fig. 40.2** Plantar callosities

## Operative Treatment

### Anesthesia

- Regional or general anesthesia with nerve blocks
- Antibiotic prophylaxis according to the hospital protocol
- Antibiotic administration prior to tourniquet inflation

### Table/Equipment

- Surgical table
- Small fragment set and K-wires
- Thigh tourniquet
- Image intensifier available

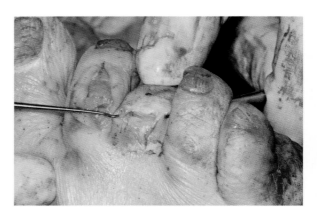

**Fig. 40.3** Oval incision

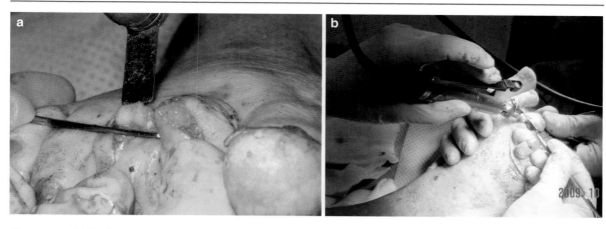

**Fig. 40.4** (**a**, **b**) Flexion and removal of proximal phalanx's head

**Fig. 40.5** (**a**) Antegrade insertion of the K-wire to the middle and distal phalanges. (**b**) Retrograde insertion of the K-wire through the remaining portion of the shaft of the proximal phalanx

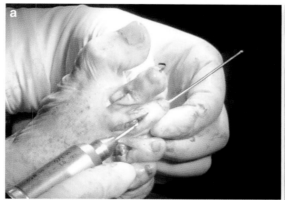
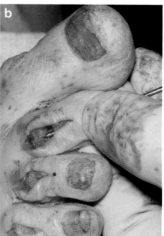

## Patient Positioning

- Supine position.
- Inflate thigh tourniquet to 300 mmHg.

## Marking and Draping

- Mark an oval incision over the apex of the flexed proximal interphalangeal joint. Include the callosity.
- Extensive below-knee skin preparation with the use of antiseptic solutions (alcoholic povidone/iodine). Extra care in the web spaces between the toes.

## Surgical Exposure

- Make an oval small incision avoiding the neuro-vascular bundles at the edges of the incision (Fig. 40.3).
- Remove the callosity together with the skin.
- Hyperflex the PIP joint to facilitate head and neck removal of the proximal phalanx (Fig. 40.4a, b).
- In case of PIP joint arthrodesis, additional removal of the base of the middle phalanx is mandatory.
- Based on the pathology's severity, lengthening of EDL, tenotomy of EDB, or other soft tissue procedures may be necessary.

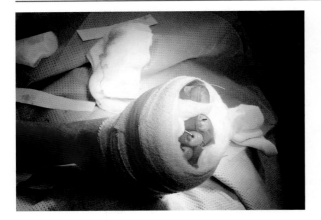

**Fig. 40.6** Wound dressing

- Insert a 1.6 K-wire antegrade through the middle and distal phalanges, exiting in the midline 2–3 mm plantar to the nail. Reverse the K-wire to drive it in a retrograde fashion through the remaining portion of the shaft of the proximal phalanx, and forward it into the metatarsal (Fig. 40.5a, b).
- Cut and bend the wire 1 cm from the skin.
- Severe deformity with dislocation of the metatarsophalangeal joint is difficult to correct. Usually, a decompression of the metatarsophalangeal joint is required (resection arthroplasty).

## Closure

- Release tourniquet and check for bleeding.
- Closure with a horizontal mattress stitch in the center and simple sutures on each side.
- Wound dressing and wool application. Use swabs in between the toes at the web spaces (Fig. 40.6).

## Postoperative Care/Rehabilitation

- Antibiotics (as per hospital protocol).
- Start mechanical VTE prophylaxis at admission and continue until the patient no longer has significantly reduced mobility, based on an assessment of risks. Start pharmacological VTE prophylaxis after surgery and continue until the patient no longer has significantly reduced mobility.

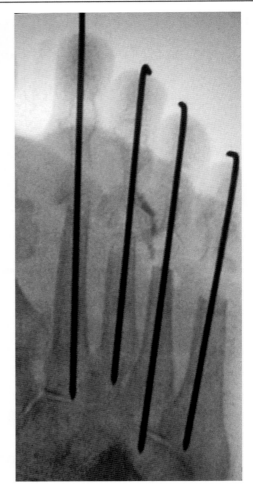

**Fig. 40.7** Postoperative AP X-ray

- Wound inspection within 48 h.
- Obtain radiographs AP/lateral of forefoot (Fig. 40.7).
- A wooden-soled shoe usually is worn for 4 weeks.
- Weight bearing as tolerated is allowed after the first 48–72 h.
- The use of crutches is optional.
- K-wire removal after 4 weeks time.

## Complications

- Wound infection
- Fracture
- Delayed union and nonunion

## Follow-Up

- Outpatients follow-up at 4, 8 weeks for clinical and radiological assessment.

## Further Reading

Bayod J, Losa-Iglesias M, de Bengoa-Vallejo RB, Prados-Frutos JC, Jules KT, Doblaré M. Advantages and drawbacks of proximal interphalangeal joint fusion versus flexor tendon transfer in the correction of hammer and claw toe deformity. A finite-element study. J Biomech Eng. 2010;132(5): 051002.

Schrier JC, Verheyen CC, Louwerens JW. Definitions of hammer toe and claw toe: an evaluation of the literature. J Am Podiatr Med Assoc. 2009;99(3):194–7.

Saltzman CL, Johnson KA, Donnelly RE. Surgical treatment for mild deformities of the rheumatoid forefoot by partial phalangectomy and syndactylization. Foot Ankle. 1993; 14(6):325–9.

# Index